HUMAN RESOURCES IN HEALTHCARE: MANAGING FOR SUCCESS

SECOND EDITION

HUMAN RESOURCES IN HEALTHCARE: MANAGING FOR SUCCESS

SECOND EDITION

Bruce J. Fried, Myron D. Fottler, and James A. Johnson
Editors

Health Administration Press, Chicago
AUPHA Press, Washington, DC

AUPHA

HAP

Your board, staff, or clients may also benefit from this book's insight. For more information on quantity discounts, contact the Health Administration Press Marketing Manager at (312) 424-9470.

10   09   08   07   5   4   3

Library of Congress Cataloging-in-Publication Data

Human resources in healthcare: managing for success / Bruce J. Fried, Myron D. Fottler, and James A. Johnson, editors.— 2nd ed.
     p. cm.
     Includes bibliographical references and index.
     ISBN 1-56793-243-6 (alk. paper)
     1. Medical personnel.   2. Personnel management.   3. Public health personnel.   I. Fried, Bruce, 1952—   II. Fottler, Myron D. III. Johnson, James A., 1954—
     RA410.6.H85 2005
     362.1'068'3—dc22   2005050220

The paper used in this publication meets the minimum requirements of American National Standard for Information Sciences-Permanence of Paper for Printed Library Materials, ANSI Z39.48-1984. ⊗™

Project manager: Jane Calayag Williams; Acquisition manager: Audrey Kaufman; Cover designer: Trisha Lartz

Health Administration Press   Association of University Programs
A division of the Foundation   in Health Administration
   of the American College of   2000 N. 14th Street
   Healthcare Executives   Suite 780
One North Franklin Street   Arlington, VA 22201
Suite 1700   (703) 894-0940
Chicago, IL 60606
(312) 424-2800

CONTENTS

DETAILED CONTENTS

FOREWORD

Health services administration is the most challenging and consequential management responsibility in modern society. It is challenging because of the complexity of the healthcare organization, which encompasses medical care; public health; public policy; economics; social ethics; and the application of management competencies in such areas as human resources, law, financing, marketing, and more. It is consequential because the practice of health services administration directly affects the quality of life in communities.

Healthcare, first and foremost, comprises people. It is a labor-intensive enterprise, complicated not only by the number of people involved in delivering health services but also by the number of occupations and the complexity of their relationships with the healthcare organization. The occupations that are essential to the hospital number in the hundreds, ranging from food service and equipment maintenance workers to physicians, physicists, and physical therapists. Each holder of that occupation contributes his or her skills to the successful performance of the organization in the service of the public.

Healthcare organizations are under tremendous pressure to attract and retain a skilled workforce, while continually improving their health and financial outcomes. Those who manage health services, at all levels of the organization, devote a substantial portion of their time and efforts to creating the conditions that encourage each healthcare worker to be successful in meeting his or her personal and professional objectives and those of the organization.

Effective human resources management is a priority strategic objective of successful healthcare organizations. When organizations do not achieve high performance results, or, even worse, when they fail altogether, the problem can often be attributed to the mismanagement or more often the "undermanagement" of their human resources. Executive leadership has failed to align human resources with strategic objectives, taking a short-term view by focusing on immediate problems at the expense of long-term workforce development. Such management has often delegated human resources management, instead of put the function squarely in the center of the senior management process and responsibility.

Organizational performance, which in simple terms means the performance of people, is the driving managerial concept in healthcare. A healthcare organization's increasing external accountabilities for continual quality improvement, patient safety, better outcomes, and transparency all direct attention to the performance of its workforce. No changes in organizational structure, financing, or technology are more important to achieving those results than is the performance of the people who work in and around the organization. There is much work to be done to bring the practice of human resources management up to meeting the mandate of those accountabilities. We in healthcare are preoccupied with financial pressures, emerging demographic and disease patterns, and changing technology. However, the response to all of these pressures is dependent on the people whose efforts are summed up in the word "performance."

Strategic human resources management must now be recognized as a core competency of health services administration and for which every executive should be held accountable. It is a much broader concept than the traditional approach to personnel administration, which is essential but not sufficient.

This book describes the full breadth and depth of the human resources management challenge. The issues that are described herein are not temporary; they are the predictable sequelae of social, political, economic, and professional changes emanating from the broader society and focusing on the hospital. The successful health services administrator is knowledgeable about these trends and their implications for the organization and is equipped to engage them strategically.

The authors have identified and described, with comprehensiveness and clarity, the issues and the management tools to help administrators engage these issues. This is at once a textbook for the future executive and a guide for senior executives, clinical leaders, trustees, and regulators. This book puts the field on notice that the days of delegating responsibility for human resources management are past. More encouragingly, the book demonstrates that there is a body of knowledge and skills that provides the foundation for the core competence of strategic human resources management.

Gary L. Filerman, Ph.D., professor and chairman,
Health Systems Administration,
Georgetown University, Washington, DC

PREFACE

Healthcare underwent remarkable changes in the last decades as a result of numerous factors, including advances in technology, availability of information, and new forms of organizations and financing mechanisms. Despite these changes, healthcare remains, and will always remain, a people-oriented enterprise. Healthcare customers are people, and regardless of the transformation in the way healthcare is provided, the central players in the delivery of care—whether preventive, diagnostic, curative, chronic, or rehabilitative—are still people.

As healthcare managers, we know (or think we know) about dealing with people. However, the manner by which we manage people in our organizations remains rather primitive. One of the reasons for this is that many healthcare professionals become managers as a result of their success in clinical or technological areas. Physicians, nurses, and laboratory technicians who are highly effective in their particular discipline are frequently rewarded by promotion into the managerial ranks. The erroneous assumption behind those promotions is that the same skills required of the clinician or technician are applicable and relevant at the managerial level.

Human Resources in Healthcare: Managing for Success is written for healthcare management students and healthcare professionals who have, or in the future will have, responsibility for managing people in healthcare organizations. This target audience includes virtually every formal leader—from supervisors to senior managers—in hospitals, health departments, physician practices, home care agencies, and other healthcare systems. Although the human resources department plays a key role in overseeing various employee affairs, that department does not "own" human resources management and is not capable of ensuring that the human resources practices implemented by managers are fair and equitable, effective and efficient, ethical, and legal. Human resources management is carried out at all levels in the organization and throughout the workday. In that sense, all healthcare managers are also human resources managers.

This book discusses the importance of systematic and strategic thinking about the organization's human resources function, focuses on ways to effectively implement human resources practices, and explores the traditions and beliefs that often stand in the way of implementation.

Chapter Overview

Our goal in this second edition is the same as in the first: to share the wealth of information that healthcare executives must know to become effective managers of people. In assembling material for this book, we again were forced to make choices about which among the many human resources concepts to include and exclude. This edition addresses topics that were not covered in the first edition:

- Workforce planning, from a macro perspective
- Staff diversity
- Nurse workload measurement
- Human resources budgeting

Discussion on these topics can be found in generic literature on human resources management but is limited. Therefore, their inclusion here adds breadth to the book.

As in the first edition, diverse professionals from academia, health administration practice, law, business, medicine, and consulting contributed their expertise to this book. As a result, this edition concisely covers the major themes in healthcare human resources management and is written to make specific areas more accessible to a wider set of audience.

Chapter 1, written by Myron Fottler, explores strategic human resources management. For many years, human resources was synonymous with "personnel," which in turn had a reputation for being passive and at times obstructionist in its relationship with internal customers. Fottler presents a proactive approach to human resources management that links human resources practices with organizational mission, strategies, and goals.

Chapter 2 is new to this edition and written by Tom Ricketts, an internationally respected researcher in healthcare workforce planning. Most human resources texts focus exclusively on internal human resources issues. In Chapter 2, human resources is addressed from the broader perspective of states, provinces, regions, and nations. Objectives and methods of healthcare workforce planning are discussed as well as the ambiguity of healthcare workforce supply requirements.

Healthcare organizations employ a diverse set of professionals, each of whom presents unique management challenges. Chapter 3 authors Kenneth White, Dolores Clement, and Kristie Stover take us through the world of healthcare professionals, discussing the functions, education, licensure, changing roles, and management implications of various healthcare professions.

Human resources management operates within a highly complex and changing web of legal and regulatory requirements. Chapter 4, written by Beverly Rubin and Bruce Fried, examines employee rights, discipline and privacy, HIPAA, and equal employment opportunity. Given the changing nature of human resources and healthcare law, being completely current in the legal requirements and court decisions in these areas is impossible. The authors, however, provide a framework for management practice that is based on aspects of the law that they see as robust and unlikely to change dramatically in the foreseeable future.

Chapter 5, contributed by Rupert Evans, explores the challenges and opportunities presented by a healthcare workforce that is becoming increasingly diverse. Evans points out that diversity involves more than race and ethnicity, categorizing it into three kinds: human diversity, cultural diversity, and systems diversity. The author then recommends ways to develop an effective diversity program.

Job analysis and job design are central to human resources management; in fact, they affect everything we do in managing our workforce. Chapter 6, by Myron Fottler, explains the processes of and provides useful approaches to conducting a job analysis, creating job descriptions, and writing job specifications. Fottler contends that the deliberate structuring of work can lead to improved individual, group, and organizational performance.

Our understanding of job requirements leads us to Chapter 7, authored by Bruce Fried. In this chapter, Fried discusses the recruitment process and enumerates innovative methods of attracting and retaining people. Issues of validity in selection tools as well as the relative reliability of measuring different human attributes are explored. This second edition includes additional discussion on retention strategies, distinguishing between strategies that are likely to improve retention and those that, while may increase morale, have not demonstrated success.

Training and employee development are vital functions, not just to improve morale but also to ensure that the workforce is knowledgeable and skilled for both current and future organizational needs. In the past, training was often viewed as a "frill." The perspective in Chapter 8, contributed by James Johnson, Gerald Ledlow, and Bernard Kerr, on the other hand, is that staff training and development are a key part of an organization's competitive strategy. The importance of the learning organization is emphasized, and the learning cycle necessary to improve individual and organizational performance is described.

Performance management is the process of assessing performance, providing feedback to employees, designing strategies for improvement, and evaluating the effectiveness of those strategies. Chapter 9, by Bruce Fried, presents a variety of approaches for evaluating performance, including the 360-degree strategy. Fried argues that performance appraisal and management should be viewed as positive, rather than punitive. In many instances, achieving this ideal perspective first requires an examination of the dominant organizational culture, which frequently views performance appraisal in a negative manner.

Reward and compensation systems can result in employee motivation, retention, and high performance. In Chapter 10, authors Howard Smith, Bruce Fried, Derek van Amerongen, and John Crisafulli provide an overview of rewards and examine the purpose of an organization's compensation policy. Incentive plans and the pros and cons of pay-for-performance schemes are discussed, as well as the problems of redesigning physician compensation in different types of organizational settings. This topic is important because physicians are increasingly moving into employee and quasi-employee relationships with organizations.

Ensuring the health and safety of workers during work hours is a continuing concern for healthcare organizations, particularly given the litigiousness of the U.S. society and the fact that the healthcare environment teems with medical threats. Michael Ryan and Anne Kilpatrick submit in Chapter 11 a framework for implementing health and safety strategies in the workplace. These authors describe how such strategies can be integrated into ongoing continuous quality improvement initiatives.

Unionization came relatively late to healthcare, but healthcare is now the biggest area of growth for the labor movement. Donna Malvey, author of Chapter 12, discusses unions, the unionization process, and labor-management relations. She gives particular attention to developments in the unionization of physicians and nurses and the implications of unionization for healthcare organizations.

Among the most important challenges facing healthcare managers is how to best deploy a key professional group, the nursing staff. Designing a deployment method is an area of considerable controversy and ambiguity, and the decision to maintain or deploy nurses is further complicated by nurse shortages. New to the second edition, Chapter 13, contributed by Cheryl Jones and George Pink, reviews the key aspects and measurement of nursing workload and offers nurse staffing metrics and calculation tools.

Eileen Hamby, writer of Chapter 14, introduces another new topic to this edition: human resources budgeting and productivity measurement. Given the size of the labor budget in healthcare organizations, methods are needed to accurately determine staffing levels, develop a labor budget, and analyze productivity using appropriate metrics. Hamby addresses out-sourcing and the impact of mergers and other changes on labor costs and productivity.

Paying attention to customers is a concept that came relatively late to healthcare, but certainly the concept contributes to improved quality and competitiveness. In Chapter 15, coauthors Myron Fottler and Robert Ford define customer focus and argue that human resources policies and practices need to change to support the healthcare organization's customer-focus strategies.

Bruce Fried and Myron Fottler close out the second edition. Chapter 16 enumerates ten trends that will have an impact on healthcare organizations and their workforces in the future.

Acknowledgments

Bruce Fried thanks, first and foremost, all of the authors who contributed to this book. All willingly and generously shared their knowledge and time and steadfastly responded to requests for clarification. Donna Cooper, my long-time assistant and friend, in the department of health policy and administration at the University of North Carolina at Chapel Hill (UNC), worked endlessly to edit drafts and to keep me organized. Audrey Kaufman, acquisitions manager at Health Administration Press, kept this project moving forward, using her well-developed human resources skills to patiently but firmly keep us as close to schedule as possible. Also at Health Administration Press, Jane Williams helped immeasurably in editing and achieved the difficult goal of consistency in style in a multiauthored book. Peggy Leatt and Laurel Files, chair and associate chair of the department of health policy and administration at UNC, provided a work environment conducive to creativity. My wife, Nancy, always provides emotional and substantive support, and my children—Noah, Shoshana, and Aaron—help me keep all of this in perspective. Finally, I thank my parents, Pearl and George Fried, who faithfully support me in all aspects of life.

Myron Fottler thanks Samantha Gottschalch, a student assistant and master's student in health services administration at the University of Central Florida. Her assistance and patience with typing various versions of my book chapters, sending out permission forms, and facilitating communications with editorial colleagues and chapter authors were invaluable and very much appreciated. My gratitude also goes to my wife, Carol, for her support on this and other projects over the years. Finally, I thank Diane Jacobs, chair of the department of health professions at the University of Central Florida, for her support of this project.

James Johnson thanks his colleagues at Central Michigan University and the Medical University of South Carolina.

Conclusion

We encourage you to think about how the concepts discussed in this book apply to the changing healthcare scene and to the healthcare organization in which you work or have worked. It may also be worthwhile for you to regularly consult the literature for changes and innovations in human resources management. Additional information and updates on this topic are posted on the Health Administration Press web site (http://www .ache.org/PUBS/fried2.cfm). Consult this web page occasionally, either to find or to share information relevant to the subject matter.

Often, issues concerning finance, operations, and technology are thought of as the "hard" organizational problems. Meanwhile, human resources dilemmas are viewed as the "soft," easily managed challenges. We disagree with this designation. People-management problems are hard problems. If people's concerns are not addressed and their needs not met, they are not motivated to perform and not committed to and supportive of the organization. Without this motivation and support, all of the organization's plans become compromised. Designing and implementing solutions to people problems are possible with the help of human resources management concepts and tools. We hope that this book gives you some of these tools and opens your eyes to alternative ways of managing people in healthcare organizations.

Bruce J. Fried, Ph.D.
University of North Carolina at Chapel Hill

Myron D. Fottler, Ph.D.
University of Central Florida

James A. Johnson, Ph.D.
Central Michigan University

STRATEGIC HUMAN RESOURCES MANAGEMENT

Myron D. Fottler, Ph.D.

Learning Objectives

After completing this chapter, the reader should be able to

- define strategic human resources management,
- outline key human resources functions,
- discuss the significance of human resources management to present and future healthcare executives, and
- describe the organizational and human resources systems that affect organizational outcomes.

Introduction

Like most other service industries, the healthcare industry is very labor intensive. One reason for healthcare's reliance on an extensive workforce is that it is not possible to produce a "service" and store it for later consumption. In healthcare, the production of the service that is purchased and the consumption of that service occur simultaneously. Thus, the interaction between healthcare consumers and healthcare providers is an integral part of the delivery of health services. Given the dependence on healthcare professionals to deliver service, the possibility of heterogeneity of service quality must be recognized within an employee (as skills and competencies change over time) and among employees (as different individuals or representatives of various professions provide a service).

The intensive use of labor for service delivery and the possibility of variability in professional practice require that the attention of leaders in the industry be directed toward managing the performance of the persons involved in the delivery of services. The effective management of people requires that healthcare executives understand the factors that influence the performance of individuals employed in their organizations. These factors include not only the traditional *human resources management* (HRM) activities (i.e., recruitment and selection, training and development, appraisal, compensation, employee relations) but also the environmental and other organizational aspects that impinge on HR activities.

Strategic human resources management (SHRM) refers to the comprehensive set of managerial activities and tasks related to developing and maintaining a qualified workforce, which then contributes to organizational effectiveness as defined by the organization's strategic goals. SHRM occurs in a complex and dynamic milieu of forces within the organizational context. A significant trend that started within the last decade is for human resources (HR) managers to adopt a strategic perspective of their job and to recognize critical linkages between organizational strategy and HR strategies (Fottler et al. 1990; Greer 2001).

This book explains and illustrates the methods and practices for increasing the probability that competent personnel will be available to provide the services delivered by the organization and that these personnel will perform necessary tasks appropriately. Implementing these methods and practices means that requirements for positions must be determined, qualified persons must be recruited and selected, employees must be trained and developed to meet future organizational needs, and adequate rewards must be provided to attract and retain top performers. This chapter emphasizes that HR functions are performed within the context of the overall activities of the organization. These functions are influenced or constrained by the environment, the organizational mission and strategies that are being pursued, and the systems indigenous to the institution.

Why study SHRM? How does this topic relate to the career interests or aspirations of present or future healthcare executives? Staffing the organization, designing jobs, building teams, developing employee skills, identifying approaches to improve performance and customer service, and rewarding employee success are as relevant to line managers as they are to HR managers. A successful healthcare executive needs to understand human behavior, work with employees effectively, and be knowledgeable about numerous systems and practices available to put together a skilled and motivated workforce. The executive also has to be aware of economic, technological, social, and legal issues that facilitate or constrain efforts to attain strategic objectives.

Healthcare executives do **not** want to hire the wrong person, to experience high turnover, to manage unmotivated employees, to be taken to court for discrimination actions, to be cited for unsafe practices, to have poorly trained staff undermine patient satisfaction, or to commit unfair labor practices. Despite their best efforts, executives often fail at human resources management as a result of hiring the wrong people or not motivating or developing their staff. The material in this book can help executives avoid mistakes and achieve great results with their workforce.

Healthcare organizations can gain a competitive advantage over competitors by effectively managing their human resources. This competitive advantage may include cost leadership (i.e., low-cost provider) and product differentiation (i.e., higher levels of service quality). A 1994 study examined the HRM practices and productivity levels of 968 organizations across 35 industries (Huselid 1994). The effectiveness of each organization's HRM practices was rated based on the presence of such benefits as incentive plans, employee grievance systems, formal performance appraisal systems, and employee participation in decision making. The study found that organizations with high HRM effectiveness ratings clearly outperformed those with low ones. A similar study of 293 publicly held companies reported that productivity was highly correlated with effective HRM practices (Huselid, Jackson, and Schuler 1997).

Based on "extensive reading of both popular and academic literature, talking with numerous executives in a variety of industries, and an application of common sense," Jeffrey Pfeffer (1995) identifies in his book the 13 HRM practices (12 of which are relevant to healthcare) that enhance an organization's competitive advantage. These practices seem to be present in organizations that are effective in managing their human resources, and they recur repeatedly in studies. In addition, these themes are interrelated and mutually reinforcing; it is difficult to achieve much positive result by implementing just one practice on its own. See Figure 1.1 for a list of the 12 HRM themes relevant to healthcare.

The bad news about achieving competitive advantage through the workforce is that it inevitably takes time to accomplish (Pfeffer 1995). The good news is that, once achieved, this type of competitive advantage is likely to be more enduring and more difficult for competitors to duplicate. Measurement is a crucial component for implementing the 12 HR practices. Failure to evaluate the impact of HR practices dooms them to second-class status, neglect, and potential breakdown. Feedback from such measurement is essential in further development of or changes to practices as well as in monitoring how each practice is achieving its intended purpose.

Most of the above HR practices are described in more detail throughout the book. Although the evidence presented in the literature shows that effective HRM practices can strongly enhance an organization's competitive advantage, it fails to indicate why these practices have such an influence. In this chapter, we describe a model—the SHRM—that attempts to explain this phenomenon. First, however, a discussion on environmental trends is in order.

FIGURE 1.1
12 HRM
Practices for
Healthcare
Organizations

1. *Employment Security.* This signals a long-standing commitment by the organization to its workforce. Norms of reciprocity tend to guarantee that this commitment is repaid by employees. Alternately, an employer who indicates through word and deed that its employees are dispensable is not likely to generate employee loyalty, commitment, or willingness to expend extra effort on behalf of the organization. Security enhances employee involvement because employees do not fear that they, or their coworkers, would lose their jobs. Both employer and employee also have a greater incentive to invest in training because the employee will likely stay long enough to earn a return on the resources invested in his or her training.

2. *Selectivity in Recruiting.* Providing employment security requires the employer to be careful in choosing the right employee for every position. Studies on a wide range of workers indicate that the most productive employees are about twice as good as the least productive ones. An employee who goes through a rigorous selection process will feel that he or she is joining an elite organization. High expectations for performance are instilled in employees, and the organization sends a message that people matter.

3. *High Wages.* High wages tend to attract more applicants, permitting the organization to be more selective in finding people who are trainable and can become committed to the organization. High wages also send a message that the organization values its people. Providing high wages is not necessarily associated with incurring high labor costs if it results in enhanced customer service, skill, and innovation.

4. *Incentive Pay.* Employees who contributed to enhanced levels of economic and noneconomic performance will want to share in the benefits. Many successful organizations seek to reward performance with some form of contingent compensation. Successful incentive plans usually involve a broad performance evaluation rather than simplistic approaches.

5. *Information Sharing.* If employees are to be a source of competitive advantage, they must have access to information necessary to perform their tasks successfully. Withholding information prevents employees from helping the organization achieve its competitive goals.

6. *Participation and Empowerment.* Sharing information is a prerequisite for encouraging the decentralization of decision making, broader worker participation in processes, and employee empowerment in controlling their own work process. Evidence shows that workforce participation results in both employee satisfaction and productivity.

7. *Self-Managed Teams.* Many successful organizations have assigned teams of workers to be responsible for hiring, purchasing, job assessments, and production. This system has reduced levels of management and service problems, and it has enhanced productivity and profitability. Self-managed teams appear to work because peers and coworkers are in charge of coordinating and monitoring jobs.

FIGURE 1.1
(continued)

8. *Training and Skill Development.* An integral part of most new work systems is a greater commitment to training and skill development along with a change in the work structure that permits both managers and employees to employ their learned skills. If no change in the work structure is done to permit application of new skills, training alone will have little effect on productivity or quality.

9. *Cross-Utilization and Cross-Training.* Training employees to do multiple jobs presents a number of potential benefits for both the employer and the employee. Variety is one of the core job dimensions that affect how people respond to their work. It permits a change of pace, a change of activity, and a change in people, which together makes work life more interesting and challenging. In healthcare, cross-trained individuals are known as multiskilled health practitioners. Multiskilling is a useful adjunct to policies that promise employment security. It is easier to keep people at work if they have multiple skills and can do different things.

10. *Symbolic Egalitarianism.* Important barriers to decentralizing decision making, using self-managed teams, and eliciting employee commitment and participation are the symbols within institutions that separate people from each other. Examples include executive washrooms or dining rooms and reserved spaces in the parking lot. Many of the organizations that are known for achieving competitive advantage through their workforce display various forms of symbolic egalitarianism—that is, ways of signaling to both insiders and outsiders that there is comparative equality among employees. Reducing the number of social categories tends to decrease the relevance of various hierarchies and diminishes the "us versus them" mentality.

11. *Wage Compression.* Large differences in rewards can often result in employees spending excessive time and energy on aligning themselves with their supervisors or trying to change the allocation criteria. A more compressed distribution of salaries can produce higher overall performance. When the wage structure is compressed, pay is likely to be deemphasized, enhancing other bases of work satisfaction and building a culture focused on other factors of employee success.

12. *Promotion from Within.* Promotion from within is a useful accompaniment to many of the other 12 HR practices. It encourages training and skill development because it binds workers to the organization and vice versa. It facilitates decentralization, participation, and delegation because it helps promote trust across all levels of the workforce. It offers employees an incentive for performing well and persuades managers to learn about the business operations.

Source: Pfeffer, J. 1995. "Producing Sustainable Competitive Advantage Through the Effective Management of People." *Academy of Management Executive* 9 (1): 55–69.

Environmental Trends

Among the major environmental trends that affect healthcare institutions are changing financing arrangements, emergence of new competitors, advent of new technology, low or declining inpatient occupancy rates, changes in physician-organization relationships, transformation of the demography and increase in diversity of the workforce, shortage of capital, increasing market penetration by managed care, heightened pressures to contain costs, and greater expectations of patients. The results of these trends have been increased competition, the need for higher levels of performance, and concern for institutional survival. Many healthcare organizations are closing facilities; undergoing corporate reorganization; instituting staffing freezes and/or reductions in workforce; allowing greater flexibility in work scheduling; providing services despite fewer resources; restructuring and/or redesigning jobs; outsourcing many functions; and developing leaner management structures, with fewer levels and wider spans of control.

Various major competitive strategies are being pursued by organizations to respond to the current turbulent healthcare environment, including offering low-cost health services, providing superior patient service through high-quality technical capability and customer service, specializing in key clinical areas (e.g., becoming centers of excellence), and diversifying within or outside healthcare (Coddington and Moore 1987). In addition, healthcare organizations are entering into strategic alliances (Kaluzny, Zuckerman, and Ricketts 1995) and establishing integrated delivery systems (Shortell et al. 1993). Regardless of which strategies are being pursued, all healthcare organizations are experiencing a decrease in staffing levels in many traditional service areas and an increase in staffing in new ventures, specialized clinical areas, and related support services (Wilson 1986). Staffing profiles in healthcare today are characterized by a limited number of highly skilled and well-compensated professionals. Healthcare organizations are no longer "employers of last resort" for the unskilled. At the same time, however, most organizations are experiencing shortages of various nursing and allied health personnel.

The development of appropriate responses to the ever-changing healthcare environment has received much attention during the past decade so that HRM planning is now well accepted in healthcare organizations. However, implementation of such plans has often been problematic. The process often ends with the development of goals and objectives and does not include strategies or methods of implementation and ways to monitor results. Implementation appears to be the major difficulty in the overall management process (Porter 1980).

A major reason for this lack of implementation has been failure of healthcare executives to assess and manage the various external, interface, and internal stakeholders whose cooperation and support are necessary to successfully implement any business strategy (i.e., corporate, business, or functional) (Blair and Fottler 1990). A stakeholder is any individual or group with a "stake" in the organization. *External stakeholders* include patients and their families, public and private regulatory agencies, and third-party payers. *Interface stakeholders* are those who operate on the "interface" of the organization in both the internal and external environments; these stakeholders may include members of the medical staff who have admitting privileges or who are board members at several institutions. *Internal stakeholders* are those that operate within the organization, such as managers, professionals, and nonprofessional employees.

Involving supportive stakeholders such as employees and HR managers is crucial to the success of any HRM plan. If HR executives are not actively involved, then employee planning, recruitment, selection, development, appraisal, and compensation necessary for successful plan implementation are not likely to occur. McManis (1987, 19) notes that "While many hospitals have elegant and elaborate strategic plans, they often do not have supporting human resource strategies to ensure that the overall corporate plan can be implemented. But strategies don't fail, people do." Despite this fact, the healthcare industry as a whole spends less than one-half the amount that other industries are spending on human resources management (*Hospitals* 1989).

The SHRM Model

A strategic approach to human resources management includes the following (Fottler et al. 1990):

- Assessing the organization's environment and mission
- Formulating the organization's business strategy
- Identifying HR requirements based on the business strategy
- Comparing the current HR inventory—in terms of numbers, characteristics, and practices—with future strategic requirements
- Developing an HR strategy based on the differences between the current inventory and future requirements
- Implementing the appropriate HR practices to reinforce the business strategy and to attain competitive advantage

Figure 1.2 provides some examples of possible linkages between strategic decisions and HRM practices.

Strategic Decision	Implications on HR Practices
Pursue low-cost competitive strategy	Provide lower compensation Negotiate give-backs in labor relations Provide training to improve efficiency
Pursue service-quality differentiation competitive strategy	Provide high compensation Recruit top-quality candidates Evaluate performance based on patient satisfaction Provide training in guest relations
Pursue growth through acquisition	Adjust compensation Select candidates from acquired organization Outplace redundant workers Provide training to new employees
Pursue growth through development of new markets	Promote existing employees based on an objective performance-appraisal system
Purchase new technology	Provide training in using and maintaining the technology
Offer new service/product line	Recruit and select physicians and other personnel
Increase productivity and cost effectiveness through process improvement	Encourage work teams to be innovative Take risks Assume a long-term perspective

SHRM has not been given as high a priority in healthcare as it has in many other industries. This neglect is particularly surprising in a labor-intensive industry that requires the right people in the right jobs at the right times and that often undergoes shortages in various occupations (Cerne 1988). In addition, the literature in the field offers fairly strong evidence that organizations that use more progressive HR approaches achieve significantly better financial results than comparable, although less progressive, organizations do (Gomez-Mejia 1988; Huselid 1994; Huselid, Jackson, and Schuler 1997; Kravetz 1988).

Figure 1.3 illustrates some strategic HR trends that affect job analysis and planning, staffing, training and development, performance appraisal, compensation, employee rights and discipline, and employee and labor relations. These trends are discussed in more detail in upcoming chapters. The bottom line of Figure 1.3 is that organizations are moving to higher levels of flexibility, collaboration, decentralization, and team orientation. This transformation is driven by the environmental changes and the organizational responses to those changes discussed earlier.

The SHRM Process

As illustrated in Figure 1.4, a healthcare organization is made up of systems that require constant interaction within the environment. To remain viable, an organization must adapt its strategic planning and thinking to extend to external changes. The internal components of the organization are affected by these changes, so the organization's plans may necessitate modifications in terms of the internal systems and HR process systems. There must be harmony among these systems. The characteristics, performance levels, and amount of coherence in operating practices among these systems influence the outcomes achieved in terms of organizational and employee-level measures of performance. HR goals, objectives, process systems, culture, technology, and workforce must be aligned both with each other (i.e., internal alignment) and with the various levels of organizational strategies (i.e., external alignment).

Internal and External Environmental Assessment

Environmental assessment is a crucial element of SHRM. As a result of changes in the legal/regulatory climate, economic conditions, and labor-market realities, healthcare organizations face constantly changing opportunities and threats. These opportunities and threats make particular services or markets more or less attractive in the organization's perspective. Among the trends currently affecting the healthcare environment are increasing diversity of the workforce, aging of the workforce, labor shortages, changing worker values and attitudes, and advances in technology. Healthcare executives have responded to these external environmental pressures through various internal, structural changes. Among these are the development of network structures, membership in healthcare systems, mergers and acquisitions, development of work teams, implementation of continuous quality improvement, telecommuting, employee leasing, and greater utilization of temporary or contingent workers.

Healthcare executives need to assess not only their organizational strengths and weaknesses but also their internal systems; human resources' skills, knowledge, and abilities; and portfolio of service markets. Management

FIGURE 1.3
Strategic
Human
Resources
Trends

Old HR Practices	Current HR Practices
Job Analysis/Planning	
Explicit job descriptions	→ Broad job classes
Detailed HR planning	→ Loose work planning
Detailed controls	→ Flexibility
Efficiency	→ Innovation
Staffing	
Supervisors make hiring decisions	→ Team makes hiring decisions
Emphasis on candidate's technical qualifications	→ Emphasis on "fit" of applicant within the culture
Layoffs	→ Voluntary incentives to retire
Letting laid-off workers fend for themselves	→ Providing continued support to terminated employees
Training and Development	
Individual training	→ Team-based training
Job-specific training	→ Generic training emphasizing flexibility
"Buy" skills by hiring experienced workers	→ "Make" skills by training less-skilled workers
Organization responsible for career development	→ Employee responsible for career development
Performance Appraisal	
Uniform appraisal procedures	→ Customized appraisals
Control-oriented appraisals	→ Developmental appraisals
Supervisor inputs only	→ Appraisals with multiple inputs
Compensation	
Seniority	→ Performance-based pay
Centralized pay decisions	→ Decentralized pay decisions
Fixed fringe benefits	→ Flexible fringe benefits (i.e., cafeteria approach)
Employee Rights and Discipline	
Emphasis on employer protection	→ Emphasis on employee protection
Informal ethical standards	→ Explicit ethical codes and enforcement procedures
Emphasis on discipline to reduce mistakes	→ Emphasis on prevention to reduce mistakes
Employee and Labor Relations	
Top-down communication	→ Bottom-up communication and feedback
Adversarial approach	→ Collaboration approach
Preventive labor relations	→ Employee freedom of choice

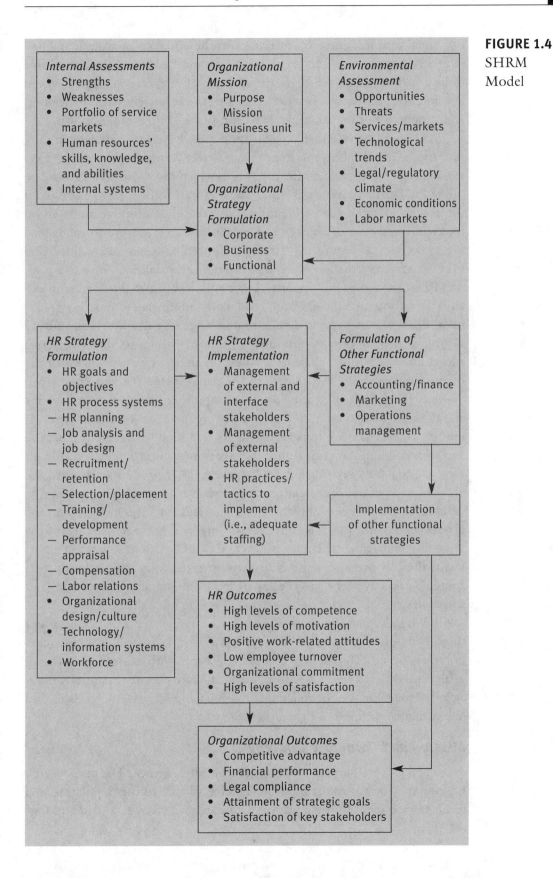

FIGURE 1.4
SHRM
Model

of human resources involves attention to the effect of environmental and internal components on the HR process system. Because of the critical role of health professionals in delivering services, healthcare managers should develop HR policies and practices that are closely related to, influenced by, and supportive of the strategic goals and plans of their organization.

Organizations, either explicitly or implicitly, pursue a strategy in their operations. Deciding on a strategy means determining the products or services that will be created and the markets to which the chosen services will be offered. Once the selection is made, the methods to be used to compete in the chosen market must be identified. The methods adopted are based on internal resources available, or potentially available, for use by managers.

Looking at Figure 1.4, strategies should be based on consideration of environmental conditions and organizational capabilities. To be in a position to take advantage of opportunities that are anticipated to occur, as well as to parry potential threats from changed conditions or competitor initiatives, managers must have detailed knowledge of the current and future operating environment. Cognizance of internal strengths and weaknesses allows managers to develop plans based on an accurate assessment of the organization's ability to perform in the marketplace at the desired level.

SHRM does not occur in a vacuum; rather, it occurs in a complex and dynamic constellation of forces in the organization's context. One significant trend has been for HR managers to adopt a strategic perspective and to recognize the critical links between human resources and organizational goals. As seen in Figure 1.4, the SHRM process starts with the identification of the organization's purpose, mission, and business unit, as defined by the board of directors and the senior management team. The process ends with the HR function serving as a strategic partner to the operating departments. Under this new view of human resources management, the HR manager's job is to help operating managers achieve their strategic goals by serving as the expert in all employment-related activities and issues.

When human resources is viewed as a strategic partner, talking about the single best way to do anything makes no sense. Instead, the organization must adopt HR practices that are consistent with its strategic mission, goals, and objectives. In addition, **all** healthcare executives are HR managers. Management of people depends on having effective supervisors and line managers throughout the organization.

Mission and Corporate Strategy

An organization's *purpose* is its basic reason for existence. The purpose of a hospital may be to deliver high-quality clinical care to the population in a given service area. An organization's *mission*, created by its board and senior managers, specifies how the organization intends to manage itself to most effectively fulfill its purpose. The mission statement often provides subtle clues on the importance the organization places on its human resources. The purpose and mission affect HR practices in obvious ways. A nursing home, for example, must employ nursing personnel, nurse aides, and food service workers to meet the needs of its patients.

The first step in formulating a corporate and business strategy is doing a *SWOT* (strengths, weaknesses, opportunities, and threats) *analysis*. The managers then attempt to use the organization's strengths to capitalize on environmental opportunities and to cope with environmental threats. Human resources play a fundamental role in SWOT analysis because the nature and type of people who work within an organization and the organization's ability to attract new talent represent significant strengths and weaknesses.

Most organizations formulate strategy at three basic levels: the corporate level, the business level, and various functional levels. *Corporate strategy* is a set of strategic alternatives that an organization chooses from as it manages its operations simultaneously across several industries and markets. *Business strategy* is a set of strategic alternatives that an organization chooses from to most effectively compete in a particular industry or market. *Functional strategies* consider how the organization will manage each of its major functions (i.e., marketing, finance, and human resources).

A key challenge for HR managers when the organization is using a corporate growth strategy is recruiting and training large numbers of qualified employees, who are needed to provide services in added operations. New-hire training programs may also be needed to orient and update the skills of incoming employees. In Figure 1.4, the two-way arrows leading from Organizational Strategy Formulation to HR Strategy Formulation and Implementation and vice versa indicate that the impact from the HR function should also be considered in the initial formulation of organizational strategy. When human resources is a true strategic partner, all parties consult with and support one another.

HR Strategy Formulation and Implementation

Once the organization's corporate and business strategies have been determined, managers can then develop an HR strategy. This strategy commonly includes a staffing strategy (planning, recruitment, selection, and placement), a developmental strategy (performance management, training, development, career planning), and a compensation strategy (salary structure, employee incentives).

A *staffing strategy* refers to a set of activities used by the organization to determine its future HR needs, recruit qualified applicants with an interest in the organization, and select the best of those applicants as new employees. This strategy should be undertaken only after a careful and systematic development of the corporate and business strategies so that staffing activities mesh with other strategic elements of the organization. For example, if retrenchment is part of the business strategy, the staffing strategy will focus on determining which employees to retain and what process to use in termination.

A *developmental strategy* helps the organization enhance the quality of its human resources. This strategy must also be consistent with the corporate and business strategies. For example, if the organization wishes to follow a strategy of differentiating itself from competitors through customer focus and service quality, then it will need to invest heavily in training its employees to provide the highest-quality service and to ensure that performance management focuses on measuring, recognizing, and rewarding performance—all of which lead to high levels of service quality. Alternatively, if the business strategy is to be a leader in providing low-cost services, the developmental strategy may focus on training to enhance productivity to keep overall costs low.

A *compensation strategy* must also complement the organization's other strategies. For example, if the organization is pursuing a strategy of related diversification, its compensation strategy must be geared toward rewarding employees whose skills allow them to move from the original business to related businesses (i.e., inpatient care to home health care). The organization may choose to pay a premium to highly talented individuals who have skills that are relevant to one of its new businesses. When formulating and implementing an HR strategy and the basic HR components discussed above, managers must account for other key parts of the organization such as organizational design, corporate culture, technology, and the workforce (Bamberger and Fiegelbaum 1996).

Organizational design refers to the framework of jobs, positions, groups of positions, and reporting relationships among positions. Most healthcare organizations use a *functional design* whereby members of a specific occupation or role are grouped into functional departments such as OB-GYN, surgery, and emergency services. Management roles are also divided into functional areas such as marketing, finance, and human resources. The top of the organizational chart is likely to reflect positions such as chief executive officer and vice presidents of marketing, finance, and human resources. To operate efficiently, and allow for seamless service, an organization with a functional design requires considerable coordination across its various departments.

Many healthcare organizations have been moving toward a flat organizational structure or *horizontal corporation*. Such an organization is created by eliminating levels of management, reducing bureaucracy, using wide spans of control, and relying heavily on teamwork and coordination to get work accomplished. These horizontal corporations are designed to be highly flexible, adaptable, streamlined, and empowered. The HR function in such organizations is typically diffused throughout the system so that operating managers take on more of the responsibility for HR activities and the HR staff plays a consultative role.

Corporate culture refers to the set of values that help members of that culture understand what they stand for, how they do things, and what they consider important. Because culture is the foundation of the organization's internal environment, it plays a major role in shaping the management of human resources, determining how well organizational members will function together and how well the organization will be able to achieve its goals.

There is no ideal culture for all organizations, but a strong and well-articulated culture enables employees to know what the organization stands for, what it values, and how to behave. A number of forces shape an organization's culture, including the founder or founders, institutional affiliations, shared experiences, symbols, stories, slogans, heroes, and ceremonies. It is important for managers to recognize the importance of culture and take appropriate care to transmit that culture to others in the organization. Culture can be transmitted through orientation, training, consistent behavior (i.e., walking the talk), corporate history, and the telling and retelling of stories.

Culture may facilitate the work of either HR managers or line managers. If the organization has a strong, well-understood, and attractive culture, attracting and retaining qualified employees become easier. If the culture is perceived as weak or unattractive, recruitment and retention become problematic. Likewise, the HR function can reinforce an existing culture by selecting new employees who have values that are consistent with that culture.

Technology also plays a role in the formulation and implementation of an HR strategy. Healthcare organizations are quite different from manufacturing organizations in terms of how they perform HR activities (e.g., different criteria for hiring employees and methods of training employees). Healthcare organizations typically emphasize educational credentials. Other aspects of technology are also important to human resources in all settings. For example, automation of certain routine functions may reduce demand for certain human resources but may increase it for others. Computers and robotics are important technological elements that affect human resources management, and rapid changes in technology affect employee selection, training, compensation, and other areas.

Appropriately designed management information systems provide data to support planning and management decision making. HR information is a crucial element of such a system, as such information can be used for both planning and operational purposes. For example, strategic planning efforts may require data on the number of professionals in various positions who will be available to fill future needs. Internal planning may require HR data in categories such as productivity trends, employee skills, work demands, and employee turnover rates. The use of an intranet (an internal Internet that is available to all members of an organization) can improve service to all employees, help the HR department, and reduce many routine administrative costs (Gray 1997).

Finally, *workforce composition* and trends also affect HR strategy formulation and implementation. The American workforce has become increasingly diverse in numerous ways; it has seen growth in the number of older employees, women, Hispanics, Asians, African Americans, the disabled, single parents, gays, lesbians, and people with special dietary preferences (Cox and Blake 1991). Previously, most employers observed a fairly predictable employee pattern: people entered the workforce at a young age, maintained stable employment for many years, and retired at the usual age—on or around 65. Obviously, such a pattern has changed and continues to evolve as a result of demographic factors, improved health, and abolition of mandatory retirement.

The successful implementation of an HR strategy generally requires the identification and management of key stakeholders (Blair and Fottler 1990, 1998). These stakeholders may be internal (i.e., employees), interface (i.e., physicians who are not employees), or external (i.e., third-party payers). The HR strategy, as all other strategies, can only be implemented through people; therefore, such implementation requires motivational and communication processes, goal setting, and leadership. Specific practices or tactics are also necessary to implement the HR strategy. For example, if a healthcare organization's business strategy is to differentiate itself from competitors through its high-level focus on meeting customer (patient) needs, then it may formulate an HR strategy to provide all employees with training in guest relations. However, that training strategy alone will not accomplish the business objective. Methods for implementation also need to be decided, such as should this training be provided in-house or through external programs such as those available through the Disney Institute? How will each employee's success in applying the principles learned be measured and rewarded? The answers to such questions provide the specific tactics needed to implement the HR strategy in response to the business goal of differentiation through customer service.

Obviously, the organization will also develop and implement other functional strategies in accounting/finance, marketing, operations management, and other areas. Positive or negative organizational outcomes are also determined by how well these functional strategies are formulated and implemented.

Outcomes

The outcomes achieved by a healthcare organization depend on its environment, its mission, the strategies it is pursuing, its HR process systems, its internal systems and how consistent the operating practices are across these systems, and how well it is executing all of the above factors. The appropriate methods for organizing and relating these factors are determined by the outcomes desired by managers and other major stakeholders of the organization. Although numerous methods exist for conceptualizing organizational performance and outcomes (Cameron and Whetten 1983; Goodman and Pennings and Associates 1977), the outcomes that may be useful in this discussion can be thought of as HR Outcomes and Organizational Outcomes (see Figure 1.4).

Numerous HR outcomes are associated with HR practices. An organization should provide its workforce with job security, meaningful work, safe conditions of employment, equitable financial compensation, and a satisfactory quality of work life. Organizations will not be able to attract and retain the number, type, and quality of professionals required to deliver health services if the internal work environment is unsuitable. In addition, employees are a valuable stakeholder group whose concerns are important because of the complexity of the service they provide. Job satisfaction (Starkweather and Steinbacher 1998), commitment to the organization (Porter et al. 1974), motivation (Fottler et al. 2005), levels of job stress (DeFrank and Ivancevich 1998), and other constructs can be used as measures of employee attitudes and psychological condition.

For long-term survival, a healthcare organization must have a balanced exchange relationship with the environment. An equitable relationship must exist because the exchange is mutually beneficial to the organization and to the elements of the environment with which it interacts. A number of outcome measures can be used to determine how well the organization is performing in the marketplace and is producing a service that will be valued by consumers, such as growth, profitability, return on investment, competitive advantage, legal compliance, attainment of strategic objectives, and satisfaction of key stakeholders. The latter may include such indices as patient satisfaction, cost per patient day, and community perception.

The mission and objectives of the organization are reflected in the outcomes that are stressed by management and in the strategies, general tactics, and HR practices that are chosen. Management makes decisions that, combined with the level of fit achieved among the internal systems, determine the outcomes the institution can achieve. For example, almost all healthcare organizations need to earn some profit for continued viability. However, some organizations refrain from initiating new ventures that may be highly profitable if the ventures do not fit their overall mission of providing quality services needed by a defined population group. Conversely, an organization may start some services that are acknowledged to be break-even propositions at best because those services are viewed as critical to its mission and the needs of the target market.

The concerns of such an organization are reflected not only in the choice of services it offers but also in the HR approaches it uses and the outcome measures it views as important. This organization likely places more emphasis on assessment criteria for employee performance and nursing unit operations that stress the provision of quality care than on criteria concerned with efficient use of supplies and the maintenance of staffing ratios. This selection of priorities does not mean that the organization is ignoring efficiency of operations; it just signals that the organization places greater weight on the former criteria. The outcome measures used to judge the institution should reflect its priorities.

Another institution may place greater emphasis on economic return, profitability, and efficiency of operations. Quality of care also is important to that organization, but the driving force for becoming a low-cost provider causes the organization to make decisions that reflect its business strategy; therefore, it stresses maintenance or reduction of staffing levels and strictly prohibits overtime. Its recruitment and selection criteria stress identification and selection of employees who will meet minimum job requirements and expectations and, possibly, will accept lower pay levels.

In an organization that strives to be efficient, less energy may be spent on "social maintenance" activities designed to meet employee needs and to keep them from leaving or unionizing. The outcomes in this situation will reflect, at least in the short run, higher economic return and lower measures of quality of work life.

Human Resources and the Joint Commission

The Joint Commission on Accreditation of Healthcare Organizations (JCAHO) initiated a pilot project to assess the relationship between adequate staffing and clinical outcomes (Lovern 2001). The project was led by a 20-member national task force comprising hospital leaders, clinicians, and technical experts, among others (JCAHO 2002). The task force submitted its recommendations, which became a standard and was implemented in January 2004. The new standard requires healthcare organizations to assess their staffing effectiveness by continually screening for potential issues that can arise from inadequate staffing.

Under JCAHO Standard HR 1.30 (which at the time of this writing is under review for next year), a healthcare organization uses data on clinical/service indicators in combination with HR screening indicators to assess staffing effectiveness. An example of a clinical/service screening indicator is adverse drug events, and examples of HR screening indicators are overtime and staff vacancy rates. *Staffing effectiveness* is defined as the number, competency, and skill mix of staff related to the provision of needed care, treatment, and services. The Joint Commission's focus is on the linkage between HR strategy implementation (i.e., adequate staffing) and organizational outcomes (i.e., clinical outcomes)—see these two boxes in Figure 1.4.

The rationale for this standard is that multiple screening indicators related to patient outcomes, including clinical/service and HR screening indicators, may be indicative of staffing effectiveness. Under this standard, the facility selects a minimum of four screening indicators—two for clinical/service and two for human resources. The idea behind using two sets of indicators is to understand their relationship with one another; it also emphasizes that no indicator, in and of itself, can directly demonstrate staffing effectiveness.

The facility has to choose at least one indicator for each clinical/service and HR categories from the Joint Commission's list, and additional screening indicators can be selected based on their unique characteristics, specialties, and services. This selection also defines the expected impact that the absence of direct and indirect caregivers may have on patient outcomes. The data collected on these indicators are analyzed to identify potential staffing-effectiveness issues when performance varies from expected targets—that is, ranges of performance are evaluated, external comparisons are made, and improvement goals are assessed. The data are analyzed over time against the screening indicators to identify trends, patterns, or the stability of a process. At least once a year, managers report to the senior management team regarding the aggregation and analysis of data related to staffing effectiveness and about any actions taken to improve staffing.

HR screening indicators include the following:

- Overtime
- Staff vacancy rates
- Staff turnover rates

- Understaffing, as compared to the facility's staffing plan
- Nursing hours per patient day
- Staff injuries on the job
- On-call per diem use
- Sick time

Clinical/service screening indicators include the following:

- Patient readmission rates
- Patient infection rates
- Patient clinical outcomes by diagnostic category

A Strategic Perspective on Human Resources

Managers at all levels are becoming increasingly aware that critical sources of competitive advantage include appropriate systems for attracting, motivating, and managing the organization's human resources. Adopting a strategic view of human resources involves considering employees as human "assets" and developing appropriate policies and programs to increase the value of these assets to the organization and the marketplace. Effective organizations realize that their employees have value, much as the organization's physical and capital assets have value.

Viewing human resources from an investment perspective, rather than as variable costs of production, allows the organization to determine how to best invest in its people. This leads to a dilemma. An organization that does not invest in its employees may be less attractive to both current and prospective employees, which causes inefficiency and weakens the organization's competitive position. However, an organization that does invest in its people needs to ensure that these investments are not lost. Consequently, an organization needs to develop strategies to ensure that its employees stay on long enough so that it can realize an acceptable return on its investment in employee skills and knowledge.

Not all organizations realize that human assets can be strategically managed from an investment perspective. Management may or may not have an appreciation of the value of its human assets relative to its other assets such as brand names, distribution channels, real estate, and facilities and equipment. Organizations may be characterized as human-resources oriented or not based on the answers to the following:

- Does the organization see its people as being central to its missions and strategy?

- Do the organization's mission statement and strategy objectives mention or espouse the value of human assets?
- Does the management philosophy encourage the development of any strategy that prevents the depreciation of its human assets, or are these human assets viewed as costs to be minimized?

An HR investment perspective often is not adopted because it involves making a longer-term commitment to employees. Because employees can leave and most organizations are infused with short-term measures of performance, investments in human assets often are ignored. Organizations that are performing well may feel no need to change their HR strategies. Those that are not doing as well usually need a quick fix to turn things around and therefore ignore longer-term investments in people. However, although investment in human resources does not yield immediate results, it yields positive outcomes that are likely to last longer and difficult to duplicate by competitors.

Summary

The intensive reliance on professionals to deliver services requires health-care executives to focus attention on the strategic management of human resources and to understand the factors that influence the performance of all employees. To assist them in understanding this relationship, this chapter presents a model that explains the association among corporate strategy, selected organizational-design features, HRM activities, employee outcomes, and organizational outcomes.

The outcomes achieved by the organization are influenced by numerous HR and non-HR factors. The mission determines the direction that is being taken by the organization and the goals it desires to achieve. The amount of integration of mission, strategy, HR functions, behavioral components, and non-HR strategies defines the level of achievement that is possible.

References

Bamberger, P., and A. Fiegelbaum. 1996. "The Role of Strategic Reference Points in Explaining the Nature and Consequences of Human Resource Strategy." *Academy of Management Review* 21 (4): 926–58.

Blair, J. D., and M. D. Fottler. 1990. *Challenges in Healthcare Management: Strategic Perspectives for Managing Key Stakeholders.* San Francisco: Jossey-Bass.

———. 1998. *Strategic Leadership for Medical Groups.* San Francisco: Jossey-Bass.

Cameron, K. S., and D. A. Whetten. 1983. *Organizational Effectiveness: A Comparison of Multiple Models.* New York: Academic Press.

Cerne, F. 1988. "CEO Builds Employee Morale to Improve Finances." *Hospitals* 62 (11): 100.

Coddington, D. C., and K. D. Moore. 1987. *Market-Driven Strategies in Healthcare.* San Francisco: Jossey-Bass.

Cox, T. H., and S. Blake. 1991. "Managing Cultural Diversity: Implications for Organizational Competitiveness." *Academy of Management Executive* 16 (1): 45–56.

DeFrank, R. S., and J. M. Ivancevich. 1998. "Stress on the Job." *Academy of Management Executives* 12 (3): 55–65.

Fottler, M. D., J. D. Blair, R. L. Phillips, and C. A. Duran. 1990. "Achieving Competitive Advantage Through Strategic Human Resource Management." *Hospital & Health Services Administration* 35 (3): 341–63.

Fottler M. D., S. J. O'Connor, T. D'Aunno, and M. Gilmartin. 2005. "Motivating People." In *Healthcare Management, 5th Edition*, edited by S. M. Shortell and A. D. Kaluzny. Albany, NY: Delmar.

Gomez-Mejia, L. R. 1988. "The Role of Human Resources Strategy in Expert Performance." *Strategic Management Journal* 9: 493–505.

Goodman, P. S., and J. M. Pennings and Associates. 1977. *New Perspectives on Organizational Effectiveness.* San Francisco: Jossey-Bass.

Gray, F. 1997. "How to Become Intranet Savvy." *HR Magazine* (4): 66–71.

Greer, C. R. 2001. *Strategic Human Resource Management.* Upper Saddle River, NJ: Prentice-Hall.

Hospitals. 1989. "Human Resources." *Hospitals* 63: 46–47.

Huselid, M. A. 1994. "Documenting HR's Effect on Company Performance." *HR Magazine* (1): 79–85.

Huselid, M. A., S. E. Jackson, and R. S. Schuler. 1997. "Technical and Strategic Human Resources Management Effectiveness as Determinants of Firm Performance." *Academy of Management Journal* 40 (1): 171–88.

Joint Commission on Accreditation of Healthcare Organizations. 2002. *Healthcare at the Crossroads: Strategies for Addressing the Evolving Nursing Crisis.* [Online publication; accessed 7/12/05.] www.jcaho.org/about+us/public+policy+initatives/health+care+at+the+crossroads.pdf.

Kaluzny, A., H. Zukerman, and T. Ricketts. 1995. *Partners for the Dance: Forming Strategic Alliances in Healthcare.* Chicago: Health Administration Press.

Kravetz, D. J. 1988. *The Human Resources Revolution: Implementing Progressive Management Practices for Bottom Line Success.* San Francisco: Jossey-Bass.

Lovern, E. 2001. "JCAHO to Study Staffing Issues." *Modern Healthcare* 31 (3): 6–8.

McManis, G. L. 1987. "Managing Competitively: The Human Factor." *Healthcare Executive* 2 (6): 18–23.

Pfeffer, J. 1995. "Producing Sustainable Competitive Advantage Through the Effective Management of People." *Academy of Management Executive* 9 (1): 55–69.

Porter, L. W., R. M. Steers, R. T. Mowday, and P. V. Boulian. 1974. "Organizational Commitment, Job Satisfaction, and Turnover Among Psychiatric Technicians." *Journal of Applied Psychology* 59: 603–09.

Porter, M. E. 1980. *Competitive Strategy*. New York: The Free Press.

Shortell, S. M., R. R. Gilles, D. A. Anderson, J. B. Mitchell, and K. L. Morgan. 1993. "Creating Organized Delivery Systems: The Barriers and the Facilitators." *Hospital & Health Services Administration* 38 (4): 447–66.

Starkweather, R. A., and C. L. Steinbacher. 1998. "Job Satisfaction Affects the Bottom Line." *HR Magazine* (9): 110–12.

Wilson, T. B. 1986. *A Guide to Strategic Human Resource Planning for the Healthcare Industry*. Chicago: American Society for Healthcare Human Resource Administration, American Hospital Association.

Discussion Questions

1. Distinguish between corporate, business, and functional strategies. How does each relate to human resources management? Why?

2. How may an organization's human resources be viewed as either a strength or a weakness when doing a SWOT analysis? What could be done to strengthen human resources in the event it is viewed as a weakness?

3. List factors under the control of healthcare managers that contribute to the reduction in the number of people applying to health professions schools. Describe the steps that healthcare providers can take to improve this situation.

4. What are the organizational advantages of integrating strategic management and human resources management? What are the steps involved in such an integration?

5. Robert Levering and Milton Moskowitz recently published a best-selling book entitled *The Best 100 Companies to Work for in America*, which is based on their review of HR practices in many organizations. Among these organizations is Beth Israel Hospital in Boston. Use a search engine to locate Beth Israel's web site, and review the information contained on the web site. What specific information interested you as a potential employee? How would you use this exercise to design a web site for a future employer, and why?

Experiential Exercises

Exercise 1   Prior to class, obtain the annual report of any healthcare organization of your choice. Review the material
presented and the language used. Write a one-page memo that assesses
that organization's philosophy regarding its human resources.

During the class period, arrange yourselves in small groups of
four or five students and compare the similarities and differences among
the organizations your group members investigated.

- How can you differentiate those who merely "talk the talk" from
  those who also "walk the walk"?
- What factors do you believe influence how a healthcare organization perceives its human resources?
- How do the "better" healthcare organizations perceive their human
  resources?
- What did you learn from this exercise?

Exercise 2   Prior to class, review the 12 HR practices, developed
by Jeffrey Pfeffer, discussed in this chapter. Consider
how well your current or most recent employer follows any three of
Pfeffer's 12 practices. Ask yourself, how compatible were your employer's
management practices with each of the three practices for managing
people. Write a 1–2 page summary listing each of the three practices
and the compatibilities (or incompatibilities) with your employer's HR
practices.

During the class session, form a group of four or five students
and share your perceptions of the HR practices at your present or most
recent employer.

- What similarities or differences did you find among the practices
  followed by the other employers in your group?
- Which of the 12 practices seem to be least prevalent, and why?

HEALTHCARE WORKFORCE PLANNING

Thomas C. Ricketts, III, Ph.D.

Learning Objectives

After completing this chapter, the reader should be able to

- trace the history of workforce planning;
- understand why and when workforce planning is undertaken;
- briefly describe the five major strategies used in workforce planning;
- understand the key concepts of benchmarking, adjusted needs, and demand as they apply to workforce planning;
- develop a simple estimate of the future supply of a profession for a population; and
- interpret the results of workforce planning reports as they relate to individual healthcare organizations and delivery systems.

Introduction

Most of this book views human resources management (HRM) from the perspective of the healthcare organization. Chapters focus on such topics as job design, recruitment and retention, and evaluation of individual performance. However, organizations are also affected by the larger external environment in which they are situated. In HRM, broad workforce and labor-market factors, which are external aspects, affect an organization's ability to attract and retain employees. An organization may have a theoretically sound recruitment program for nurses, but if sufficient numbers of nurses are not being trained, the program will likely prove unsuccessful. This chapter's focus is unique among the chapters in this book in that it addresses workforce planning for communities, regions, states, countries, and other jurisdictions. It devotes attention to societywide healthcare workforce needs rather than the needs of particular organizations.

Healthcare workforce planning deals with questions such as the following:

- How do we determine the number of surgeons needed in a particular geographic area?

- What factors help us to best anticipate future supply and need for various types of healthcare workers?
- What techniques are used to project future workforce needs? What are the strengths and weaknesses of different techniques, and how may they be most effectively applied?

This chapter, therefore, takes a macro-level perspective on the healthcare workforce and examines concepts and methodologies that are useful in projecting workforce requirements for communities and larger regions. Much of the remainder of this book focuses on internal strategies for managing human resources, which we can view as micro-level approaches, and addresses workforce concerns from the perspective of a single organization.

Workforce planning is the assessment of needs for human resources. This process can be very formal or "back-of-the-envelope" estimates and can be applied to small organizations or practices as well as to national and international healthcare delivery systems. Workforce planning fits in with overall health systems planning and human resources development and management. One conceptualization sees workforce planning as one of three steps in workforce development (De Geyndt 2000):

1. Planning is the quantity concern.
2. Training is the quality concern.
3. Managing is the performance and output concern.

The Australian Medical Workforce Advisory Committee (2003) describes workforce planning succinctly: "ensuring that the right practitioners are in the right place at the right time with the right skills." However, the consensus remains that workforce planning is "not an exact science" (Fried 1997).

Workforce planning is used to support decision making and policy development for a wide range of concerns. For healthcare organizations to meet their goals and objectives, they must effectively deploy and support workers of all kinds, and doing so requires that the numbers and types of workers match the needs of the patients, regulators, and payers who make up the functional environment of a healthcare organization. For state, provincial, and regional or national systems, policymakers also require information from planning processes. Functionally, workforce planning does several things:

- Defines and identifies shortages and surpluses
- Interprets tasks and roles
- Establishes education and training needs

- Describes the dynamics of the workforce
- Describes and disseminates information about workforce and workplace change

The History of Healthcare Workforce Planning

Daniel Fox (1996) describes healthcare workforce policy in the United States as "contentious and uncertain" and characterizes its history as a process that moved from "piety, to platitudes, to pork." His observations apply mostly to the ongoing debate over whether government should directly support the education and preparation of physicians, or indirectly through some levy on social insurance, or not at all. Fox tracked the history of policies that were discussed and applied over time to support medical education. His analysis pertains to the development of policy that depends on workforce planning, but he did not speak specifically of that development process.

Fox's observations provide useful context for understanding why we would or would not plan for a healthcare workforce in the United States. These reasons have implications for whether planning should be supported. By calling the initial stage of workforce policymaking the result of "pious" thinking, Fox implies that policymakers knew exactly the "right thing to do" and needed no or little specific guidance or planning to assist them. The subsequent dependence on "platitudes" about the reality of need and supply of physicians and nurses was made by using "accepted wisdom," which again meant that there was little need for either planning or research. The culmination of the policy stream with "pork" meant that resources were distributed according to political power with little regard for the "facts"—again, a situation that does not require the development of information and specific planning.

Healthcare workforce policy has traditionally been driven by a perception of a shortage of one or more of the healthcare professions. The history of concern over shortages may have started with physicians, but nurses were also considered a special part of the healthcare workforce and subject to policy attention. The Nurse Training Act of 1941 attempted to expand nursing schools during wartime to provide nurses for the military. An apparent shortage of nurses in the late 1950s generated the very first federal legislation to support training of healthcare professionals for the "market," not for some specific federal role. Subsidies for nursing education and public health traineeships were included in the Health Amendments Act of 1956, beginning an incremental expansion of federal government support for healthcare workforce training.

What followed were a series of healthcare professions laws that encouraged the creation of training programs, supported faculty, expanded schools, or provided special aid for programs to redistribute the workforce. The Health Professional Educational Assistance Act of 1963 (PL 88-129) provided construction money for healthcare professions schools, funds tied to increase enrollment requirements to assist with the school's operating expenses, as well as loans and scholarship programs. It authorized support to medical schools for the first time and firmly established the presence of the federal government in health-related educational institutions. This was followed by an almost annual succession of laws that added support for nurses, created loan-repayment plans, and paid for construction. In 1970, the National Health Service Corps was created, which put the federal government in a role as a direct provider of healthcare professional service for the general population.

The precedent had been set for federal involvement in workforce policy in 1956, but early in the twentieth century many states took on healthcare professions education and regulation as an extension of their responsibility for public education and their implied "police powers" to protect the health, safety, and welfare of their citizens. Assuming a combination of power over both education and entry into the healthcare professions seems to suggest that the conditions were ripe for some form of planning on the part of the states that were investing substantial resources in medical and other health-professions schools and that had ready policy levers to control the supply of practitioners. However, the politics of the healthcare professions were clearly dominated by the professions themselves, and the dominant culture was to support the market for a highly paid elite physician workforce assisted by less well-paid nurses and other caregivers (Starr 1982). According to Weissert and Silberman (1998), not until the 1990s did the states began to "send a message that the medical schools have a responsibility to the state and its citizens." For some reason, the states were not overly concerned with healthcare workforce supply and needs until the beginning of the twenty-first century.

Workforce planning can be considered a subtopic in the general area of healthcare planning, but the two do not necessarily share a common history and important differences exist in the way they are approached. Planning is usually initiated when there is a perception that there are limited resources to meet all possible needs and that the market will not adequately distribute the available benefits.

The Rationale for Healthcare Workforce Planning

History tells us that policy and political pressures are generated when either the market or activated citizens signal a shortage of some type of basic good or service. In the case of healthcare workforce, the shortage is of healing practitioners and their necessary supporting trades and professions. The case for formal planning, however, is often made in a more abstract and value-free context. Advocates for workforce planning sometimes appeal to a need for "rational policymaking," but the stimulus for formal activity often comes when people simply cannot get what they want or feel they need or deserve. In the United States today, the perception that there are shortages of nurses and a potential shortage of physicians is stimulating demand for workforce planning. In Canada and the United Kingdom, there are queues for certain types of care, and these conditions are drawing attention to workforce planning.

Overview of Workforce Planning Methodologies

There are five basic strategies used in workforce planning: (1) population-based estimating, (2) benchmarking, (3) needs-based assessment, (4) demand-based assessment, and (5) training-output estimating. Each approach has its strengths and weaknesses, depending on the goal of the planning exercise and the context in which it is to be applied.

The strategies may be used separately or in combination. For national health systems, the population-based estimating approach may be more applicable in combination with training-output estimating. The goal may be to balance investments in training with overall population needs for healthcare. For organizations, benchmarks may provide useful information on how to staff a hospital or clinic to achieve productivity compared to that of peer institutions. Combined with demand analysis, planning can allow managers to anticipate the effects of changes in requirements for staff after increased marketing efforts or proactive modifications to product mix (Schnelle et al. 2004).

Population-Based Estimating

This approach rests on presumed appropriate or normative ratios of personnel and professionals to population. These ratios are not always generated from epidemiological analysis or careful study of productivity and utilization, but they often come from rules of thumb or from the current state of balance of practitioners to population. In the United States, several proposals for the most appropriate ratio of physician to population have been based on observations of current and past ratios. For example, the indicator of a shortage for primary care services in the United States—the Health Professional Shortage Area criterion—sees a ratio of one full-time equivalent primary care physician for every 3,500 people as indicating a severe level of need. A ratio of 1:3,000 accompanied by elevated population-risk indicators, such as infant mortality and a high proportion of people older than 65 years in a "rational service" area, also signal high need, making the area or population eligible for designation.

In a description of the origins of the Health Manpower (now Professional) Shortage Area criteria, a federal report suggested that the primary-care-physician-to-population ratio of 1:3,500 was selected because it was determined to have been 1.5 times the mean-population-to-primary-care-physician ratio by county for 1974, and because it qualifies a quarter of all counties with the worst ratios (Bureau of Health Manpower 1977). That report indicated that the ratio of 1:2,500 was selected as a measure of relative adequacy, being close to the primary-care-physician-to-population median ratio for all U.S. counties in 1974.

Many ratios have been suggested as indicative of adequate supply. Figure 2.1 summarizes 16 such "ideal" or "adequate" ratios. The ratios are drawn from work by David Kindig (1994) and the Council on Graduate Medical Education (1996, 1999). The wide variation in ratios points to the weaknesses inherent in the population-based approaches. Variability can be the result of differences in assumptions concerning the productivity of practitioners, the needs for services in the population, and even miscalculations caused by poor data in surveys and practice lists. Nevertheless, analysts as well as planners persist in using ratios as standard indicators of desired staffing or as guides to their studies of professional supply.

Benchmarking

The benchmarking approach takes into consideration existing ratios but adds a test of efficiency to the analysis. The most prominent example focuses on the physician workforce in the United States, where regional, population-based ratios have been estimated and compared to organizational ratios (Schroeder 1996; Goodman et al. 1996). In this case, regional ratios for hospital-referral areas generated for the Dartmouth Atlas of Healthcare were compared to the ratio in a large managed care system and selected market-area ratios where there was intense or few managed care. This approach to setting national standards is much more controversial than its use for organizations (Malone 1997; Wholey, Burns, and Lavizzo-Mourey 1998). The ratios used in the Goodman analysis included an adjusted HMO staffing ratio (1:1908) and the actual generalist ratio for the Wichita, Kansas (1:1,527), and Minneapolis, Minnesota (1:1,316), hospital referral regions (see Figure 2.1). Across the United States, using the hospital-referral regions to calculate denominators, 96 percent of the population lived in areas with more generalist physicians than the HMO benchmark, 60 percent lived in areas that exceeded the Wichita standard, and 27 percent lived in areas that exceeded the Minneapolis standard. Advocates of the benchmarking approach

FIGURE 2.1
Summary
of Population-
to-Physician
Ratios,
Suggested as
Standards

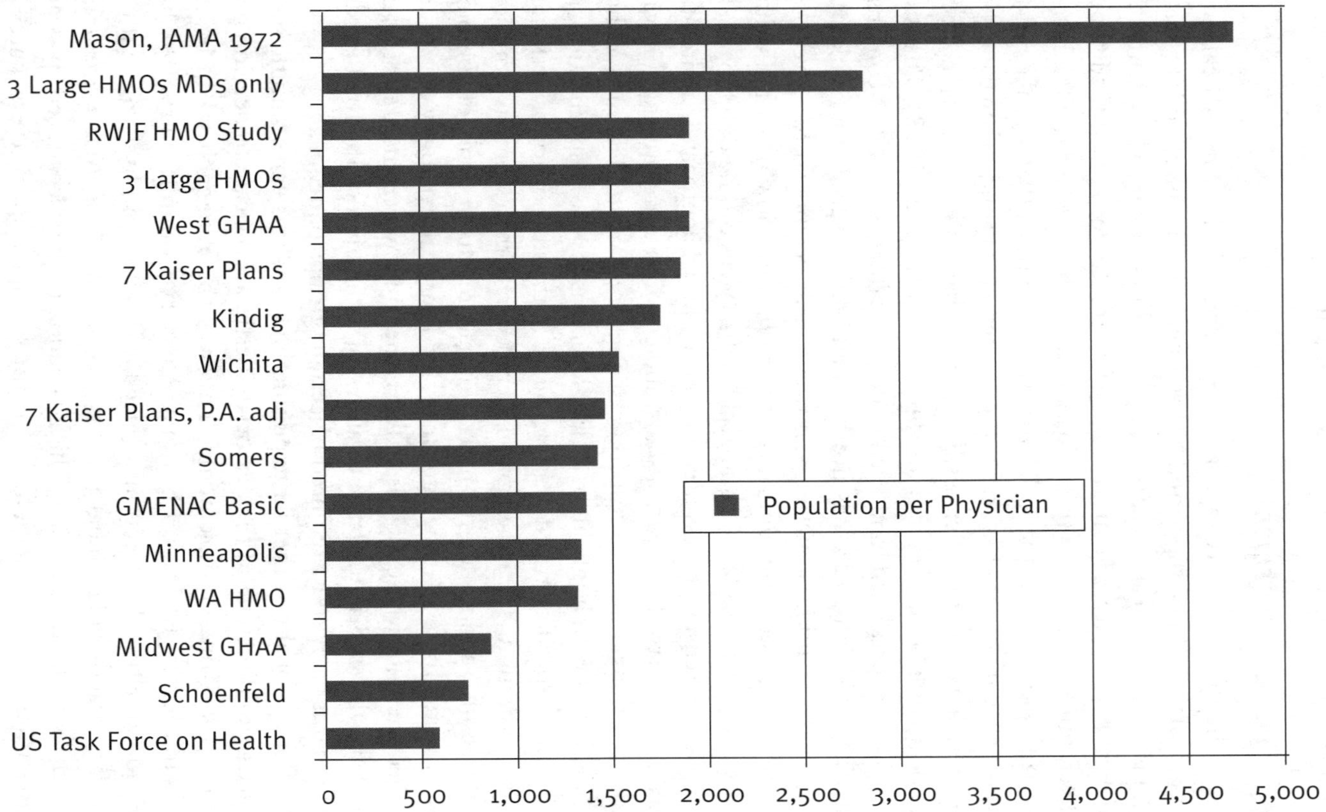

Sources: Council on Graduate Medical Education [COGME]. 1996. *Eighth Report: Patient Care Physician Supply and Requirements: Testing COGME Recommendations.* Washington, DC: Division of Medicine, Bureau of Health Professions, HRSA; COGME. 1999. *Fourteenth Report: COGME Physician Workforce Policies: Recent Developments and Remaining Challenges in Meeting National Goals.* Washington, DC: Bureau of Health Professions, HRSA; Kindig, D. A. 1994. "Counting Generalist Physicians." *JAMA* 271 (19): 1505–07.

see these ratios as achievable, optimal ratios and accept the implication that these ratios describe the most efficient supply of practitioners.

The benchmarking approach has become a part of the workforce-analysis process, and the growing influence of the Dartmouth Atlas of Healthcare in guiding policy debate may make this approach more important. However, there has been little acceptance of the specific standards applicable for policy targets or for setting standards for underservice.

Needs-Based Assessment

Perhaps the most obvious approach to determining how many healthcare professionals should be supported in a system or an organization is to match the consensus healthcare needs of the population or client base with their biological need for care. Unfortunately, healthcare need is a difficult thing to determine and is subject to much variation. The substantial difference in physician opinions over the indicators and conditions that signal need for various procedures—such as carotid endarterectomy and coronary bypass graft operations, among other costly and specialized interventions—has been well documented (Birkmeyer et al. 1998; Wennberg et al. 1998). That variation has been persistent, and even concerted efforts to develop consensus on need for specialist care has not been altogether successful (Fink et al. 1984). Those consensus methods, however, can be applied to more localized situations, and useful guidance for determining how many individuals in a population are likely to require selected services can be developed.

The consensus process used in a needs-based approach is an iterative process, where lists of indicators, signs, and conditions are presented in various combinations and where "expert" clinicians are asked to determine if these combinations are high, medium, or low-level reasons for hospitalization, for conducting a specific procedure, for course of therapy, or for prescribing a specific medication. The expert panel members rate these combinations, discuss the results, and re-rate them. This usually results in a mix of combinations for which there is strong agreement for a particular pathway of care and for other situations where there is less agreement. However, the area of agreement is usually sufficiently large to allow for estimation of the total burden of care that is likely to be required by certain groups of people.

For national or other large populations, analysts can combine separate classes of diseases and their associated estimates of care to develop projections of staffing requirements. This was the approach taken by the Graduate Medical Education National Advisory Committee (1980) when it developed national projections of need and supply of physicians and primary care practitioners. That process was called an *adjusted needs-based approach* to workforce planning. This adaptation of the needs-based approach has been used since its development for specialty-specific estimates of requirements (Elisha, Levinson, and Grinshpoon 2004). Even for very specific specialties, the task of determining even supply is very difficult: "The actual number of FTE [full-time equivalent] neurosurgeons in practice is more difficult to determine, because the number is constantly changing as a result of death, retirement, modification of practice habits and mix of clinical practice versus other professional activities" (Popp and Toselli 1996).

The use of a needs-based approach to plan for staffing is supported by more carefully structured studies for some sectors of the healthcare system than for others; an example includes the development of appropriate ratios of practitioners for dental care (DeFriese and Barker 1982). Practical applications in healthcare organizations and bounded delivery systems require a focus on a particular type of need related to a specific type of organizational form—for example, the need in relation to staffing for outpatient mental health clinics, where those clinics are managed centrally and few alternative sources of this type of care exist (Elisha, Levinson, and Grinshpoon 2004).

Demand-Based Assessment

This approach to workforce planning is explicitly economic in nature and is based largely on past patterns of service utilization. Demand is considered to be somewhat independent of need for care in that some individuals may seek care when they are not ill, either misreading symptoms or desiring to be treated regardless of medical need. In practice, need and demand are considered very closely tied. In an economic sense, demand is equal to utilization (what is consumed *is* what is demanded)—that is, there is a balance in supply and demand in the market that is regulated by the price of the goods and services that are consumed. However, often the case is that demand and supply are not in balance in a sector such as healthcare because prices are not easily determined by either the purchaser or the supplier. Still, utilization can be a strong indicator of demand in a system where there are few barriers to care caused by restrictions on access. An open argument in the United States is whether or not the government restricts access by market rationing, which is opposite the explicit budget rationing in countries such as the United Kingdom and Canada.

A good example of the use of the demand-based model is provided in studies commissioned by the American Medical Association (Marder et al. 1988). Any mathematical model that projects the supply or demand for healthcare professionals must include certain assumptions about the future. For example, knowing that there will be a substantial growth in the number and population proportion that is very old allows the planner to anticipate much higher levels of utilization. These increased levels of demand will be reflected in increased supplies of practitioners who are trained to care for the elderly, provided the training system is able to respond. In an application of this principle at a very macro level, Cooper and colleagues (2002) have attempted to demonstrate that overall economic activity is what determines the future supply of physicians in the United States. Their assumption is that the supply of medical practitioners is determined by the degree to which demand can be expressed in a relatively open market for care.

Training-Output Estimating

This is perhaps the most common approach used to anticipate supply of practitioners. Essentially it makes use of the data that come from training programs: the numbers of enrollees, anticipated graduates, and trends in applications. It has been used to anticipate trends in the general supply of physicians (Cooper, Stoflet, and Wartman 2003), general surgeons (Jonasson, Kwakwa, and Sheldon 1995), internists (Andersen et al. 1990), pediatricians (Bazell and Salsberg 1998), and allied health professionals (DePoy, Wood, and Miller 1997).

Estimations of the supply of nurse practitioners and physician assistants rely heavily on trends in enrollment in training programs (Hooker and Cawley 2002; Buerhaus, Staiger, and Auerbach 2000). Anticipating the characteristics of the future workforce in relation to current training patterns is important to understand how well the practitioners will meet clinical as well as social needs in the future. This issue has become very important in the United States, as national policy has shifted toward having a workforce that matches the racial and ethnic structure of the population (Fiscella et al. 2000).

Challenges and Difficulties of Workforce Planning

The fundamental challenge to workforce planning is that any credible analysis that points to an impending shortage or surplus of practitioners is likely to result in a policy or organizational response that precludes that scenario from occurring. Retrospective analyses of "how well we did" often emphasize how poorly projections performed rather than how much reaction they generated (Cooper et al. 2002). Those retrospectives are, disappointingly, applied only to national estimates of the state of the workforce at some unspecified future time. In planning for physician supply, rarely are organizational or delivery system studies discussed and critiqued, except as the basis for making national estimates (Weiner 2004, 1994, 1987; Hart et al. 1997).

In the field of planning for nursing staffing, there is much more organizational emphasis because such planning is considered a "staffing" problem subject to management, rather than a need to anticipate a market response (Seago et al. 2001). Nursing staffing, however, is also subject to broad-scale analyses to anticipate local conditions (Cooper and Aiken 2001).

International Perspectives

National-level healthcare workforce planning is practiced more often in countries other than the United States. This is a function of the political economy of these countries' healthcare systems, in which central direction and planning is the norm. In other countries, most ministries or departments of health include a human resources division or section that, in turn, is responsible for the planning function. The planning that goes on is applicable to the overall system, where decisions are made concerning the number of practitioners and support staff to be trained or allowed into the country. Organizational planning for specific staffing needs of institutions often takes place within the same part of the bureaucracy, but sometimes delineation is made between strategic planning for national needs and strategic planning for policy and institutional planning for staffing and management decision making.

Canada, for example, has recently developed the Pan-Canadian Health Human Resources (HHR) Planning Initiative intended to bring more evidence-based methods to the work of Health Canada. This is a consortium effort that relies on external research and analysis groups as well as on internal staff. The task of the Canadian HHR planning group is focused on assessing the future staffing and contracting needs of Health Canada and the provincial ministries and departments, as that nation attempts to reform the Canadian healthcare system in response to the 2003 First Ministers' Accord on Health Care Renewal. The Canadian 2003 federal budget allocated $90 million over five years to strengthen healthcare human resources planning and coordination. The national work and interprovincial planning activities are coordinated through the Advisory Committee on Health Delivery and Human Resources, which has assigned a planning subcommittee to develop evidenced-based recommendations on education strategies, especially interprofessional education, and on establishing a workforce that can respond to a patient-centered healthcare system.

In 1995, Australia developed formal structures in its Department of Health to oversee planning activities for its healthcare workforce. For political and practical reasons, the oversight of planning functions were divided between two committees—one for medical positions (Australian Medical Workforce Advisory Committee) and one for all other professions and occupations (Australian Health Workforce Advisory Committee). The central technical task of these committees is to estimate the "required health work-force to meet future health service requirements and the development of strategies to meet that need" (Australian Medical Workforce Advisory Committee 2003).

The World Health Organization supports the Human Resources for Health program, which has invested heavily in developing skills of personnel who can do workforce planning for national and regional health-care systems (see www.wpro.who.int/rd/chapter3_2.asp for an example of work done in the western Pacific). Australia, for example, has committed substantial resources and energy in the development of plans for its rural and remote workforce, and more recently it has developed a national public health workforce plan (see www.nphp.gov.au/workprog/workforce/index.htm). In New Zealand, the notion of central, policy-driven work-force planning is out of favor with the government. The government holds that system managers can help direct workforce resources to the proper places and into the proper roles (see www.asms.org.nz/publications/work-plan.html).

Barriers to healthcare-workforce development in all countries have included a failure to specify health goals, limited liaison between the health and education sectors, and resource constraints. Other factors that have complicated a strategic approach to workforce development in the health-care sector include the diversity and rapid evolution of health services, the long training period for most healthcare professions, and the increasing mobility of the healthcare workforce. Political ideology can also be of major importance. In New Zealand, the market-oriented health reforms of the 1990s created a competitive rather than a collaborative environment, in which workforce development was not a priority (Hornblow 2002).

One international development that is likely to have widespread effects on workforce planning and planning in a management context is the European Union's Working Time Directive (Roche-Nagle 2004; Paice and Reid 2004). This rule applies to a wide range of healthcare professionals and sets limits on the amount of time an individual is allowed to work in a day and over a work week.

Workforce Supply Metrics

Measuring the supply of healthcare professionals is not as straightforward as it seems. A doctor is what a doctor does, but when considering the over-all professional supply needed for a specific area or organization the dis-tinction is harder to make. For example, in counting primary care physicians, most experts and policies consider a family physician as dedicated to primary care, which is defined as the kind of healthcare most people need most of the time. A primary care practitioner then takes care of the most common complaints and coordinate the care needs of a patient—be it specialty or inpatient. However, is a psychiatrist or an OB-GYN a primary care physician? Each may be the patient's first contact with the medical system, and each may coordinate the care for many individuals, but the practice of a psychiatrist and an OB-GYN is limited to certain aspects of human health and illness. To add more confusion, in many states and under certain federal regulations, these practitioners are considered primary care physicians.

The extent of detail involved in creating an inventory of primary care physicians is indicative of the complexity of any process that tries to ascertain how well the supply of healthcare professionals meets a population's or an organization's needs. This challenge often deters managers as well as planners from attempting to balance their anticipated needs for healthcare professionals with likely scenarios for supply. Sufficient models are available on how to approach workforce planning that can make the effort well worthwhile in reducing overall costs of staffing or training and the costs associated with mismatches of needs and resources.

Summary

Workforce planning is the anticipation of how many practitioners and support workers that an organization or a system will require to achieve its mission. The development of effective workforce plans depends on the use of accurate and reliable data that describe current supply, pattern of entry and exit from professions and positions, and the number of incoming workers from training programs and schools. Healthcare workforce planning at the national level also requires an understanding of major economic and social trends as well as a keen sense of the politics involved in labor and professions.

Five basic strategies are used in workforce planning: (1) population-based estimating, (2) benchmarking, (3) needs-based assessment, (4) demand-based assessment, and (5) training-output estimating. Each approach offers strengths depending on the context in which it is applied. The institutional planner can make use of all these at some time to assist in the development of staffing plans, prepare for turnover and transitions, and position the organization to compete effectively for resources.

References

Andersen, R. M., C. Lyttle, C. H. Kohrman, G. S. Levey, K. Neymarc, and C. Schmidt. 1990. "National Study of Internal Medicine Manpower: XVII.

Changes in the Characteristics of Internal Medicine Residents and Their Training Programs, 1988–1989." *Annals of Internal Medicine* 113 (3): 243–49.

Australian Medical Workforce Advisory Committee. 2003. Specialist Medical Workforce Planning in Australia. North Sydney, Australia: Australian Medical Workforce Advisory Committee. www.healthworkforce.health. nsw.gov.au/amwac/amwac/plan_proc.html.

Bazell, C., and E. Salsberg. 1998. "The Impact of Graduate Medical Education Financing Policies on Pediatric Residency Training." *Pediatrics* 101 (4 Pt 2): 785–92; discussion 793–94.

Birkmeyer, J. D., S. M. Sharp, S. R. Finlayson, E. S. Fisher, and J. E. Wennberg. 1998. "Variation Profiles of Common Surgical Procedures." *Surgery* 124 (5): 917–23.

Buerhaus, P. I., D. O. Staiger, and D. I. Auerbach. 2000. "Implications of an Aging Registered Nurse Workforce." *JAMA* 283 (22): 2948–54.

Bureau of Health Manpower. 1977. *Report on Development of Criteria for Designation of Health Manpower Shortage Areas*. Rockville, MD: Health Resources Administration.

Coffman, J. M., J. A. Seago, and J. Spetz. 2002. "Minimum Nurse-to-Patient Ratios in Acute Care Hospitals in California." *Health Affairs (Millwood)* 21 (5): 53–64.

Cooper, R. A., and L. H. Aiken. 2001. "Human Inputs: The Healthcare Workforce and Medical Markets." *Journal of Health Politics, Policy & Law* 26 (5): 925–38.

Cooper, R. A., T. E. Getzen, H. J. McKee, and P. Laud. 2002. "Economic and Demographic Trends Signal an Impending Physician Shortage." *Health Affairs* 21 (1): 140–54.

Cooper, R. A., S. J. Stoflet, and S. A. Wartman. 2003. "Perceptions of Medical School Deans and State Medical Society Executives About Physician Supply." *JAMA* 290 (22): 2992–95.

Council on Graduate Medical Education. 1996. *Eighth Report: Patient Care Physician Supply and Requirements: Testing COGME Recommendations*. Washington, DC: Bureau of Health Professions, HRSA.

———. 1999. *Fourteenth Report: COGME Physician Workforce Policies: Recent Developments and Remaining Challenges in Meeting National Goals*. Washington, DC: Bureau of Health Professions, HRSA.

DeFriese, G. H., and B. D. Barker. 1982. *Assessing Dental Manpower Requirements: Alternative Approaches for State and Local Planning, Issues in Dental Health Policy*. Cambridge, MA: Ballinger.

DePoy, E., C. Wood, and M. Miller. 1997. "Educating Rural Allied Health Professionals: An Interdisciplinary Effort." *Journal of Allied Health* 26 (3): 127–32.

De Geyndt, W. 2000. "Health Workforce Development in the NIS." In *NIS (New Independent States)/US Health Workforce Planning 2000*, edited by G. L. Filerman. Washington, DC: American International Health Alliance.

Elisha, D., D. Levinson, and A. Grinshpoon. 2004. "A Need-Based Model for Determining Staffing Needs for the Public Sector Outpatient Mental Health Service System." *Journal of Behavioral Health Services Research* 31 (3): 324–33.

Fink, A., J. Kosecoff, M. Chassin, and R. H. Brook. 1984. "Consensus Methods: Characteristics and Guidelines for Use." *American Journal of Public Health* 74 (9): 979–83.

Fiscella, K., P. Franks, M. R. Gold, and C. M. Clancy. 2000. "Inequalities in Racial Access to Healthcare." *JAMA* 284 (16): 2053.

Fox, D. M. 1996. "From Piety to Platitudes to Pork: The Changing Politics of Health Workforce Policy." *Journal of Health Politics, Policy and Law* 21 (4): 825–44.

Fried, B. J. 1997. "Physician Resource Planning in an Era of Uncertainty and Change." *Canadian Medical Association Journal* 157 (9): 1227–28.

Goodman, D. C., E. S. Fisher, T. A. Bubolz, J. E. Mohr, J. F. Poage, and J. E. Wennberg. 1996. "Benchmarking the US Physician Workforce. An Alternative to Needs-Based or Demand-Based Planning." *JAMA* 276 (22): 1811–17.

Graduate Medical Education National Advisory Committee. 1980. *Report of the Graduate Medical Education National Advisory Committee to the Secretary, Department of Health and Human Services, Volume 1.* Washington, DC: Office of Graduate Medical Education.

Hart, L. G., E. Wagner, S. Pirzada, A. F. Nelson, and R. A. Rosenblatt. 1997. "Physician Staffing Ratios in Staff-Model HMOs: A Cautionary Tale." *Health Affairs (Millwood)* 16 (1): 55–70.

Hooker, R., and J. F. Cawley. 2002. *Physician Assistants in American Medicine, 2nd Edition.* Philadelphia, PA: W. B. Saunders.

Hornblow, A. 2002. Second NCETA Workforce Development Symposium, Adelaïde, Australia, May 1.

Jonasson, O., F. Kwakwa, and G. F. Sheldon. 1995. "Calculating the Workforce in General Surgery." *JAMA* 274 (9): 731–34.

Kindig, D. A. 1994. "Counting Generalist Physicians." *JAMA* 271 (19): 1505–07.

Malone, S. 1997. "Staffing to Volume in Integrated Delivery Networks." *Journal of AHIMA* 68 (9): 42, 44, 46–48.

Marder, W. D., P. R. Kletke, A. B. Silberger, and R. J. Willke. 1988. *Physician Supply and Utilization by Specialty: Trends and Projections.* Chicago: American Medical Association.

Paice, E., and W. Reid. 2004. "Can Training and Service Survive the European Working Time Directive?" *Medical Education* 38 (4): 336–38.

Popp, A. J., and R. Toselli. 1996. "Workforce Requirements for Neurosurgery." *Surgery and Neurology* 46: 181–85.

Roche-Nagle, G. 2004. "The European Working Time Directive: A Survey of Surgical Specialist Registrars." *International Medical Journal* 97 (6): 175–78.

Schnelle, J. F., S. F. Simmons, C. Harrington, M. Cadogan, E. Garcia, and M. Bates-Jensen. 2004. "Relationship of Nursing Home Staffing to Quality of Care." *Health Services Research* 39 (2): 225–50.

Schroeder, S. A. 1996. "How Can We Tell Whether There Are Too Many or Too Few Physicians?" The Case for Benchmarking [editorial; comment]." *JAMA* 276 (22): 1841–34.

Seago, J. A., M. Ash, J. Spetz, J. Coffman, and K. Grumbach. 2001. "Hospital Registered Nurse Shortages: Environmental, Patient, and Institutional Predictors." *Health Services Research* 36 (5): 831–52.

Starr, P. 1982. *The Social Transformation of American Medicine*. New York: Basic Books.

Weiner, J. P. 1987. "Primary Care Delivery in the United States and Four Northwest European Countries: Comparing the 'Corporatized' with the 'Socialized'." *Milbank Quarterly* 65 (3): 426–61.

———. 1994. "Forecasting the Effects of Health Reform on US Physician Workforce Requirement. Evidence from HMO Staffing Patterns." *JAMA* 272 (3): 222–30.

———. 2004. "Prepaid Group Practice Staffing and U.S. Physician Supply: Lessons for Workforce Policy." *Health Affairs (Millwood)* (Suppl Web Exclusives): W4, 43–59.

Weissert, C. S., and S. L. Silberman. 1998. "Sending a Policy Signal: State Legislatures, Medical Schools and Primary Care Mandates." *Journal of Health Politics, Policy and Law* 23 (5): 743–45.

Wennberg, D. E., F. L. Lucas, J. D. Birkmeyer, C. E. Bredenberg, and E. S. Fisher. 1998. "Variation in Carotid Endarterectomy Mortality in the Medicare Population: Trial Hospitals, Volume, and Patient Characteristics." *JAMA* 279 (16): 1278–81.

Wholey, D. R., L. R. Burns, and R. Lavizzo-Mourey. 1998. "Managed Care and the Delivery of Primary Care to the Elderly and the Chronically Ill." *Health Services Research* 33 (2 Pt II): 322–53.

Discussion Questions

1. What are the major types of healthcare workforce planning? Provide examples of situations where each strategy would be more appropriate than the others.

2. Healthcare workforce planning is often done after a shortage in a particular profession is recognized. How could planning help avert those shortages?

3. Counting healthcare professionals as part of healthcare workforce planning is not always straightforward. For a specific profession—nursing, dentistry, or medicine—describe how the practice patterns of the professionals may change the effective supply of that profession.

Experiential Exercise

Case   In 1999, California became the first state to pass a law requiring minimum staffing ratios for nurses in acute care hospitals (Coffman, Seago, and Spetz 2002). California Assembly Bill 394 (AB 394) mandated the Department of Health Services to create "minimum, specific, and numerical nurse-to-patient ratios by licensed nurse classification and by hospital unit for the inpatient parts of general hospitals in the state."

In January 2004, those regulations came into effect, requiring, for example, that there be no more than four patients per nurse in an emergency room or that nurses on post-operative surgical units care for no more than six. The national nursing supply-and-demand model indicates the following trajectory of supply for registered nurses (RNs) in general acute care hospitals in North Carolina (see Table E2.1).

The North Carolina General Assembly is considering implementing a mandatory staffing ratio that matches the California rules for emergency rooms and post-op units. This required staffing rule will increase the demand for nurses in emergency rooms in North Carolina's 125 hospitals by 4 percent and for post-op units by 6 percent in the first year of implementation, and this demand will remain steady for the next 15 years. The North Carolina Hospital Association found that across all hospitals, the emergency room accounted for 8 percent of RN staffing and the post-op units for 11 percent of RNs. Overall, hospital RNs account for 48 percent of all active RNs in North Carolina.

Case Exercise

Estimate the change in demand for nurses through the year 2020, if the North Carolina law is put into effect on January 1, 2005. The use of emergency rooms and post-op units is expected to rise in direct proportion to the overall use of hospitals measured by inpatient days.

TABLE E2.1
Projected
Supply of RNs
and Inpatient
Hospital
Days, North
Carolina,
2004–2020

Year	RNs	Inpatient Days
2004	31,584	4,024,336
2005	32,153	4,058,776
2006	32,726	4,093,069
2007	33,320	4,129,125
2008	33,976	4,170,419
2009	34,576	4,205,502
2010	35,186	4,241,959
2011	35,751	4,273,354
2012	36,574	4,328,715
2013	37,334	4,377,928
2014	38,077	4,424,951
2015	38,820	4,471,687
2016	39,568	4,518,369
2017	40,350	4,567,598
2018	41,180	4,621,497
2019	41,994	4,672,401
2020	42,828	4,724,685

HEALTHCARE PROFESSIONALS

Kenneth R. White, Ph.D., FACHE; Dolores G. Clement, Dr.P.H.; and

Kristie G. Stover, M.B.A., CHE

Learning Objectives

After completing this chapter, the reader should be able to

- understand the role of healthcare professionals in the human resource management function of healthcare organizations;
- define the elements of a profession, with an understanding of the theoretical underpinnings of the healthcare professions in particular;
- describe the healthcare professions, which include the majority of healthcare workers, and the required educational levels, scopes of practice, and licensure issues for each;
- relate knowledge of the healthcare professions to selected human resources management issues and systems development; and
- comprehend the changing nature of the existing and emerging healthcare professions in the healthcare workforce, particularly the impact of managed care.

Introduction

Healthcare professionals are central to the delivery of high-quality health services. Extensive training, education, and skills are essential in meeting the needs and demands of the population for safe, competent healthcare. These specialized techniques and skills that healthcare professionals acquired through systematic programs of intellectual study are the basis for socialization into their profession. Additionally, the healthcare industry is labor intensive and is distinguished from other service industries by the number of licensed and registered personnel that it employs and the variety of healthcare fields that it produces. These healthcare fields have emerged as a result of the specialization of medicine, development of public health, increased emphasis on health promotion and prevention, and technological development and growth.

Because of this division of labor within medical and health services delivery, many tasks that were once the responsibility of medical providers have been delegated to other healthcare personnel. Such delegation of duties raises important questions for the industry. Should healthcare providers other than those specifically trained to practice medicine be considered professionals in their own right? To what extent should their scope of practice be extended?

In this chapter, we respond to the aforementioned questions by defining key terms, describing the healthcare professions and labor force, explaining the role of human resources in healthcare, and discussing key human resources issues that affect the delivery of healthcare.

Professionalization

Although the terms occupation and profession often are used interchangeably, they can be differentiated. An *occupation* enables workers to provide services, but it does not require skill specialization. An occupation is the principal activity that supports one's livelihood. However, it is different from a profession in several ways. An occupation typically does not require higher skill specialization. An individual in an occupation is usually supervised, adheres to a defined work schedule, and earns an hourly wage rate. An individual in an occupation may be trained for a specific job or function and, as a result, is less able to move from one organization to another.

A *profession* requires specialized knowledge and training that enable professionals to gain more authority and responsibility and to provide service that adheres to a code of ethics. A professional usually has more autonomy in determining the content of the service he or she provides and in monitoring the workload needed to do so. A professional generally earns a salary, requires higher education, and works with more independence and mobility than do nonprofessionals.

The distinction between an occupation and a profession is important as the evolving process of healthcare delivery requires professionals who are empowered to make decisions in the absence of direct supervision. The proliferation of knowledge and the skills needed in the prevention, diagnosis, and treatment of disease have required increasing levels of education. Undergraduate- or graduate-level degrees are now required for entry into virtually every professional field. Some professions, such as pharmacy and physical therapy, are moving toward professional doctorates (i.e., Pharm.D. and D.P.T., respectively) for practice.

A countervailing force against the increasing educational requirements of the healthcare professions is ongoing change in the mechanisms for delivery and payment for services. With consolidation of the healthcare system and the rise of managed care, along with its demands for efficiency, fewer financial resources are available. As a result, healthcare organizations are pressured to replace highly trained, and therefore more expensive, healthcare professionals with unlicensed support personnel. Fewer professionals are being asked to do more, and those with advanced degrees are required to supervise more assistants who are functionally trained for specified organizational roles.

Functional training produces personnel who can perform tasks but who may not know the theory behind the practice; understanding theory is essential to becoming fully skilled and being able to make complex management and patient care decisions. Conversely, knowing the theory without having the experience also makes competent practice difficult. When educating potential healthcare professionals, on-the-job training or a period of apprenticeship is needed, particularly in addition to basic coursework. Dreyfus and Dreyfus (1996) contend that both theoretical knowledge and practiced response are needed in the acquisition of skill in a profession. They lay out five stages of abilities that an individual passes as he or she develops a skill:

1. *Novice.* At this stage, the novice learns tasks and skills that enable him or her to determine actions based on recognized situations. Rules and guidelines direct the novice's energy and action at this stage.
2. *Advanced beginner.* At this stage, the advanced beginner has gained enough experience and knowledge that certain behaviors become automatic, and he or she can begin to learn when tasks should be addressed.
3. *Competent.* At this stage, the competent individual has mastered the practiced response of definable tasks and processes and acquired the ability to deal with the unexpected events that may not conform to plans.
4. *Proficient.* At this stage, the proficient individual has developed the ability to discern a situation, intuitively assess it, plan what needs to be done, decide on an action, and perform the action more effortlessly than possible in the earlier stages.
5. *Expert.* At this stage, the expert can accomplish the goals without realizing that rules are being followed because the skill and knowledge required to reach the goal have become second nature to him or her.

Theoretical understanding is melded with practice in each progressive stage. Functional training can help an individual progress through the first three stages and provide the individual with calculative rationality or inferential reasoning ability to be able to apply and improve theories and rules learned. For skill development at the proficient and expert levels, deliberative rationality or ability to challenge and improve theories and rules learned is required. Healthcare professionals need to become experts in fields where self-direction, autonomy, and decision making for patient care may be required (Dreyfus and Dreyfus 1996).

Healthcare Professionals

The healthcare industry is the largest and most powerful industry in the United States. It constitutes over 6.5 percent of the total labor force and nearly 15 percent of the gross domestic product. Healthcare professionals include physicians, nurses, dentists, pharmacists, optometrists, psychologists, nonphysician practitioners such as physician assistants and nurse practitioners, healthcare administrators, and allied health professionals. Allied health professionals are a huge group that consists of therapists, medical and radiologic technologists, social workers, health educators, and other ancillary personnel. Healthcare professionals are represented by professional associations; Table 3.1 provides a sample of professional associations.

Healthcare professionals work in a variety of settings, including hospitals; ambulatory care centers; managed care organizations; long-term care organizations; mental health organizations; pharmaceutical companies; community health centers; physician offices; laboratories; research institutions; and schools of medicine, nursing, and allied health professions. According to the National Center for Health Statistics (Bureau of Labor Statistics 2004), healthcare professionals are employed by the following:

- Hospitals (40.9 percent)
- Nursing and personal and residential care facilities (22.1 percent)
- Physician offices and clinics (15.5 percent)
- Dentist offices and clinics (5.9 percent)
- Chiropractic offices and clinics (1.4 percent)
- Other health service sites (14.1 percent)

The U.S. Department of Labor recognizes about 400 different job titles in the healthcare sector; however, many of these job titles are not included in our definition of healthcare professionals. For example, almost one-third of those employed in the healthcare sector probably belong in the support staff category—that is, employees who are part of the patient care team or are involved in delivering health services. These approximately 2.2 million nursing aides, home health aides, and personal attendants are critical to the delivery of healthcare services (HRSA 2004).

Organization	Target Audience	Web Site
Health Professions		
Pew Health Professions Commission	Future healthcare professionals	www.futurehealth. ucsf.edu
Health Management Careers	Future healthcare managers and administrators	www.healthmanage mentcareers.org
Accrediting Organizations		
Accreditation Association for Ambulatory Health Care	Ambulatory healthcare	www.aaahc.org
Accreditation Council for Graduate Medical Education	Graduate medical education	www.acgme.org
American Osteopathic Association (AOA)	Osteopathic hospitals and health systems	www.aoa-net.org
Commission on Accreditation of Rehabilitation Facilities (CARF)	Rehabilitation facilities	www.carf.org
Joint Commission on Accreditation of Healthcare Organizations (JCAHO)	Hospitals and health systems	www.jcaho.org
National Committee for Quality Assurance (NCQA)	Managed care plans	www.ncqa.org
American Association of Blood Banks (AABB)	Blood banks	www.aabb.org
American College of Surgeons	Surgeons	www.facs.org
American College of Surgeons Commission on Cancer	Cancer programs	www.facs.org/dept/ cancer/coc/liaison. html
College of American Pathologists (CAP)	Clinical laboratories	www.cap.org
Professional Associations		
American College of Healthcare Executives (ACHE)	Healthcare executives	www.ache.org
National Association of Health Services Executives (NAHSE)	African-American healthcare executives	www.nahse.org

TABLE 3.1
Resource Guide for the Healthcare Professional

TABLE 3.1
(continued)

Organization	Target Audience	Web Site
Institute for Diversity in Health Management (IFD)	Healthcare managers	www.diversity connection.org
Medical Group Management Association (MGMA)	Physician practice managers and executives	www.mgma.com
American Society for Healthcare Human Resource Administration	Healthcare HR executives	http://www.hospital connect.com/ ashhra/aboutus/ aboutusindex.html
American College of Physician Executives (ACPE)	Physician executives	www.acpe.org
American College of Health Care Administrators (ACHCA)	Long-term care administrators	www.achca.org
American Association for Medical Transcription (AAMT)	Medical transcriptionists	www.aamt.org
American Association of Nurse Anesthetists (AANA)	Nurse anesthetists	www.aana.com
American Association for Respiratory Care (AARC)	Respiratory therapists	www.aarc.org
American Health Information Management Association (AHIMA)	Medical records and information management professionals	www.ahima.org
American Medical Technologists (AMT)	Medical technologists	www.amt1.com
American Nurses Association (ANA)	Nurses	www.ana.org
American Association for Homecare	Homecare administrators	www.aahomecare. org
American Occupational Therapy Association, Inc. (AOTA)	Occupational therapists	www.aota.org
American Organization of Nurse Executives (AONE)	Nurse executives	www.aone.org
National League of Nursing	Nurses	www.nln.org
American Physical Therapy Association (APTA)	Physical therapists	www.apta.org

TABLE 3.1
(continued)

Organization	Target Audience	Web Site
American Society of Clinical Pathologists (ASCP)	Pathologists and medical technologists	www.ascp.org
American Society of Health-System Pharmacists (ASHP)	Pharmacists	www.ashp.org
American Society of Radiologic Technologists (ASRT)	Radiologic technologists	www.asrt.org
American Speech-Language-Hearing Association (ASHA)	Speech therapists, audiologists, and speech pathologists	www.asha.org
Healthcare Financial Management Association (HFMA)	Comptrollers, CFOs, and accountants	www.hfma.org
Health Information and Management Systems Society (HIMSS)	Health information managers	www.himss.org
National Cancer Registrars Association (NCRA)	Cancer program registrars	www.ncra-usa.org
Trade Associations		
American Hospital Association (AHA)	Hospitals, health systems, and personal membership groups	www.aha.org
Federation of American Hospitals (FAHS)	Investor-owned hospitals and health systems	www.fahs.com
Association of American Medical Colleges (AAMC): Council of Teaching Hospitals and Health Systems (COTH)	Academic medical centers	www.aamc.org/about/coth/start.htm
Catholic Health Association of the United States (CHA)	Catholic hospitals and health systems	www.chausa.org
American Association of Health Plans (AAHP)	Health plans	www.aahp.org

The primary reasons for the increased supply and demand for healthcare professionals include the following interrelated forces:

- Technological growth
- Specialization

- Changes in third-party coverage
- The aging of the population
- The proliferation of new and diverse healthcare delivery settings

This chapter focuses primarily on nurses, pharmacists, selected allied health professionals, and healthcare administrators. Table 3.1 provides a sampling of healthcare professional organizations as well as related organizations.

Nurses

The art of caring, combined with the science of healthcare, is the essence of nursing. Nurses focus not only on a particular health problem, but on the whole patient and his or her response to treatment. Nurses work in many different areas, but the common thread of nursing is the nursing process. This process involves five steps (ANA 2004):

1. *Assessment:* collecting and analyzing physical, psychological, and sociocultural data about a patient
2. *Diagnosis:* making a judgment on the cause, condition, and path of the illness
3. *Planning:* creating a care plan that sets specific treatment goals
4. *Implementation:* supervising or carrying out the actual treatment plan
5. *Evaluation:* continuously assessing the plan

Nurses also serve as patient advocates, multidisciplinary team members, managers, executives, researchers, and entrepreneurs.

Nurses comprise the largest group of licensed healthcare professionals in the United States. According to the "National Sample Survey of Registered Nurses" (HRSA 2001), the United States has 2.6 million registered nurses (RNs), over 2.2 million (82 percent) of whom are employed in healthcare organizations. Approximately 60 percent of employed RNs, or 1.3 million, work in hospitals, while 18 percent, or 468,000, work in community or public health settings. Complementing this workforce are 720,000 licensed practical nurses (LPNs), or licensed vocational nurses (LVNs) as they are known in some states (Bureau of Labor Statistics 2004).

According to the demographic profiles compiled by the National League for Nursing (2004) and the "National Sample Survey of Registered Nurses," most nurses are women. In 2001 the average age of a nurse was 45.2 years old, nearly a year older than in 1997 when the average age was 44.5 years. The aging of the workforce is also reflected in the demographics of nurses: the RN population under 30 dropped from 25 percent in 1980 to 9 percent in 2001. Only 5.4 percent of RNs are men, although 13 percent of enrolled nursing students in 2000 were men, and only 12 percent of RNs come from racial/ethnic minority backgrounds.

All U.S. states require nurses to be licensed to practice. The licensure requirements include graduation from an approved nursing program and successful completion of a national examination. Educational preparation distinguishes the two levels of nurses from each other.

Registered Nurses and Licensed Practical Nurses

RNs must complete an associate's degree in nursing (ADN), a diploma program, or a baccalaureate degree in nursing (BSN) to qualify for the licensure examination. ADN programs generally take two years to complete and are offered by community and junior colleges, and hospital-based diploma programs can be completed in about three years. The fastest growing avenue for nursing education is the baccalaureate preparation, which typically can be completed in four years and is offered by colleges and universities. Licensed practical nurses (LPNs), on the other hand, must complete a state-approved program in practical nursing and must achieve a passing score on a national examination. Each state maintains regulations and practice acts that delineate the scope of nursing practice for RNs and LPNs.

Among employed RNs, about 40 percent hold associate degrees, 30 percent have hospital-based program diplomas, and 30 percent possess BSN degrees. In 2001, only 9 percent of nurses reported having a master's degree, with only 1 percent of nurses being doctorally prepared (HRSA 2001). In addition to licensure and educational achievements, some nurses obtain certification in specialty areas such as critical care, infection control, emergency nursing, surgical nursing, and obstetrical nursing. The nursing field comprises many specialties and subspecialties; certification in these areas requires specialty education, practical experience, and successful completion of a national examination. Some nurses obtain certification in these specialty areas because certification helps them maintain their professional associations. To remain certified, continued employment, continuing education units, or reexamination may be required.

An advanced practice nurse (APN) possesses particular skills and credentials, which typically include basic nursing education; basic licensure; graduate degree in nursing; experience in a specialized area; professional certification from a national certifying body; and, if required in some states, APN licensure (National Council of State Boards of Nursing 2004). The APN specializes as a nurse practitioner (NP), certified nurse midwife (CNM), certified registered nurse anesthetist (CRNA), or clinical nurse specialist (CNS).

Advanced Practice Nurses

The APN role is defined by seven core competencies or skillful performance areas. The first core competency of direct clinical practice is central to and informs all of the others as follows (Hamric, Spross, and Hanson 2005):

- Direct clinical practice (central)
- Expert guidance and coaching of patients, families, and other care providers
- Consultation
- Research skills, including use and implementation of evidence-based practice, evaluation, and conduct
- Clinical and professional leadership, which includes competence as a change agent
- Collaboration
- Ethical decision-making skills

Additional core competencies may be needed in each specialty area that an APN pursues. The largest number of APNs comprises NPs, who may further specialize in acute care or community settings or for particular client groups such as adults, children, women, or psychiatric/mental health populations.

Each state maintains its own laws and regulations regarding recognition of an APN, but the general requirements in all states include licensure as a registered nurse and successful completion of a national specialty examination. Some states permit certain categories of APNs to write prescriptions for certain classes of drugs. This prescriptive authority varies from one state to another and may be regulated by boards of medicine, nursing, pharmacy, or allied health. Some states require physician supervision of APN practices, although some managed care plans now include APNs on their lists of primary care providers.

APN specialization   Certified nurse midwives (CNMs) specialize in low-risk obstetrical care, including all aspects of the prenatal, labor and delivery, and postnatal processes. Certified registered nurse anesthetists (CRNAs) complete additional education to specialize in the administration of various types of anesthesia and analgesia to patients and clients. Often, nurse anesthetists work collaboratively with surgeons and anesthesiologists as part of the perioperative care team. Clinical nurse specialists (CNSs) hold master's degrees, have successfully completed a specialty certification examination, and are generally employed by hospitals as nursing "experts" in particular specialties. The scope of the CNS is not as broad as that of the NP. CNSs work with a specialty population under a somewhat circumscribed set of conditions, and the management authority of patients still rests with physicians. In contrast, NPs have developed an autonomous role in which their collaboration is encouraged, and they generally have the legal authority to implement management actions.

Pharmacists

In the foreseeable future, the pharmacy profession will continue to undergo extensive change. Until the latter part of the past decades, pharmacists performed the traditional role of preparing drug products and filling prescriptions. In the 1980s, however, pharmacists expanded that role. Pharmacists now act as experts for clients and patients on the effects of specific drugs, drug interactions, and generic drug substitutions for brand-name drugs.

To be eligible for licensure, pharmacists must graduate from an accredited baccalaureate program in pharmacy, successfully complete a state board examination, and obtain practical experience or complete a supervised internship. After passing a national examination, a registered pharmacist (R.Ph.) is permitted to carry out the scope of practice outlined by state regulations. The trend in pharmacy has been to broaden education to include the terminal degree Doctor of Pharmacy (Pharm.D.). Many pharmacy schools offer this program for those interested in research careers, teaching, higher administrative responsibility, or as members of the patient care team. This educational preparation also requires successful completion of a state board examination and other practical clinical experience, as outlined by state laws.

Allied Health Professionals

The term allied health professional is generally not well understood because of its ambiguous definition (O'Neil and Hare 1990) and a lack of consensus about what such a role constitutes. In general, allied health professionals complement the work of physicians and other healthcare providers, although one may also be a provider. The U.S. Public Health Service (Health Professions Education Extension Amendments of 1992, Section 701 PHS Act) defines an allied health professional as:

> . . . a health professional (other than a registered nurse or a physician assistant) who has received a certificate, an associate's degree, a bachelor's degree, a master's degree, a doctoral degree, or post-baccalaureate training in a science related to health care; who shares in the responsibility for the delivery of health care services or related services, including (1) services relating to the identification, evaluation and prevention of disease and disorders, (2) dietary and nutrition services, (3) health promotion services, (4) rehabilitation services, or (5) health systems management services;

and who has not received a degree of doctor of medicine, a degree of doctor of osteopathy, a degree of doctor of veterinary medicine or equivalent degree, a degree of doctor of optometry or equivalent degree, a degree of doctor of podiatric medicine or equivalent degree, a degree of bachelor science in pharmacy or equivalent degree, a graduate degree in public health or equivalent degree, a degree of doctor of chiropractic or equivalent degree, a graduate degree in health administration or equivalent degree, a degree of doctor of clinical psychology or equivalent degree, or a degree in social work or equivalent degree.

A debate on the exclusiveness and inclusiveness of the U.S. Public Health's definition continues. Some observers of healthcare consider nursing, public health, and social work to fall under the umbrella of allied health, but they are often categorized as separate professional groups. Figure 3.1 lists the major categories that comprise the allied health profession and the job titles that frequently fall under each category.

According to the "1999 National Occupational and Wage Estimates" for healthcare personnel, the allied health profession constitutes 40.6 percent of the healthcare workforce in the United States (Bureau of Labor Statistics 2001). This number excludes physicians, nurses, dentists, pharmacists, veterinarians, chiropractors, and podiatrists. The allied health profession is the most heterogeneous of the personnel groupings in healthcare.

The National Commission on Allied Health (1995) broadly divided allied health professionals into two categories of personnel: (1) therapists/technologists and (2) technicians/assistants. Some of the job titles presented in Figure 3.1 may not fit into these two categories. In general, the therapist/technologist category represents those with higher-level professional training and who are often responsible for supervising those in the technician/assistant category. Therapists/technologists usually hold baccalaureate and higher degrees, and they are trained to evaluate patients, understand diagnoses, and develop treatment plans in their area of expertise. On the other hand, the technicians/assistants are most likely to have two years or less postsecondary education, and they are functionally trained with procedural skills for specified tasks.

Educational and training programs for the allied health profession are sponsored by a variety of organizations in different academic and clinical settings. They range from degree offerings at colleges and universities to clinical programs in hospitals and other health facilities. Prior to 1990, one-third of the allied health programs were housed in hospitals, although hospitals graduated only 15 percent of their students (O'Neil and Hare 1990). Junior or community colleges, vocational or technical schools, and

Behavioral Health Services

Substance abuse counselor   Community health worker
Home health aide   Mental health assistant
Mental health aide

Clinical Laboratory Sciences

Laboratory associate   Laboratory technician
Laboratory microbiologist   Chemist (biochemist)
                                   Microbiologist
                                   Associate laboratory microbiologist

Dental Services

Dental assistant   Dental laboratory technologist
Dental hygienist

Dietetic Services

Dietitian   Assistant director of food service
Dietary assistant   Associate supervising dietitian

Emergency Medical Services

Ambulance technician   Emergency medical technician

Health Information Management Services

Director of medical records   Senior medical record systems analyst
Assistant director of medical record Health information manager
  service   Data analyst
Medical record specialist   Coder

Medical and Surgical Services

Electroencephalograph technician   Medical equipment specialist
Electroencephalograph technologist Electrocardiograph technician
Operating room technician   Dialysis technologist
Biomedical equipment technician   Surgical assistant
Biomedical engineer   Ambulatory care technician
Cardiovascular technologist

FIGURE 3.1

Major
Categories
of the Allied
Health
Profession and
Professional
Titles

FIGURE 3.1
(continued)

Occupational Therapy

Occupational therapist
Occupational therapy assistant

Occupational therapy aide

Ophthalmology

Ophthalmic dispenser
Optometric aide

Optometric technologist

Physical Therapy

Physical therapist

Physical therapy assistant

Radiological Services

Nuclear medicine technician
Radiation technician
Ultrasound technician
Medical radiation dosimetry

Nuclear medicine technologist
Diagnostic medical sonographer
Radiologic (medical) technologist

Rehabilitation Services

Art therapist
Exercise physiologist
Recreational therapist
Recreation therapy assistant
Addictions counselor
Addictions specialist
Psychiatric social health technician

Music therapist
Dance therapist
Rehabilitation counselor
Rehabilitation technician
Sign-language interpreter

Orthotics/Prosthetics

Orthopedic assistant

Respiratory Therapy Services

Respiratory therapist
Respiratory therapy assistant

Respiratory therapy technician

Speech-Language Pathology/Audiology Services

Audiology clinician
Staff Speech pathologist

Staff audiologist
Speech clinician

Other Allied Health Services

Central supply technician
Podiatric assistant
Health unit coordinator
Home health aide

Medical illustrator
Veterinary assistant
Chiropractic assistant

academic health centers can all sponsor allied health programs. These programs can also be stand-alone when aligned with an academic health center, or they could be under the auspices of the school of medicine or nursing if a specific school of allied health professions does not exist. Dental and pharmacy technicians or assistants may or may not be trained in their respective schools or in a school of allied health professions.

A vast number of the undergraduate allied health programs are accredited by the Commission on Accreditation of Allied Health Educational Programs (CAAHEP), a freestanding agency that replaced the American Medical Association's Committee on Allied Health Education and Accreditation in 1994. The formation of CAAHEP was intended to simplify the accrediting process, to be more inclusive of allied health programs that provide entry-level education, and to serve as an initiator of more far-reaching change. Some key allied health graduate programs, such as physical therapy and occupational therapy, are accredited through specialty professional accreditation organizations.

Healthcare Administrators

Healthcare administrators organize, coordinate, and manage the delivery of health services; provide leadership; and organize the strategic direction of healthcare organizations. The variety and numbers of healthcare professionals they employ; the complexity of healthcare delivery; and environmental pressures to provide access, quality, and efficient services make healthcare institutions among the most complex organizations to manage.

Healthcare administration is taught at the undergraduate and graduate levels in a variety of settings, and these programs lead to a number of different degrees. The settings include schools of medicine, public health, healthcare business, and allied health professions. A bachelor's degree in health administration will allow individuals to pursue positions such as nursing home administrator, supervisor, or middle manager in healthcare organizations. Most students who aspire to have a career in healthcare administration will go on to receive a master's degree. (For a detailed description of various career paths and options, see Haddock, McLean, and Chapman 2002).

Graduate education programs in healthcare administration are accredited by the Commission on Accreditation of Healthcare Management Education, formerly known as the Accrediting Commission on Education for Health Services Administration. Most common degrees include the master of health administration (MHA), master of business administration (MBA, with a healthcare emphasis), master of public health (MPH), or master of public administration (MPA). However, the MHA degree, or its equivalent, has been the accepted training model for entry-level managers in the various sectors of the healthcare industry. The MHA program, when compared to the MPH program, offers core courses that focus on building business management (theory and applied management), quantitative, and analytical skills and that emphasize experiential training. In addition, some MHA programs require students to complete three-month internships or 12-month residencies as part of their two- or three-year curricula. Some graduates elect to complete post-graduate fellowships that are available in selected hospitals, health systems, managed care organizations, consulting firms, and other health-related organizations.

Physicians and other clinicians represent a growing number of healthcare administrators. As evidence, membership in the American College of Physician Executives has increased to more than 10,000 in 2004, up from 5,700 in 1990. Physicians, nurses, and others refocus their clinical careers on the business of healthcare and get involved in the strategy, decision making, resource allocation, and the operations of healthcare organizations. A traditional role for physician executives is chief medical officer (or a similar position) in a hospital, managing the medical staff and serving as a liaison between clinical care and administration. Likewise, a typical career path for nurses is the chief nursing officer role, with responsibility for clinical care provided by the employed professional staff. Chief medical officers typically enjoy a career practicing medicine, slowly transitioning into the operations of a healthcare organization. However, physician executives work at every level and in every setting in healthcare. Many physician executives earn a graduate degree such as an MHA or MBA when they are interested in pursuing a formal educational program in healthcare administration and management. As of 2004, 42 medical schools offer a combined MD/MBA program, and one medical school offers an MD/MHA degree (AAMC 2004). Whether a physician begins his or her career as an administrator or shifts to a physician executive after clinical practice, being a physician executive provides doctors an alternative way to make an impact on the delivery of healthcare.

Nursing home administrator programs require students to pass a national examination administered by the National Association of Boards of Examiners for Nursing Home Administrators. This examination is a standard requirement in all states, but the educational preparation needed to qualify for this exam varies from state to state. Although more than one-third of states still require less than a bachelor's degree as the minimum academic preparation, approximately 70 percent of the practicing nursing home administrators have, at a minimum, a bachelor's degree. As the population continues to live longer, the demand and educational requirements for long-term care administrators is estimated to increase, along with the growth of educational programs specific to this sector of the healthcare industry.

Considerations for Human Resources Management

The role of human resources management (HRM) in healthcare organizations is to develop and implement systems, in accordance with regulatory guidelines and licensure laws, that ensure selection, evaluation, and retention of healthcare professionals. In light of this role, human resources (HR) personnel should be aware that each of the healthcare professions, and often the subspecialties within those professions, has specific requirements that allow an individual to qualify for an entry-level job in his or her chosen profession. The requirements of national accrediting organizations (e.g., the Joint Commission), regulatory bodies (e.g., the Centers for Medicare & Medicaid Services), and licensure authorities (e.g., state licensure boards) should be considered in all aspects of HRM. We briefly discuss some of the issues that a healthcare organization's HR department must consider when dealing with healthcare professionals.

Qualifications

In developing a comprehensive employee-compensation program, HR personnel must include the specific skill and knowledge required for each job in the organization. Those qualifications must be determined and stated in writing for each job. The job description usually contains the level of education, experience, judgment ability, accountability, physical skills, responsibilities, communication skills, and any special certification or licensure requirements. HR personnel need to be aware of all specifications for all job titles within their organizations. This knowledge of healthcare professionals is necessary to ensure that essential qualifications of individuals coincide with job specifications, and it is also necessary for determining wage and salary ranges (see Chapter 6).

Licensure and Certification

An HR department must have policies and procedures in place that describe the way in which licensure is verified on initial employment. Also, the department must have a system in place for tracking the expiration dates of licenses and for ensuring licensure renewal. Therefore, the department must be conscientious about whether the information it receives is a *primary verification* (in which the information directly comes from the licensing authority) or a *secondary verification* (in which a candidate submits a document copy that indicates licensure has been granted, including the expiration date). Certifications must be verified during the selection process, although certifications and licenses are generally not statutory requirements. Many organizations accept a copy of a certification document as verification. If the certification is a job requirement, systems must be in place to track expiration dates and to access new certification documents.

Career Ladders

In selecting healthcare professionals, HR personnel must consider past employment history, including the explanation of gaps in employment. To assess the amount of individual experience, evaluating the candidate's breadth and depth of responsibility in previous jobs is essential. Many organizations have career ladders, which are mechanisms that advance a healthcare professional within the organization. Career ladders are based on the Dreyfus and Dreyfus model of novice to expert (explained earlier in the chapter), and experience may be used as a criterion for assignment of an individual to a particular job category. In addition, organizations may conduct annual reviews of employees with leadership and management potential. This review entails the HR department working with senior management to assess the competency, ability, and career progression of employees on an ongoing basis.

Educational Services

Healthcare professionals require continuous, lifelong learning. Organizations must have in-house training and development plans to ensure that their healthcare professionals achieve competency in new technologies, programs, and equipment and are aware of policy and procedure changes. Certain competencies must be renewed annually in areas such as cardiopulmonary resuscitation, safety and infection control, and disaster planning.

In addition to developing specific training programs, organizations should provide orientation for all new employees. Such organization-specific training enables the leadership to share the values, mission, goals, and policies of the institution. Such clear communication often serves as a retention tool that enables employees to better understand the organization and to be successful. Similarly, some professions and licensing jurisdictions may require continuing education that is profession specific.

An organization can provide training and development in a variety of ways. On one end of the spectrum, training and development can be outsourced to a firm that specializes in conducting educational programs. Conversely, another option is to consolidate all training and developing in-house, which is typically managed by the HR department. Regardless of how each organization provides continuing education, training and development should be a priority. Strong programs can be viewed as recruitment and retention tools. As such, healthcare organizations must be cognizant of fiscal resources necessary to support these educational requirements.

Practitioner Impairment

Healthcare professionals are accountable to the public for maintaining their high professional standards, and the governing body of healthcare organizations is by statute responsible for the quality of care rendered in the organization. This quality is easily jeopardized by an impaired practitioner. An *impaired practitioner* is a healthcare professional who is unable to carry out his or her professional duties with reasonable skill and safety because of a physical or mental illness, including deterioration through aging, loss of motor skill, or excessive use of drugs and alcohol.

The HR department must periodically evaluate the performance of all healthcare professionals in the organization to ensure their competence (which is the basic education and training necessary for the job) and proficiency (which is the demonstrated ability to perform job tasks). Mechanisms must be in place to identify the impaired practitioner, such as policies and procedures that describe how the organization will handle investigations, subsequent recommendations for treatment, monitoring, and employment restrictions or separation. Hospitals, for instance, usually have a process in place for the board of directors to review provider credentials and performance and to oversee any employment actions, as the governing board has ultimate responsibility for the quality of patient care. Each national or state licensing authority maintains legal requirements for reporting impaired practitioners.

In the coming decades, new challenges and opportunities, such as the issues described above, will face the HR department of each organization as a result of ever-increasing changes in the healthcare professions.

Changing Nature of the Healthcare Professions

In the 1990s we entered a new era of uncertainty in healthcare, one faced with a quickening pace of change (Begun and White 1999). Within this framework, new ways of thinking are rewarded as the meaning of health is redefined, the boundaries of healthcare professionals are reshaped, and the outcomes of healthcare professional interventions are measured in terms of quality of life. Changes in the organization and financing of healthcare services have shifted delivery from the hospital to outpatient facilities, the home, long-term care facilities, and the community. This is largely the result of three major forces: (1) a shift in managed care reimbursement to outpatient settings and a focus on cost containment, (2) technological advances such as telemedicine and the electronic medical record, and (3) medical innovation—the science of medicine has progressed to the point that complicated procedures that once required several-nights stay as an inpatient can now be treated with a simple procedure or even solely with medication. These changes are intended to improve the delivery of healthcare while reducing cost and increasing access for patients.

As the setting for the delivery of care continued to change, so did arrangements between providers and healthcare organizations. For instance, physicians can function as individual providers (either solo practitioners or in a group practice) and refer patients to the hospital. These "private-practice doctors" typically have admitting privileges to the hospital but are not governed by the hospital, do not serve as attending physicians, and infrequently participate on hospital committees. Physicians considered on staff at any hospital are those who refer and treat patients at that hospital. They are credentialed by the hospital credentialing committee (usually managed through the chief-of-staff office) and are governed by the medical-staff bylaws. This is a common type of hospital-provider arrangement.

However, there has been a growing trend toward hospitals employing physicians. In this arrangement, the providers are on hospital staff and refer and treat their patients only at the hospital where they are employed. These providers are considered employees and, as such, are held to the HR policies of the organization separate from and in addition to being governed by the medical-staff bylaws. Physicians employed by the hospital can also maintain a private practice.

Finally, the field of hospitalists is also growing. These physicians are employed by the hospital but typically do not have their own practice. Hospitalists work full time for the hospital and are trained in delivering specialized inpatient care. Regardless of the type of arrangement, most hospitals have a chief medical officer, or a similar position, who oversees the roles and responsibilities of the providers as a member of the medical staff; the providers' employee issues and responsibilities are typically managed by the HR department. These relationships grow more complex within academic medical centers, which must integrate the roles and responsibilities of the providers, the hospital, and the medical school.

As a result of the changing environment and decreased reimbursement, more primary care physicians are joining or forming group practices. Large physician-owned group practices offer several advantages to physicians, including competitive advantage with vendor and manufacturers, improved negotiating power with managed care organizations, shared risk and decision making, and improved flexibility and choice for patients. Physicians usually own or share ownership in the group practice and therefore are responsible for the business operations. Typically, group practices employ an office manager who works closely with the physicians to manage the day-to-day operations. Often a full-time administrator is also on staff not only to manage day-to-day issues but also to formulate strategies and oversee personnel, billing and collection, purchasing, patient flow, and other functions. Many group practices opt to outsource the business functions, including human resources, to specialized firms. For complete details on medical practice management, go to www.mgma.org.

These shifts in the various healthcare settings and arrangements have changed the roles, functions, and expectations of the healthcare workforce and gave way to the emergence of the following issues.

Supply and Demand

Throughout the twentieth century, the nursing labor market cycled through periods of shortages and surpluses (Aiken et al. 2002; Kovner 2002; Coile 2001; Jones 2001; Buerhaus, Staiger, and Auerbach 2000). The beginning of the twenty-first century brought the nursing and allied health professions the challenge of keeping pace with the demand for their services. Indicators of demand include the number of position vacancies and turnover and a rise in salaries. To fill positions, hospitals—the largest employers of nurses and allied health professionals—have raised salaries, provided scholarships, and given other incentives such as sign-on bonuses and tuition reimbursement.

The supply of nurses and allied health professionals is reflected in the number of students in educational programs and those available for the healthcare workforce. Future supply of such professionals continues to be threatened by the following:

- *Aging of the nursing workforce* (Buerhaus and Staiger 1999). According to an AACN (2003) survey, the average age of a master's- and doctoral-prepared nurse faculty is 48.8 and 53.5, respectively.
- *Decline in available educational resources.* Almost two-thirds (64.8 percent) of the nursing schools responding to the AACN survey identified faculty shortages as a reason for not accepting all qualified applicants into entry-level baccalaureate programs. The survey also noted lack of classroom space and clinical facilities and budgetary restraints (AACN 2003).
- *Decline in nursing school enrollees.* From 1995 through 2000, enrollment decreased 21 percent. From 2000 through 2001, there was a 3.6 percent increase, but the overall enrollment numbers remained below 1995 levels (AACN 2003).

As a result, recruitment of nursing and allied health professions students has become a major focus of practitioners, professional associations, and academic institutions. In response, healthcare organizations are developing innovative ways (in addition to increasing salaries) to recruit and retain nurses and allied health professionals. Such developments include opening or sponsoring new schools, offering shorter and more flexible shifts, and providing child care.

Alternative Therapies

Alternative therapies have gained more popularity, judging by the growing number of related titles on the topic in the lay press and academic literature. A turning point in the acceptance and increased respectability of alternative therapies (Weber 1996) was noted in a sentinel study of the prevalence in use of alternative or unconventional therapies (Eisenberg et al. 1993). In the study, Eisenberg and colleagues concluded that one in three adults relied on treatments and interventions that are not widely taught at medical schools in the United States; examples of these alternative interventions included acupuncture and chiropractic and massage therapies. In a follow-up study, Eisenberg and colleagues (1998) determined that there was a 47.3 percent increase in visits to alternative medicine practitioners from 1990 to 1997. Additionally, a 1998 study (Wetzel, Eisenberg, and Kaptchuk 1998) reported that 75 (64 percent) of 125 medical schools surveyed offered a course in complementary or alternative medicine. As the use of alterative therapies continues to gain acceptance and to be integrated in medical school curriculum, this specialty area may be more and more considered an emerging healthcare profession field.

Nonphysician Practitioners

With the advent of managed care, greater reliance has been placed on nonphysician practitioners. Collaborative practice models with nurse practitioners, physician assistants, pharmacists, and other therapists are appropriate to both acute and long-term healthcare delivery. Strides have been made in the direct reimbursement for some nonphysician provider services, which is an impetus for further collaboration in practice.

The consolidation and integration of the healthcare delivery system has not, however, eliminated slack and duplication of services. Although the changes attributed to managed care have led to the promotion and use of less-costly sites for care delivery, a larger impact on the division of labor among all healthcare professionals, and thus on health professions, may yet occur.

Licensure and Certification

The use of nonphysician practitioners at various sites may be viewed as an opportunity for the growth of nursing, pharmacy, allied health professions, and health administration. Alternatively, Hurley (1997) contends that it may lead to concerted efforts to repeal professional licensure and certification in healthcare. If policymakers jump on the bandwagon, this deregulation may lead to the demise of some healthcare professions and may also lead to the proliferation of functionally trained, unlicensed personnel. The use of less highly educated personnel will have greater implications for the existence and growth of educational programs in academic medical centers.

The use of unlicensed support personnel poses concerns about the intensity and quality of healthcare delivered. When fewer highly trained professionals are employed for oversight, the potential for adverse outcomes increases. Aiken, Sochalski, and Anderson (1996) found that, although the percentage of registered nurses increased overall, fewer nurses per patient were available in the mid-1990s than a decade earlier to provide care for more acutely ill patients. The net effect was a relative increase in nonclinical personnel, which added stress for those who were expected to supervise unlicensed staff and to care for sicker patients.

Recruitment and Retention

Recruitment and retention of healthcare professionals are important for healthcare organizations as shortages have continued among key healthcare professions, including nursing and allied health professions. The RN vacancy rate was projected to be 15 percent by 2003 and 20 percent by 2020 (Buerhaus, Staiger, and Auerbach 2000; Heinrich 2001). One in five nurses plan to leave the profession within the next five years (Letvak 2002), with turnover costs up to two times a nurse's salary. Similarly, the American Hospital Association (2005) reported shortages among other healthcare professionals, such as pharmacists, laboratory technologists, and imaging technicians, that range from 4.3 percent to 7 percent. These shortages require current professionals to treat more patients and to work longer hours. Such conditions can contribute to emergency department diversions, increased patient wait times, and decreased patient safety.

In response, healthcare organizations need to develop and execute recruitment and retention programs. These programs require senior management support and dedicated financial and human resources. Such programs should focus on building "a culture of professional satisfaction" (JCAHO 2002). While salary is an important aspect, leadership support, ability to contribute to the organization and provide quality care to patients, degree of autonomy, relationship with direct supervisors and peers, working conditions, and enabling work-life balance are all important in attracting and keeping employees satisfied. Additional tools to retain employees include employee engagement surveys, mentoring, and training programs.

One innovative way to differentiate a hospital, which helps in recruitment and retention, is to achieve magnet status. The American Nurses Credentialing Center's Magnet Nursing Services Recognition Program was developed in 1993 as a way to specifically recognize excellence in nursing services at the institutional level and to benchmark best practices to be disseminated throughout the industry. Hospitals that apply for and achieve magnet status have created and demonstrated a professional practice environment that ensures quality outcomes. These hospitals are recognized for their best practices in nursing care, improved patient outcomes, and increased workplace satisfaction. The actual evaluation process is based on nine magnet standards, the completion of an intensive written application, and a two-day site visit by a team of nurse scholars. Hospitals that do not wish to engage in the application process can benefit greatly from using magnet strategies to create a culture based on excellence in nursing and patient care (Pieper 2003). For more information on magnet status, see http://nursingworld.org/ancc/magnet.html.

Entrepreneurship

Given the bureaucratic nature of organizations, the regulation of the healthcare industry, and additional constraints by payers and managed care, many healthcare professionals are choosing to pursue opportunities on their own. The service economy coupled with knowledge-based professions may encourage pursuit of new and different ventures for individuals who have the personality, skills, and tenacity to go into their own business. An entrepreneur must have a mix of management skills and the means to depart from a traditional career path to practice on one's own.

White and Begun (1998) characterize the entrepreneurial personality traits of a profession in terms of its willingness to take the risks associated with undertaking new ventures. Each profession may be categorized either as defending the status quo and therefore entails little risk (defender professions) or as looking for new and different opportunities with greater risk (prospector professions). White and Begun view the more entrepreneurial professions as more diversified in terms of processes and services delivered. The accrediting bodies of such entrepreneurial professions encourage educational innovation that may extend to nontraditional careers. Each of the healthcare professions has, to greater or lesser extents, defender and prospector aspects.

Workforce Diversity

Each of the healthcare professions must continue to monitor and encourage diversity in its membership because the demographic shifts that the United States is going through will have an impact on this nation's workforce composition in the coming decades. Although workforce diversity is a broad concept, it focuses on our differences in gender, age, and race; these aspects not only reflect the population that healthcare serves but also the people who provide the services. Some professions are dominated by one gender or the other, which is illustrated by the predominantly female field of nursing or the historically predominantly male field of healthcare administration. The healthcare administration profession, however, has made strides during the past decade as more females have entered the field. Labor shortages and employee turnover are common in the healthcare professions. Consequently, healthcare executives need to balance the needs of new entrants into the profession with those already in the profession.

Changes in the ethnic and racial composition of the workforce are proportional to the changes in the size and age of the entire population (D'Aunno, Alexander, and Laughlin 1996). Because many healthcare professionals are racial/ethnic minorities, a concerted effort needs to be made to recruit and retain them because the diversity of the members of a profession should reflect the diversity of the members of the population.

Summary

Healthcare professionals make up a large segment of the U.S. labor force. Historically, the development of healthcare professionals is related to the following trends:

- Supply and demand
- Increasing use of technology
- Changes in disease and illness
- The impact of healthcare financing and delivery

The healthcare workforce is very diverse. The different levels of education, scopes of practice, and practice settings contribute to the complexity of this sector of the industry. The coming decades will be characterized by some reforms within the healthcare professions because of increasing pressures to finance and deliver healthcare with higher quality, lower cost, and measurable outcomes.

References

Aiken, L. H., J. Sochalski, and G. F. Anderson. 1996. "Downsizing the Hospital Nursing Workforce." *Health Affairs* 15 (4): 88–92.

Aiken, L. H., S. P. Clarke, D. M. Sloane, J. Sochalski, and J. H. Silber. 2002. "Hospital Nurse Staffing and Patient Mortality, Nurse Burnout, and Job Dissatisfaction." *JAMA* 288 (16): 1987–93.

American Association of Colleges of Nursing. 2003. "Thousands of Students Turned Away from the Nation's Nursing Schools Despite Sharp Increase in Enrollment." News Release. [Online article; retrieved 7/20/04.] http://www.aacn.nche.edu/Media/NewsReleases/enrl03.htm.

American Hospital Association. 2005. "Overview of the U.S. Health Care System." Data from the 2004 AHA Survey of Hospital Leaders. [Online information; retrieved 3/22/05.] http:// www.aha.org/aha/resource_ncenter/statistics/statistics.html.

American Nurses Association. 2004. "Planning a Career in Nursing." [Online article; retrieved 7/16/04.] http:www.ana.org/about/careerlt.htm.

Association of American Medical Colleges. 2004. "Combined Degree Programs." [Online article; retrieved 7/16/04.] http://services.aamc.org/currdir/section3/degree2.cfm.

Begun, J. W., and K. R. White. 1999. "The Profession of Nursing as a Complex Adaptive System: Strategies for Change." In *Research in the Sociology of Health Care*, edited by J. J. Kronenfeld. Greenwich, CT: JAI Press.

Buerhaus, P. I., and D. O. Staiger. 1999. "Trouble in the Nurse Labor Market? Recent Trends and Future Outlook." *Health Affairs* 18 (1): 214–22.

Buerhaus, P. I., D. O. Staiger, and D. I. Auerbach. 2000. "Implications of a Rapidly Aging Registered Nurse Workforce." *JAMA* 283 (22): 2948–54.

Bureau of Labor Statistics. 2001. [Online information; retrieved 7/30/01.] http://stats.bls.gov/oes.

———. 2004. *Occupational Outlook Handbook, 2004–05 Edition, Registered Nurses*. [Online information; retrieved 7/13/04.] http://www.bls.gov/oco/ocos083.htm.

Coile, R. C. 2001. "Magnet Hospitals Use Culture, Not Wages, To Solve Nursing Shortage." *Journal of Healthcare Management* 46 (3): 224–28.

D'Aunno, T., J. A. Alexander, and C. Laughlin. 1996. "Business as Usual? Changes in Health Care's Workforce and Organization of Work." *Hospital & Health Services Administration* 41 (1): 3–18.

Dreyfus, H. L., and S. E. Dreyfus. 1996. "The Relationship of Theory and Practice in the Acquisition of Skill." In *Expertise in Nursing Practice: Caring, Clinical Judgment, and Ethics*, edited by P. Benner, C. A. Tanner, and C. A. Chesla. New York: Springer.

Eisenberg, D. M., R. D. Kessler, C. Foster, R. E. Norlock, D. R. Calkins, and T. L. Delbanco. 1993. "Unconventional Medicine in the United States." *New England Journal of Medicine* 328 (24): 246–52.

Eisenberg, D. M., R. B. Davis, S. L. Ettner, S. Appel, S. Wilkey, M. Van Rompay, and R. C. Kessler. 1998. "Trends in Alternative Medicine Use in the United States, 1990–1997: Results of a Follow-Up National Survey." *New England Journal of Medicine* 280 (18): 1569–75.

Haddock, C. C., R. A. McLean, and R. C. Chapman. 2002. *Careers in Healthcare Management*. Chicago: Health Administration Press.

Hamric, A. B., J. A. Spross, and C. M. Hanson (eds.). 2005. *Advanced Practice Nursing: An Integrative Approach, 3rd Edition*, 95–96. St. Louis, MO: Elsevier Saunders.

Health Professions Education Extension Amendments of 1992, Section 701 PHS Act. Washington, DC: Government Printing Office.

Health Resources and Services Administration. 2001. "The Registered Nurse
    Population: National Sample Survey of Registered Nurses—March
    2000." U.S. Department of Health and Human Services, Bureau of
    Health Professions Division of Nursing. [Online information; retrieved
    7/20/04.] www.bhpr.hrsa.gov.

———. 2004. "Nursing Aides, Home Health Aides, and Related Health Care
    Occupations—National and Local Workforce Shortages and Associated
    Data Needs." U.S Department of Health and Human Services, Bureau of
    Health Professions National Center for Health Workforce Analyses.
    [Online information; retrieved 3/21/05.] www.bhpr.hrsa.gov.

Heinrich, J. 2001. *Nursing Workforce: Emerging Nurse Shortages Due to Multiple
    Factors.* GAO Report to Health Subcommittee on Health: GAO-01-944,
    pages i–15. Washington, DC: Government Accountability Office.

Hurley, R. E. 1997. "Moving Beyond Incremental Thinking." *Health Services
    Research* 32 (5): 679–90.

Joint Commission on Accreditation of Healthcare Organizations. 2002.
    "Healthcare at the Crossroads: Strategies for Addressing the Evolving
    Nursing Crisis." Public Policy Initiative White Paper. [Online informa-
    tion; retrieved 7/15/04.] www.jcaho.org.

Jones, C. B. 2001. "The Future Registered Nurse Workforce in Healthcare
    Delivery." In *The Nursing Profession*, edited by N. L. Chaska, 123–38.
    Thousand Oaks, CA: Sage Publications.

Kovner, C. T. 2002. "CMS Study: Correlation Between Staffing and Quality."
    American Journal of Nursing 102 (9): 65–67.

Letvak, S. 2002. "Retaining the Older Nurse." *Journal of Nursing
    Administration* 32: 387–92.

National Commission on Allied Health. 1995. *Report of the National
    Commission on Allied Health.* Rockville, MD: Health Resources and
    Services Administration.

National Council of State Boards of Nursing. 2004. [Online information;
    retrieved 7/16/04.] www.ncsbn.org.

National League for Nursing. 2004. [Online information; retrieved 7/16/04.]
    www.nln.org.

O'Neil, E. H., and D. M. Hare (eds.). 1990. "Perspectives on the Health
    Professions." In *Pew Health Professions Programs*. Durham, NC: Duke
    University.

Pieper, S. K. 2003. "Retaining Staff the Magnet Way: Fostering a Culture of
    Professional Excellence." *Healthcare Executive* 18 (3): 12–17.

Weber, D. O. 1996. "The Mainstreaming of Alternative Medicine." *Healthcare
    Forum Journal* 39 (6): 16–27.

Wetzel, M. S., D. M. Eisenberg, and T. J. Kaptchuk. 1998. "Course Involving
    Complementary and Alternative Medicine at US Medical Schools."
    JAMA 280 (9): 784–87.

White, K. R., and J. W. Begun. 1998. "Nursing Entrepreneurship in an Era of
    Chaos and Complexity." *Nursing Administration Quarterly* 22 (2): 40–47.

Discussion Questions

1. Describe the process of professionalization. What is the difference between a profession and an occupation?
2. Describe the major types of healthcare professionals (excluding physicians and dentists) and their roles, training, licensure requirements, and practice settings.
3. Describe and apply the issues for human resources management and systems development to healthcare professionals.
4. How has managed care affected the healthcare professions?
5. Who are nonphysician practitioners that provide primary care? What is their role in the delivery of health services?

Experiential Exercise

The purpose of this exercise is to give readers an opportunity to explore one healthcare profession in detail.

From all of the healthcare professions in the industry, select one for analysis. Describe the following characteristics of the profession selected:

- Knowledge base
- Collective goals
- Training
- Licensure (this will vary by state)
- Number of professionals in practice by
  1. Vertical differentiation (position, experience, education level)
  2. Horizontal differentiation (geography, practice setting, specialty)
- History and evolution of the profession
- Professional associations and their roles
- Competitor professions
- Current strategic issues facing the profession and the profession's position on these issues

To get started on this exercise, you may wish to go to the web sites (listed in Table 3.1) for professional organizations and for various state licensing boards. You may also interview members of the profession as well as leaders in the field.

THE LEGAL ENVIRONMENT OF HUMAN RESOURCES MANAGEMENT

Beverly L. Rubin, J.D., and Bruce J. Fried, Ph.D.

Learning Objectives

After completing this chapter, the reader should be able to

- understand the impact of legal considerations on key human resources management activities and functions;
- define employment-at-will and its public policy exceptions;
- enumerate the major pieces of federal equal employment opportunity legislation;
- explain the rationale for government intervention in the workplace to prevent discrimination;
- describe the strategies organizations use to prevent and identify discrimination in the workplace;
- understand the concepts of disparate impact and disparate treatment and the types of evidence required to demonstrate each form of discrimination;
- discuss the key features of the Americans with Disabilities Act, including the concepts of undue hardship and reasonable accommodation;
- understand that sexual harassment is a form of employment discrimination, and describe the legal definitions of sexual harassment law;
- address employee rights and responsibilities, and distinguish among statutory, regulatory and common-law rights;
- list employee privacy issues, including HIPAA, and realize when to consult legal counsel when privacy issues arise;
- recognize the legal backdrop for a variety of healthcare-specific employee rights and responsibilities issues;
- discuss the contractual implications of employee handbooks, employment agreements, personnel manuals, separation agreements, and disciplinary documents;
- define the concepts of dismissal for cause and due process;
- explain the concept of progressive discipline, and know the steps required for employee termination; and

- enumerate the types and role of alternative dispute-resolution methods in the workplace.

Introduction

Most people who work outside the home spend a majority of their waking hours in the workplace. In fact, Americans work an average of 43.2 hours per week (Kundu 1999). According to a 2001 study by the United Nations' International Labor Organization, Americans work longer hours than "anyone else in the industrialized world," including Canada, Germany, and Japan (Anderson 2001).

Because Americans spend so much time at work, for some people the office or job site has become a microcosm of home and family and is viewed as the source of self-esteem, social interaction, anxiety, and insecurity. The workplace, however, cannot be run like a family. Employees must perform their jobs, and employers must adhere to objective rules and requirements applicable to the workplace. The laws governing the relationship between employer and employee reflect the organization's attempt to achieve a complex balance between making an employee's job free from personal injury, prejudice, duress, and unwanted sexual advances and allowing the organization to pursue its business goals. Because labor and employment laws involve the protection of societal values, individual rights, and the pursuit of capitalism, it is a confusing and often conflicting area of law.

The healthcare workplace is a highly complex environment that operates under myriad laws and regulations that further complicate matters within that environment. It is not necessary for managers to be lawyers, but it is essential that managers are aware of key legal issues that affect human resources management (HRM), because laws and regulations govern so much of the employee-employer relationship. Managers have discretion in how they manage the workforce, but managers' adherence to legal requirements places significant constraints on their autonomy. It is particularly important that managers and supervisors in large healthcare organizations understand legal requirements and constraints. While senior managers in any organization need to understand the legal issues inherent in HRM, day-to-day application of these laws falls to line managers who may not have the same degree of awareness as senior management. This is an important consideration because senior managers and boards of directors are the ones liable for violations that occur at any level of the organization.

Perhaps an even more compelling reason for managers to understand and comply with legal requirements is this: compliance implies good management practice; this is most notably the case with regard to equal employment opportunity. While "equal opportunity" is often viewed as a regulatory challenge or at worst a quota-based scheme, adherence to mandated procedures is consistent with sound HR practices. In fact, there is evidence in the literature that many companies choose to continue affirmative action initiatives even when such programs are being dismantled through legislation and executive orders (Fisher 1994).

An important consideration concerning the legal and regulatory environment is the ambiguity of the actual laws and regulations. Virtually every employment-related law has been subject to extensive and far-reaching interpretation by the courts and quasi-judicial administrative agencies, such as the National Labor Relations Board and the Equal Employment Opportunity Commission. For this reason, employment law cannot be understood by simply reading the text of existing laws. Furthermore, as with all legislation, application of employment law may have unintended consequences. For example, implementation, interpretation, or use of a particular law may be inconsistent with the original intent of the lawmakers. One example is the Americans with Disabilities Act (ADA). The ADA was intended to increase the employment potential of individuals with disabilities. However, the majority of complaints filed under the ADA deal with on-the-job injuries of employees. After the terrorist attacks in the United States on September 11, 2001, significant changes have been made to employment law that affect employee privacy. On the flip side, the privacy requirement of the Health Insurance Portability and Accountability Act (HIPAA), which went into effect on April 14, 2003 (April 14, 2004 for smaller health plans), offers greater privacy protection for personal health information.

Because of the constantly changing legal landscape, this chapter cannot present the most current court rulings and agency regulations. However, the chapter aims to sensitize the reader to the legal framework that currently governs the workplace, communicate the importance of keeping up with such laws and regulations, and emphasize that equal employment opportunity laws and good management practices should be compatible.

Employment Laws

The respective rights and responsibilities governing the workplace are documented in federal and state statutes, administrative agency regulations, case-law interpretations of various state and federal legislation and regulations, written and verbal employment agreements, and employee handbooks. Among the most important federal statutes that directly or indirectly affect the employment setting are the Civil Rights Act of 1964, the Age Discrimination in Employment Act, the Fair Labor Standards Act, the

Health Insurance Portability and Accountability Act of 1996, and the Americans with Disabilities Act. Each of these is discussed later in the chapter. Other key laws that deal directly or indirectly with employment include the following:

- *Consolidated Omnibus Budget Reconciliation Act (COBRA)* is an amendment to ERISA (see below). COBRA gives employees and their families the right to choose to continue to receive health benefits provided by the employer's group health plan for a limited period of time in such circumstances as voluntary or involuntary job loss, reduction in hours worked, transition between jobs, death, divorce, and other life events.

- *Consumer Credit Protection Act (Title III)* prohibits an employer from discharging an employee because his or her earnings are subject to garnishment and from limiting the amount of wages that can be withheld for garnishment in a single week. *Wage garnishment* refers to a procedure whereby an employer withholds the earnings of an employee to pay a debt resulting from a court order or other procedure.

- *Drug-Free Workplace Act of 1988* requires that all organizations that receive federal grants in any amount or federal contracts of $25,000 must certify that they are providing a drug-free workplace. *Drug-free workplace certification* is a precondition of receiving a federal grant, and criteria for compliance include the organization establishing an explicit drug policy, implementing it, and publicizing it to all employees.

- *Employee Polygraph Protection Act of 1988* generally prohibits employers from using lie-detector tests either for preemployment screening or during the course of employment. A number of people are exempt from this act, including federal contractors engaged in national security intelligence or counterintelligence functions; employees suspected of involvement in an incident resulting in economic loss to the employer; employees of security firms; and prospective employees engaged in manufacturing, distributing, or dispensing controlled substances.

- *Employee Retirement Income Security Act 1974 (ERISA)* regulates private pension plans and sets minimum standards for most voluntarily established pension and health plans. ERISA requires plans to provide participants with information about plan features and funding, establishes fiduciary responsibilities for those who manage and control plan assets, orders plans to establish grievance and appeals procedures for participants, and gives participants the right to sue for benefits and breaches of fiduciary duty.

- *Equal Pay Act of 1963* (part of the Fair Labor Standards Act) requires employers to pay all employees equally for equal work, regardless of their gender. The intent of the act was to correct wage disparities experienced by women workers because of sex discrimination. Jobs are considered equal if they involve equal levels of skill, effort, and responsibility and if performed under similar conditions.

- *Executive Orders 11246 and 11375* bar discrimination on the basis of race, color, religion, and national origin in federal employment and in employment by federal contractors and subcontractors. It also requires government contractors to develop a written affirmative action program to help identify and analyze problems in workforce participation by women and minorities.

- *Family and Medical Leave Act (FMLA)* of 1993 requires employers to provide 12 weeks of unpaid leave for family and medical emergencies, childbirth, or serious health condition. FMLA is discussed further in Chapter 10.

- *Immigration Reform and Control Act of 1986* is intended to control unauthorized immigration to the United States and designates penalties for employers who hire people not authorized to work in the United States. The Act also prohibits discrimination against individuals on the basis of national origin or citizenship.

- *Occupational Safety and Health Administration* (OSHA) serves two regulatory functions: setting standards and conducting inspections to ensure that employers are providing safe and healthful workplaces. OSHA established the National Institute for Occupational Safety and Health as its research institution. OSHA addresses a broad range of health and safety issues, including exposure to toxic chemicals, excessive noise levels, mechanical dangers, heat or cold stress, and sanitation. OSHA is discussed further in Chapter 11.

- *Worker Adjustment and Retraining Notification Act* (WARN) requires employers to provide notice to employees 60 days in advance of plant closings and mass layoffs. WARN's intent is to provide workers and their families transition time to adjust to the prospective loss of employment, to seek and obtain alternative jobs and, if necessary, to enter skill training or retraining.

A number of sources exist for further information about these and other federal laws (see, for example, the U.S. Department of Labor web site at www.dol.gov).

State law covers additional rights and responsibilities for employees. For example, in North Carolina, an employer may not withhold money from an employee's paycheck if that employee owes money to the employer unless the employee was given prior notice and has authorized the transaction (see NC Gen. Stat. § 95–25.8 to 95–25.10). Other states, such as California, have enacted statutes supplemental to federal statutes—for example, in the area of pregnancy leave (see CA Govt. § 12945). An employer familiar with well-publicized federal law inadvertently may ignore non-pre-empted state law and thereby deprive an employee of protected rights.

Employment Discrimination

The legal environment affects virtually all aspects of HRM; however, this was not always the case. Traditionally, the employee-employer relationship was guided by the *employment-at-will principle*, which assumes that both employee and employer have the right to sever the work relationship at any time without notice, for any reason, no reason, or even a bad or immoral reason (Bouvier 1996). Within this context, an employee may be terminated for trying to organize a union, for being a member of a particular race/ethnic group, or for refusing to participate in illegal activities. The employment-at-will principle was strengthened in 1908 in *Adair v. United States* (208 U.S.161) and continues to be the basis for employee-employer relations in the private sector. The employment-at-will principle has been eroded dramatically by a variety of laws and regulations during the twentieth century. This principle will be discussed in more detail later in the chapter.

Before we begin our review of specific legislation, let us address two key concepts: discrimination and workplace regulation. *Illegal discrimination* means discrimination against a particular individual or group of individuals based on non-job-related characteristics such as race, ethnicity, age, gender, sexual preference, or disability. A great deal of legislation is aimed at reducing non-job-related discrimination. The passage of laws that address illegal discrimination is, in effect, a form of workplace regulation. Whenever any type of regulatory legislation is considered, the question arises about whether such legislation is, in fact, required. Put another way, can market forces perform these regulatory functions? According to some economists, illegal discrimination is ineffective and inefficient over the long haul. The organization that hires highly qualified individuals regardless of, for example, race, gender or age will win over the organization that hires individuals of its preferred race, gender, or age. According to this view, discriminating employers will lose and perhaps learn that discrimination does not serve the organization well. Presumably, such organizations will change their ways.

What leads organizations to engage in illegal discriminatory practices? Some organizations and individuals have a "taste" for discrimination and may simply not want certain types of individuals in their workplaces.

These organizations seem to be willing to pay for their preference with lower profits, diminished quality of service, and decreased market share that accompany the practice of hiring a preferred group (England 1994). Alternatively, employers may discriminate not because of their own tastes but as a result of their customers' or employees' tastes (Becker 1957; Cooter 1994).

Others see a more deliberate application of discrimination—that is, *statistical discrimination*, in which a calculated decision is made about a particular individual based on one's perceptions about the larger group to which the individual belongs. For example, if an employer believes that newly married women in their early 20s are highly likely to leave work in the near future for family reasons, this view will be applied to all female job applicants who fit this category. This view puts all members of a particular group at a disadvantage. Employers may consciously or unconsciously use statistical generalizations about the group to which an individual belongs to make hiring and other employment decisions (England 1994). If an employer uses or administers selection tools (such as those in Figure 4.1) inconsistently or differently for certain groups, then the organization may be charged with systemic discrimination.

Equal Employment Opportunity Legislation

In this section, the most important laws and regulations that deal with equal employment opportunity are outlined.

Equal employment opportunity (EEO) refers to governmental attempts to ensure that all individuals have an equal chance for employment, regardless of age, race, religion, disability, and other non-job-related characteristics. Employment is defined broadly and includes hiring, firing, fairness in promotions, compensation and benefits, training opportunities, and other employment activities. To accomplish EEO aims, the federal government has used constitutional amendments, legislation, executive orders, and courts and quasi-judicial bodies. Table 4.1 provides a summary of the major constitutional provisions, laws, and executive orders that support EEO. The table is not a comprehensive listing of relevant federal laws and does not include state and local ordinances.

The *Fourteenth Amendment* forbids the state from taking life, liberty, or property without due process of law and prevents states from denying equal protection of the laws. This amendment, passed immediately after the Civil War, was originally intended to protect blacks, but it has more recently been used in cases of alleged reverse discrimination. The most notable case was *Bakke v. California Board of Regents of the University of California* (438 U.S. 265) in 1978, in which a white applicant to a med-

FIGURE 4.1
Tools for
Screening
Candidates

- Detailed application form
- Interview
- Honesty test
- Handwriting analysis
- Drug screening
- Criminal background check
- Credit report check
- Reference check
- Motor vehicle record check
- Educational records check
- Personality tests

ical school alleged that he was not admitted because of a discriminatory quota system. The Supreme Court found in his favor, stating that the quota system had violated his right to equal protection under the law.

The 1960s was a period of significant social activism in the United States. Federal legislation was passed to extend civil rights and equal opportunity in housing, voting, education, employment, and other areas. The basic premise of all of these laws is that employment decisions, including hiring, promotion, compensation and benefits, and training opportunities, should not be based on non-job-related characteristics such as age, gender, race, or disability. As a result of the complexity of these laws, the federal government has produced a useful document entitled *Uniform Guidelines on Employee Selection Procedures* (EEOC 1978), which summarizes and synthesizes the employment-related implications of these laws. The *Uniform Guidelines* provide basic guidance on compliance in virtually every HR function and is a valuable resource for all management professionals.

The *Fair Labor Standards Act* (FLSA) was originally passed in 1938 but has been amended many times since. The major provisions of the FLSA concern the minimum wage, overtime payments, child labor, and equal pay. With respect to equal employment opportunity, the child labor and equal-pay provisions are most critical. The FLSA forbids the employment of children younger than 18 years of age in hazardous occupations such as mining, logging, woodworking, meatpacking, and certain types of manufacturing. Severe restrictions are placed on the employment of minors under

TABLE 4.1
Sources of
EEO Law

Source	Purpose	Coverage	Administration
Fifth Amendment, U.S. Constitution	Protects against federal violation of due process	All individuals	Federal courts
Thirteenth Amendment, U.S. Constitution	Abolishes slavery	All individuals	Federal courts
Fourteenth Amendment, U.S. Constitution	Provides equal protection for all citizens, and requires due process in state action	State (actions, decisions) or governmental organizations	Federal courts
Civil Rights Acts of 1866 and 1871	Establishes the rights of all citizens to make and enforce contracts	All individuals	Federal courts
Equal Pay Act of 1963	Requires that men and women performing equal jobs receive equal pay	Employers engaged in interstate commerce	EEOC* and federal courts
Civil Rights Act of 1964, Title VII, as amended in 1991	Prohibits discrimination on the basis of race, color, religion, sex, or national origin	Employers with 15 or more employees working 20 or more weeks per year; labor unions; employment agencies	EEOC

TABLE 4.1
(*continued*)

Source	Purpose	Coverage	Administration
Age Discrimination in Employment Act of 1967	Prohibits discrimination in employment against individuals 40 years of age and older	Employers with 15 or more employees working 20 or more weeks per year; labor unions; employment agencies	EEOC
Rehabilitation Act of 1973	Protects persons with disabilities against discrimination in the public sector, and requires affirmative action in the employment of individuals with disabilities	Government agencies; federal contractors and subcontractors with contracts of or greater than $2,500	OFCCP**
Americans with Disabilities Act of 1990	Prohibits discrimination against individuals with disabilities	Employers with more than 15 employees	EEOC
Executive Orders 11246 and 11375	Prohibits discrimination by contractors and subcontractors of federal agencies, and requires affirmative action in hiring women and minorities	Federal contractors and subcontractors with contracts of or greater than $10,000	OFCCP
Family and Medical Leave Act	Requires employers to provide 12 weeks of unpaid leave for family and medical emergencies, childbirth, and other serious personal events	Employers with more than 50 employees	Department of Labor

* Equal Employment Opportunity Commission

** Office of Federal Contract Compliance Program

age 16 in most other industries. Minors age 14 to 15 may work outside school hours under the following restrictions (29 CFR 570.119):

- No more than 3 hours on a school day, 18 hours in a school week, 8 hours on a non-school day, or 40 hours in a non-school week
- Work may not begin before 7 A.M. nor end after 7 P.M., except between June 1 and Labor Day, when 9 P.M. is the ending time

The *Equal Pay Act of 1963*, an amendment to the FLSA, requires that men and women in the same organization who perform equal jobs receive equal pay. This act outlaws the once-prevalent practice of paying women less because of their gender, not the work they perform. This practice was commonly defended on the theory that a married man needed a higher salary to support his family. Sometimes, determining what constitutes "equal work" may be difficult. The Equal Pay Act specifies that jobs are the same if they are equal in terms of skill, effort, responsibility, and working conditions. If pay differences are the result of differences in seniority, merit, quantity or quality of work, or any other factor other than gender, then differences in compensation are allowable (Greenlaw and Kohl 1995). Although the Equal Pay Act has been law for more than 40 years, substantial gaps in earnings between men and women still exist. In 2002, women age 35 to 44 earned 75.4 cents on the dollar of what men made, compared with 58.3 cents in 1979 (U.S. Department of Labor 2003).

Because of the difficulty in eradicating wage differences between men and women, some jurisdictions have adopted *comparable worth* legislation (Ledvinka and Scarpello 1991). Comparable worth is a concept that calls for equal or comparable pay for jobs that require similar skills, effort, and responsibility and that are performed in comparable working conditions. In the healthcare environment, this concept is particularly salient because of the large concentration of female employees in certain occupations. If the work of hospital nurses, for example, is only compared to that of other nurses, it would be difficult to remedy gender-based wage discrepancies. If, however, the wages of nurses are compared to the wages of employees whose contribution or worth is comparable to that of nurses, wage disparities may be discovered and addressed.

Title VII of the Civil Rights Act of 1964 is clearly the most far-reaching and significant of all antidiscrimination statutes. The act prohibits discrimination in a variety of areas, including voting, public accommodations, use of public facilities, public education, and employment. In terms of employment, the act bars discrimination in hiring, promotion, compensation, training, benefits, and other aspects. Discrimination is specifically prohibited on the basis of race, color, religion, gender, and national origin.

As amended by the Equal Employment Opportunity Act of 1972 and the Civil Rights Act of 1991, the jurisdiction of Title VII includes the following:

1. All private employers involved in interstate commerce that employ 15 or more employees for 20 or more weeks per year
2. State and local governments
3. Private and public employment agencies
4. Joint labor-management committees that govern apprenticeship or training programs
5. Labor unions that have 15 or more members or employees
6. Public and private educational institutions
7. Foreign subsidiaries of U.S. organizations that employ U.S. citizens
8. Federal government employees covered by section 717 of Civil Rights Act and Civil Service Reform Act

A large majority of employers in the United States are covered by the Civil Rights Act, except for U.S.-government-owned corporations, tax-exempt private clubs, religious organizations that employ persons of a specific religion, and organizations that hire Native Americans on or near a reservation. Title VII is quite specific in its definition of discrimination; section 703a states the following:

(a) It shall be an unlawful employment practice for an employer-

(1) to fail or refuse to hire or to discharge any individual, or otherwise to discriminate against any individual with respect to his compensation, terms, conditions, or privileges of employment, because of such individual's race, color, religion, sex, or national origin; or

(2) to limit, segregate, or classify his employees or applicants for employment in any way which would deprive or tend to deprive any individual of employment opportunities or otherwise adversely affect his status as an employee, because of such individual's race, color, religion, sex, or national origin.

The Civil Rights Act is a far-reaching law with strong enforcement provisions, particularly after the 1991 amendments. Prior to 1991, Title VII limited damage claims to equitable relief, such as back pay, lost benefits, front pay in some cases, and attorney's fees and costs. The 1991 amendments allow compensatory and punitive damages when intentional or reckless discrimination is proven. Compensatory damages may include future pecuniary loss, emotional pain, suffering, and loss of enjoyment of life. Punitive

damages are intended to discourage discrimination by providing for payments to the plaintiff beyond actual damages suffered. Maximum damages
are limited by the number of employees in the organization and range from
$50,000 to $300,000 (Kobata 1992).

The *Age Discrimination in Employment Act (ADEA) of 1967* forbids discrimination against men and women who are 40 years and older
by employers, unions, employment agencies, state and local governments,
and the federal government. As with Title VII of the Civil Rights Act,
enforcement of the ADEA is the responsibility of the Equal Employment
Opportunity Commission (EEOC). Most ADEA suits are brought on a
disparate treatment theory of intentional discrimination because of age.

Discrimination against individuals with disabilities was first prohibited in federally funded activities by the *Vocational Rehabilitation Act of
1973.* Because individuals with disabilities were not covered by Title VII,
they were not protected from employment discrimination. The *Americans
with Disabilities Act (ADA)*, which covers various segments of life, includes
substantial protections for disabled individuals in the work setting. It covers private-sector organizations, or a department or agency of state or local
government, that employ 15 or more employees. In sum, the ADA covers
the majority of individuals with disabilities that are employed or potentially
employable. Of the many federal EEO laws, the ADA is unique in that it
received unanimous support from both political parties—Republican and
Democrat. The ADA prohibits discrimination against individuals with disabilities in all aspects of the employee-employer relationship, including job
application procedures, hiring, termination, promotions, compensation,
and training. After the ADA's passage, the law led most large organizations
to examine their procedures and, in many cases, to modify them to ensure
compliance.

The language of the ADA, like other legislation, is somewhat vague
and open to interpretation. The Americans with Disabilities Act of 1990
§ 3(2)(a) defines a disability as "(a) a physical or mental impairment that
substantially limits one or more of the major life activities of such individual; (b) a record of such impairment; or (c) being regarded as having such
impairment." Each of these clauses is obviously open to considerable debate
and interpretation. Part (a) of this definition includes individuals who have
serious disabilities, such as epilepsy, blindness, deafness, or paralysis, that
affect their ability to carry out major life activities. Part (b) includes individuals with a history of a disability, such as history of cancer, heart disease, or mental disorder. Part (c) deals with people who are regarded as
having an impairment, such as burn victims and individuals with disfigur-
ing conditions. For example, Part (c) protects individuals who may be
denied employment because an employer feels that coworkers will have

negative reactions to that individual's physical appearance (*Employment Law Update* 1991). While these categories are rather broad, the ADA specifically *excludes* the following from the definition of a disability:

1. Homosexuality and bisexuality (State and local legislation may provide protection against discrimination based on sexual orientation.)
2. Gender-identity disorders that do not result from physical impairment or other sexual behavior disorders (e.g., transvestitism, transsexualism)
3. Compulsive gambling, kleptomania, or pyromania
4. Psychoactive substance abuse disorders
5. Current illegal use of drugs

One of the biggest areas of review by the EEOC has been the definition of a disability. In the area of obesity, for example, the EEOC has determined that only severely obese (i.e., weight in excess of 100 percent of the norm for a particular height) persons or those whose weight can be linked to a medical disorder can be covered by the ADA. In addition, because almost 13 percent of all complaints filed with the EEOC between 1993 and 1997 were related to emotional and mental disorders, the EEOC released guidelines in 1997 that deal specifically with this type of issue.

The ADA does not require an organization to hire someone who has a disability but is otherwise not qualified for a job. For an employee or prospective employee to be protected under the ADA, the person must be qualified. In the language of the ADA (42 U.S.C. § 12111[8]), "the term 'qualified individual with a disability' means an individual with a disability who, with or without reasonable accommodation, can perform the essential functions of the employment position that such individual holds or desires." This definition first of all requires that the organization have a good and defensible understanding of the essential functions of the job, with accurate and current job descriptions. The "qualified individual" definition simply implies that an employer cannot discriminate against an individual with a disability if that person can do the job with or without reasonable accommodation.

This leads us to the next dilemma in the ADA: the concept of *reasonable accommodation*. The ADA specifically states that it is the employer's responsibility to make reasonable accommodation to the physical or mental limitations of an employee with a disability, unless doing so will impose an undue hardship on the organization. Reasonable accommodation may be defined as attempts by employers to adjust, without undue hardship, the working conditions or schedules of employees with disabilities. (Note that the reasonable accommodation concept may also be applied to Civil Rights Act issues concerning individuals with religious preferences.) This rule, again, is ambiguous in that reasonable accommodation may be interpreted in many ways. Reasonableness is determined on a case-by-case basis and typically includes relatively noncontroversial accommodations such as making existing facilities accessible to individuals with disabilities. However, it may also be reasonable to restructure jobs, alter work schedules, reassign individuals to different tasks, adjust training materials, and provide readers or interpreters.

Defining reasonable accommodation depends on determining the level of undue hardship to the organization. There are no strict guidelines for determining the threshold of undue hardship, but the law suggests this: compare the cost of the accommodation with the employer's operating budget. The law also stipulates that the overall size of the organization may be considered as well as the type of operation and the nature and cost of the accommodation. The cost of most accommodations is not great. In fact, a study of Sears Roebuck & Company revealed that 69 percent of all accommodations cost nothing, 28 percent cost less than $1,000, and only 3 percent cost more than $1,000 (Reno and Thornburgh 1995). The EEOC has published *A Technical Assistance Manual*, which suggests the following process for assessing reasonable accommodation:

1. Examine the particular job involved, and determine its purpose and essential job function.
2. Consult the individual with the disability to identify potential accommodations that may be needed. If several accommodations are available and possible, deference should be given to the individual's preferred accommodation.

Supreme Court rulings have sought to curtail what many consider abuses of the ADA. Policymakers and managers should understand this law so that they can anticipate and deal with both its intended and unintended consequences.

Implementing Equal Employment Opportunity Principles

In this section, the implications of equal employment laws on HRM practices, including hiring, training, and discipline, are examined. There are two interacting aspects of implementation: (1) the legal requirements associated with compliance and (2) the mechanisms that ensure legal compliance. The first aspect involves tasks such as completion of affirmative action plans and filling out the annual AA-1 government reporting form. The second aspect deals with ensuring that the organization's human resources systems, including job design, employee selection, and performance appraisal, comply with requirements.

Interview Questions

It is important to exhibit cultural sensitivity when framing interview questions and posing them to potential employees. If the appropriateness of an interview question is inconclusive, it is prudent to avoid the question. Furthermore, the same questions should be asked of all interviewees. If a question can only be asked to a certain segment of those interviewed, the appropriateness of the question is dubious. For example, a question regarding plans for becoming pregnant or for retirement is not appropriate for two reasons: (1) it can only be asked of certain applicants (in this case, female and older candidates, respectively) and (2) it delves too deeply into personal issues that have no bearing on the candidate's ability to perform the job.

Screening

Effective screening of potential employees is a necessary step in minimizing employer liability and in preventing employee discipline in the future. The amount of screening to be performed must be balanced against the level of risk associated with the open position. Employers are expected to perform more thorough screening on candidates for positions that carry greater risk, including those that give the employee access to master keys, narcotics, finances, children, the elderly, and disabled individuals. Many preemployment screening tests (see Figure 4.1) pose risks or may be objectionable to applicants; thus, the employer must consider such screenings as well and apply them consistently and on a nondiscriminatory basis. At a minimum, employers should check for references, education, and professional license status.

Employee Selection

As noted earlier, the federal government published the *Uniform Guidelines on Employee Selection Procedures* to assist employers in the areas of hiring, retention, promotion, transfer, demotion, dismissal, and referral. The document, published in the *Federal Register*, is the most readily accessible and useful interpretation of the rules, helping employers comply with federal antidiscrimination statutes. The *Guidelines* (see www.uniformguidelines.com) define the circumstances under which an employee selection procedure may be discriminatory (EEOC 1978):

> The use of any selection procedure which has an adverse impact on the hiring, promotion, or other employment or membership

opportunities or members of any race, sex, or ethnic group will be considered to be discriminatory and inconsistent with these guidelines, unless the procedure has been validated in accordance with these guidelines (or, certain other provisions are satisfied).

This definition implies that selection processes, such as job qualifications, tests, and interview procedures, must be job related and positively associated with job success. The *Guidelines* also describe different methods of validating a test (these methods are discussed further in Chapter 7). A selection procedure may be found discriminatory if it measures factors unrelated to job success, which adversely affects an individual or group. The landmark case in this area was *Griggs v. Duke Power Company* in 1971 (401 U.S. 424), in which an employee's request for a promotion was denied because he was not a high school graduate. Griggs, an African American, claimed that this job standard was discriminatory because it did not relate to job success and because the standard had an adverse impact on a protected class. *Protected class* refers to a group of individuals that fall under the protective umbrella of a particular law (e.g., women, minorities). The Supreme Court decided in favor of Griggs and established two important principles. First, employer discrimination need not be overt or intentional to be present and illegal. Second, employment selection practices must be job related, and employers have the burden of demonstrating that employment requirements are job related or constitute a business necessity. Employment practices that had the effect of excluding protected classes was found to be illegal, even if they appeared racially neutral (Dobbin 2004). This is called *disparate impact.*

More common than discrimination based on disparate impact is disparate treatment. *Disparate treatment* exists when individuals in similar employment situations are treated differently because of race, color, religion, sex, national origin, age, or disability status. The most obvious case of disparate treatment is when an employer decides whom to hire on the basis of one of these criteria. Disparate treatment may also be more subtle, such as asking female job applicants to demonstrate a particular skill when male applicants are not asked to do the same. The defining case in this area was *McDonnell Douglas Corp. v. Green* in 1973 (411 U.S. 792), in which a member of a protected class applied for a job and was rejected, but the company continued to advertise for this position. This case established the four-part guideline for determining disparate treatment:

1. The person is a member of a protected class.
2. The person applied for a job and is qualified.
3. The person was rejected for the job.

4. The position remained open to applicants with equal or fewer quali-
    fications.

The most important difference between disparate impact and disparate
treatment is that motive is irrelevant in disparate impact cases, but in disparate treatment cases proof must exist that an intent to discriminate is present. In a disparate impact case, the plaintiff must make the case that a particular
employment practice disproportionately affects a particular group; whether
the employer intends to discriminate is not necessary to demonstrate disparate impact. In fact, disparate impact can be proven where employment
practices appear quite innocuous. A minimum height requirement, for
example, may appear quite neutral; however, height is not distributed equally
among sexes and ethnic groups, and if this requirement is not linked to
job performance, a disparate impact case can be made. With disparate treatment, it must be proven that a discriminatory intent is behind the employment procedure.

A number of legitimate defenses can be made against charges of disparate treatment. One defense is that while a qualified individual may have
had the qualifications for a particular job, the employer hired someone with
superior qualifications. Another defense is that a protected class characteristic (e.g., gender) is in fact a *bona fide occupational qualification* (BFOQ).
A clear example of a BFOQ is requiring a woman to work as an attendant
in a women's restroom. However, there is great debate on what constitutes a BFOQ, and court rulings are inconsistent in this area. The courts
have rejected the argument that because most women cannot lift 50 pounds,
all women should be eliminated from consideration for jobs that require
heavy lifting. On the other hand, citing safety concerns, the U.S. Federal
Court of Appeals upheld the Federal Aviation Administration policy of
forced retirement of pilots at age 60 (Castaneda 1977).

Generally, liability for the employee's conduct rests with the employer
and therefore with the manager. The legal concept of this relationship is
that of *agency*. The employer empowers the employee under his or her supervision to perform duties, services, and/or work in the name of the organization. The employee's conduct while in this charge is a direct reflection of
the employer or organization. Legally, the employee's actions are of potential equal liability to the employer. Specifically, the legal doctrine of *respondeat superior* (Furrow et al. 1997) holds the employer liable for the conduct
of employees because of the employer's enablement of the employee and
the employer's responsibility to manage and supervise the employee. In this
age of technology, employers may be liable even for the employee's use of
a computer for sex-related crimes and violation of securities laws (Davis
2002; see *Haybeck v. Prodigy Services*, 944 F. Supp. 326 (S.D.N.Y. 1996).

Therefore, it is of utmost importance to train employees in appropriate conduct and subsequently to supervise the conduct thereafter. An employer cannot assume that employees are knowledgeable about equal opportunity, discrimination, and sexual harassment legalities. The employer should assume the burden of employee education to promote organizational compatibility and to prevent future litigation.

Defenses Against Discrimination

A healthcare organization's best defense against lawsuits is creating and following a set of policies that are nondiscriminatory in nature. Disseminating organizational policies serves multiple purposes. First, it is an initial step in educating employees of what behavior is expected and accepted by the organization. Specifying unacceptable behavior and its consequences at the onset of employment is likely to decrease future inappropriate behavior. Second, standard policies will promote consistent employee conduct that lends itself to fair and nondiscriminatory employee treatment. In other words, employees trained with uniform methods are likely to conduct themselves in a relatively similar manner. Third, publicizing desired employee conduct to employees and the public is a preemptive step against litigation. A set of policies allows an organization, to a certain extent, to separate specific employee conduct from conduct that the organization expects of its employees. Legally, it is important to distinguish between that which the employee does through autonomous choices and that which the employee does through organizational support or inattention. A set of policies permits the organization to delineate what behavior it endorses. However, simply having a set of policies in place is not a substantial defense. Organizational policies must be monitored and enforced for them to be effective, and this is a fact recognized by the courts. Tacit, un-policed policies are ineffective defenses against discrimination.

Sexual Harassment Cases

Increased awareness of sexual harassment issues has come about as a result of feminism and the women's movement, greater societal attention to issues of diversity and accommodation in the workplace, and the increase in the number of women in the workplace. Certainly, well-publicized cases, such as that involving President Bill Clinton and Supreme Court Justice Clarence Thomas, have increased the attention given to sexual harassment. Sexual harassment has a long history in the workplace, and surprisingly it is only in the recent past that employers and courts have recognized the prevalence and impact of sexual harassment.

The major statute governing sexual harassment is Title VII of the Civil Rights Act. Under this statute, sexual harassment is considered a violation of an individual's civil rights. Several Supreme Court cases have also provided a richer understanding of sexual harassment. Many ambiguities surround sexual harassment charges. To clarify ambiguities, the EEOC has established a definition of sexual harassment to help courts, employers, and employees understand the scope of sexual harassment (see Figure 4.2).

Consistent with the EEOC's definition are two recognized types of sexual harassment: (1) quid pro quo and (2) hostile environment. *Quid pro quo sexual harassment* occurs when a job-related benefit is made contingent on an employee's submission to sexual advances. A typical case is that of the employee at the University of Massachusetts Medical Center who was awarded $1 million in 1994 after she testified that her supervisor had forced her to engage in sex once or twice a week over a 20-month period as a condition of keeping her job (BNA 1994). The second type is more subtle. *Hostile environment sexual harassment* occurs when behavior of anyone in the work setting is perceived by an employee as offensive and undesirable. While the law is not explicit about what constitutes this type of harassment, some examples may include posting of sexually explicit pictures in the workplace, using sexual-related jokes, and using sexually explicit language. While some cases of sexual harassment are relatively clear cut, other cases' clarity is contingent on the particular workplace and the individuals involved.

In a 2003 Supreme Court case, the Court stated that the distinction between quid pro quo and hostile environment is not the controlling factor for determining liability (Gabel and Mansfield 2003). The determining factor in such cases is whether there was a "tangible employment action" taken against the employee, which is an action that changes the employment status. If no tangible employment action exists, the employer may use the following affirmative defense: "(a) that the employer exercised reasonable care to prevent and correct promptly any sexually harassing behavior, and (b) that the plaintiff employee unreasonably failed to take advantage of any preventive or corrective opportunities provided by the employer or to avoid harm otherwise" (*Burlington Indus., Inc. v. Ellerth*, 524 U.S. 742, 746 [1998]). This defense is not available to the employer if tangible employment action exists in the situation.

For employers, an important concern is liability. In sexual harassment cases, courts typically address three issues in determining whether harassment occurred and whether the employer is liable. First, the plaintiff cannot have invited the sexual advances; sexual advances must be unwelcome. Courts typically have looked for repetitiveness in the harassment. A plaintiff is more likely to be successful if it can be demonstrated that the harassment was not a one-time event but was in fact persistent and perni-

FIGURE 4.2

EEOC's
Definition
of Sexual
Harassment

Unwelcome sexual advances, requests for sexual favors, and other verbal or physical contact of a sexual nature constitute sexual harassment when

1. Submission to such contact is made, either explicitly or implicitly, a term of condition of an individual's employment

2. Submission to or rejection of such conduct by an individual is used as the basis for employment decisions affecting such individual

3. Such conduct has the purpose or effect of unreasonably interfering with an individual's work performance or creating an intimidating, hostile, or offensive work environment

cious. Second, the harassment needs to have been severe enough to have altered the terms, conditions, and privileges of employment. Basically, significant consequences for the employee must have occurred. Particularly in hostile environment cases, it is often difficult to assess in an objective manner whether an environment is actually "hostile." The Supreme Court has established several questions to help courts decide on hostile environment sexual harassment cases:

*   How frequent is the discriminatory conduct?
*   How severe is the discriminatory conduct?
*   Is the conduct physically threatening or humiliating?
*   Does the conduct interfere with the employee's work performance?

Third, courts need to examine the extent of employer liability for the harassment. Two questions are typically considered here: (1) Did the employer know about the harassment, or should it have known? and (2) Did the employer take steps to stop the behavior? In most instances, if the employer knew about the harassment and the behavior did not stop, courts will decide that the employer did not act appropriately to curtail the behavior. Table 4.2 provides a summary of the most important precedent-setting court cases in the last 25 years.

For many years, sexual harassment was simply not recognized as an important workplace concern. As we learn about the extent of sexual harassment occurrence and as we use the legal system to enforce existing laws, we get a clearer picture of the magnitude of this problem in the workplace:

*   A 1991 report by the National Council for Research on Women concludes that 42 percent to 67 percent of working women can expect to be sexually harassed during their careers (Lee and Greenlaw 1995).

TABLE 4.2
Key Court
Decisions
on Sexual
Harassment in
the Workplace

Case	Key Finding and Precedent
Bundy v. Jackson, 641 F.2d934, 24 FEP 1155, D.C. Cir. (1981)	A quid pro quo harassment case, it extended the idea of discrimination to sexual harassment.
Meritor Savings Bank v. Vinson, Supreme Court of the United States, 40 FEP 1822 (1986)	The U.S. Supreme Court ruled that sexual harassment can constitute unlawful sex discrimination under Title VII if the harassment is so severe as to alter the conditions of the victim's employment and create an abusive working environment.
Ellison v. Brady, United States Court of Appeals, Ninth Circuit, 924 F.2d 872 (1991)	The Supreme Court ruled that sexual harassment must be viewed from the perspective of a "reasonable woman" and not people in general; employers must take positive action to eliminate sexual harassment from the workplace.
Harris v. Forklift Systems, Inc., 114 S. Ct. 367 (1993)	An abusive work environment can be demonstrated even when the victim does not suffer serious psychological harm; adopted the idea that harassment occurs if a "reasonable person" would find the behavior leading to a hostile or abusive working environment.
Oncale v. Sundowner Offshore Services, Inc., 523 US 75 (1998)	Same-sex harassment is actionable under Title VII.
Burlington Industries v. Ellerth, 524 U.S. 742 (1998)	Employers are vicariously liable for supervisors who create hostile working conditions for subordinates even if threats are not carried out and the harassed employee suffers no adverse, tangible effects. Employers may defend themselves by demonstrating that they acted quickly to prevent and correct harassment and that the harassed employee failed to utilize their protection.
Faragher v. Boca Raton, 524 U.S. 775 (1998)	Employers are vicariously liable under Title VII of the Civil Rights Act of 1964 for discrimination caused by a supervisor.
Lockard v. Pizza Hut, Inc., 1998 10CIR 1472, 162 F.3d 1062 (1998)	Employers can be liable when a nonemployee harasses one of their employees.

- Sexual harassment is as prevalent, or more so, in healthcare than in other industries. A study by Walsh and Borowski (1995) indicates that nearly three-fourths of women in healthcare have been sexually harassed.
- A 1990 study conducted by the American Medical Association reveals that 81 percent of female medical students in the study endured sexual slurs and 50 percent were direct targets of sexual advances, with the worst harassment occurring in academic medical centers (Decker 1997).
- *Fortune 500* companies spend an average of $1.6 million each year to manage sexual harassment claims (Sherer 1995).
- The number of sexual harassment claims filed with the EEOC increased from 5,643 in 1989 to 13,566 in 2003 (EEOC 2004).

Furthermore, courts have recently awarded damages to plaintiffs and allowed other cases to proceed based on same-sex harassment (see *Beach v. Yellow Freight System, Inc.*, 312 F.3d 391 (8th Cir. 2002); *Rene v. MGM Grand Hotel, Inc.*, 305 F.3d 1061 (9th Cir. 2002) (en banc), cert. denied, 123 S. Ct. 1573 (2003).

Although sexual harassment is unfortunately common in virtually all organizations, it is particularly problematic in healthcare organizations. The American Nurses Association's House of Delegates declared a resolution denouncing sexual harassment in the workplace and called on the industry to adopt and enforce sexual harassment policies (Mikulenak 1992). Several factors may explain why sexual harassment is so prevalent in healthcare organizations. First, sexual harassment almost always includes an important element of power and control. Because of the hierarchical nature of many healthcare organizations and the traditional gender dynamics of the doctor-nurse relationship, there is an imbalance of professional and organizational authority between men and women. From a gender perspective, hospitals are very unique in that the majority of hospital employees are women, but those in positions of authority (i.e., physicians and administrators) are, at least until relatively recently, predominantly men. This differential in authority is frequently the precursor to sexual harassment. Controlling sexual harassment in hospitals is also difficult because of the ambiguous lines of authority in hospitals. While every nurse certainly has a formal supervisor in the organization, the supervision of physicians is less clear. Second, the nature of healthcare work entails a certain amount of intimacy among care providers. Strong coworker relationships often form in the high-stress environment of healthcare, and sexual jokes and off-color humor may emerge. Indeed, discussion of the human body and sexuality is central to much of healthcare, and it is not difficult to envision how such discussion can evolve in an abusive, condescending, or suggestive manner.

The first line of defense against sexual harassment is the existence of a sexual harassment policy and strong support by management of this policy. Typically this policy includes the following (Segal 1992):

1. A statement against sexual harassment, including a definition of sexual harassment and a strong statement indicating that it will not be tolerated
2. Extensive training of all employees on the policy, with particular focus on employees with management and supervisory authority
3. Instructions on how to report complaints, including procedures to bypass a supervisor if he or she is involved
4. Assurances of confidentiality and protection against retaliation
5. A guarantee of prompt investigation
6. A statement that disciplinary action will be taken against harassers up to and including termination

Such a policy needs to be reinforced with strong communications and training. Supervisors must understand clearly the requirements of Title VII as well as their duty to provide an environment free of sexual harassment. Supervisors also need to know the investigative procedures to be used when charges occur. If a complaint arises, management needs to respond immediately; launch an investigation; and, after an investigation proves the allegations true, discipline the offender according to policy. As done with violations of any other HR policy, sexual harassment discipline has to be carried out consistently across similar cases and among managers and hourly employees alike.

Workplace Searches

Not only do employers have an interest in monitoring employees for theft and attendance, but they also may be held accountable for the misconduct of the employee (see Davis 2002). A non-public employee has limited privacy rights against the search of a desk, office, or work area. In *Schowengerdt v. General Dynamics Corp.*, a 1987 case, (823 F.2d 1328 (9th Cir.), cert. denied 117 L.Ed.2d 650), the court ruled that a private employee who has no property interest in an area searched continues to have privacy rights. Workplace searches conducted without employee consent or a search warrant may still be valid if the search meets a "standard of reasonableness under all of the circumstances" (see *O'Connor v. Ortega*, 480 U.S. 709, 720, 94 L.Ed2d714, 725, 107 S.Ct 1492 [1987]). In *O'Connor v. Ortega*, a state-employed physician's (public employee) desk and file cabinet were searched. Most of the U.S. Supreme Court justices agreed that the physician had a reasonable expectation of privacy in his office and that there was a reasonable expectation of privacy in the physician's desk and file cabinet.

Electronic Monitoring

Employers use monitoring in the workplace to investigate organizational problems, particularly loss of productivity as a result of wasted time e-mailing coworkers, friends, and family outside the workplace. Use of company computer systems to send discriminatory or harassing materials also can lead to litigation if the employer fails to take proper precautionary or corrective measures. Figure 4.3 lists some reasons that employers may choose to undertake an employee surveillance program.

Monitoring techniques that employers use can be as simple and obvious as a desk search or can involve sophisticated hidden cameras and microphones. Some employers will install such devices, for example, when an employee is suspected of a particular inappropriate act or when inventory is missing. Figure 4.4 lists some common monitoring techniques most often used by employers.

The Employee Polygraph Protection Act (EPPA) is a legislative attempt to provide direction in this area and to monitor potential for abuse. The EPPA prohibits an employer from doing the following:

* Requiring employees to take a lie-detector test
* Using the results of a lie-detector test
* Taking action against an employee for refusing to take a lie-detector test or for the results of such a test
* Retaliating against the employee for complaining about any of the above

There are significant exemptions to EPPA applicable to the healthcare industry and to the handling of controlled substances (*see* 29 U.S.C. §§ 2001–2009).

Employers' surveillance of employees is widespread and is increasing, as evidenced by research conducted by the American Management Association (AMA). In one survey, the AMA reveals that almost three-fourths of the American businesses in the study used employee-surveillance practices (Greenberg 2000). See Figure 4.5 for suggestions on how employers can reduce the likelihood of privacy violations.

Drug Testing

Employees in the healthcare industry have access to many controlled substances, which may account for significant problems with substance abuse among healthcare employees. Employers may choose to initiate a preem-

FIGURE 4.3
Why Do
Employers
Monitor
Employees?

- Ensure and promote safety
- Protect trade secrets
- Enhance productivity
- Prevent theft or other unlawful activity
- Assess the quality and regularity of customer service
- Search for drug use
- Limit employer liability by detecting and recording discriminatory or illegal behavior

ployment policy for cause and random drug-testing program. A number of states have established laws that regulate the circumstances under which an employer may test for drugs. Thus, if an employer (e.g., a multisystem organization) has employees in multiple states, it must check for the specific requirements of each state. Testing must be done on a confidential basis, and employers must determine its next steps if the employee's results reveal drug use. An employer's options include disciplining the employee, referring the employee to an employee assistance program, or ordering the employee to attend a treatment/rehabilitation program.

Employers should consult with HR personnel or legal counsel who have experience in such matters before initiating an employee drug-testing program. Employers also should use a certified laboratory and medical review officer to conduct and interpret the testing. Using a laboratory experienced in such testing will reduce the likelihood of claims by employees for invasion of privacy.

HIPAA Compliance

To protect the health and medical information of an individual, the U.S. Department of Health and Human Services promulgated new regulations under the Health Insurance Portability and Accountability Act of 1996 (HIPAA). HIPAA was enacted in 1996 to ensure that employees have health insurance coverage after leaving a job and to provide standards for electronic healthcare transactions. Effective for most entities on April 14, 2003, the HIPAA Privacy Rules regulate the use of protected health information that is electronically transmitted or maintained by health plans, healthcare clearinghouses, and healthcare providers.

The goal of the HIPAA Privacy Rules is to protect the use and disclosure of protected health information in this age of technology. Employers who provide self-insured health coverage for employees may be unaware

FIGURE 4.4

Common Surveillance and Monitoring Techniques

- Placing hidden cameras and microphones

- Monitoring e-mail, voicemail, and fax use

- Recording telephone conversations

- Monitoring incoming and outgoing mail

- Searching desk or drawers

- Examining computer use

- Searching company property such as lockers or personal property such as brief cases

Source: Ramsey, R. 1999. "The 'Snoopervision' Debate: Employer Interest Vs. Employee Privacy." *Supervision* 60 (8): 40–45.

that the complex HIPAA regulations apply to them. These organizations should seek legal assistance when releasing such information to worker's compensation carriers or other third parties.

Employment-at-Will Principle and Its Exceptions

In the United States, employment is generally at-will, which means that either party to the employment relationship may terminate the relationship for any reason, without cause, and without notice. A substantial caveat to this rule, however, is that an employer cannot terminate an employee for a reason the law has deemed illegal. Examples of illegal grounds for termination include pregnancy, race, and age, disability status, and the violation of federal and state restrictions.

Whistleblowing

An at-will employee may challenge termination based on violation of public policy. An employee, for instance, can claim wrongful discharge when terminated solely for refusing to commit perjury or for reporting the employer's violation of OSHA standards. Such challenges become difficult to handle if the employee's performance is also poor, as the employer may need to provide evidence that the termination is based solely on performance and not on the employee's whistleblowing activities.

Many wrongful discharge cases also arise from an employer asking an employee to violate federal or state law on its behalf. Courts have allowed employees to pursue such claims because there is a public interest in protecting individuals who speak up about an employer's illegal acts. Such

FIGURE 4.5

Measures to
Minimize
Litigation
Over Privacy
Violations

- Develop a policy statement that clarifies to employees that privacy in the workplace should not be assumed

- Use private information for justifiable reasons only

- Restrict the distribution of employee's personal information to company officials on a need-to-know basis

- Maintain employee medical records separate from the employee file

- Obtain a signed consent or waiver when using the employee's name or picture in an advertisement, promotional material, or training film

employers are viewed as harmful to the public in general (as in the case of unsafe practices at nuclear reactors that can pose dangers to communities) or to employees within the company (as in the case of locked fire and emergency exits that can result in injuries and deaths to workers). This public policy exception creates a cause of action for wrongful discharge when an employer fires a worker for reasons that violate or offend public policy (Yamada 1998).

A *whistleblower* is an employee who discloses or otherwise exposes to law enforcement or a government agency illegal activity in the workplace. Such illegal acts may involve, among other things, discrimination, fraud, or embezzlement. Employees who "blow the whistle" on their employers are protected by the law. It is illegal for an employer to retaliate against or mistreat an employee for whistle blowing (see example in Figure 4.6). The False Claims Act (31 U.S.C. §§ 3729–33 [1991]), only one of myriad laws in this area, governs actions in cases in which a company or individual has financially defrauded the federal government. In 1997, 54 percent of whistleblower cases were based on healthcare fraud (*Modern Healthcare* 1999). Various state whistleblower laws only provide protection to the whistleblower if the individual has reported the problem to his or her supervisor, allowing for a reasonable amount of time to correct the problem, or if the individual has reason to believe the problem will not be corrected if reported (see Title 26 Maine Revised Statutes Annotated, § 833[2]).

Whistleblowers often face an ethical and moral dilemma when trying to decide whether to disclose information. They must consider the consequences of being deemed "disloyal" to their company and whether the disclosure benefits the public. The decision by an employee to blow the whistle clearly is difficult, as the potential detriment to career and the personal stakes are high. The laws described above seek to alleviate such concerns.

FIGURE 4.6

Consider the scenario of a company that is hiring individuals who are not authorized to work in the United States. An at-will employee reports this illegal practice to the Immigration and Naturalization Service (now known as the U.S Citizenship and Immigration Services). The employer subsequently terminates the complaining employee. In this situation, the complaining employee may be successful in pursuing a claim for wrongful or bad-faith discharge based on the public policy exception.

Case Example: At-Will Employment and the Public Policy Exception

Personnel Policies

An employer's personnel policies, contained in handbooks or other policy documents, that imply promises of continued employment may restrict the employer's ability to discharge employees at will. Disciplinary documents prepared by inexperienced managers or HR personnel may contain language that implies a promise of continued employment as well. For instance, consider an employee who has been absent from work for several consecutive days without excuse. Her manager prepares a disciplinary document stating that the employee must maintain a better attendance record over the subsequent 12-month period to keep her job. This document may be interpreted as the employee can stay on the job for 12 months providing she maintains a good attendance record. One way to avoid such an implied promise is for a manager, with assistance from human resources or with legal advice, to use language such as the following: "Nothing contained herein alters the at-will nature of your employment or constitutes a promise of future employment." Employee handbooks and personnel policies must contain similar language in an acknowledgment page signed by the employee and placed in the employee's personnel file.

Employment Agreements

Another notable exception to at-will employment is the employment agreement, with a specified term of employment. The terms of these agreements are either oral or written, or a combination of both. An employer may tell an employee upon hire, transfer, or promotion that the employee has a guaranteed position for one year. However, this type of agreement is not recommended for either party. More typically, an employment agreement is in writing and signed by both parties. Depending on the employee's position, an employment agreement can range from 1 page to as many as 25 or 50 pages in length. Some standard items in employment agreements appear in Figure 4.7.

Early termination of a fixed-term employment agreement usually entitles the employee to collect severance payments or liquidated damages

FIGURE 4.7

Standard
Items in
Employment
Agreements

1. Start date

2. Job title

3. Salary

4. Reporting relationships

5. Job duties or description

6. Term of employment

7. Notice and renewal periods

8. Termination—for-cause provisions

9. Severance payments

10. Bonus information

11. Fringe benefits

12. Confidentiality and work-product provisions

13. Noncompetition and nonsolicitation provisions

14. Assignment clauses

15. Choice of law

specified under the agreement or to pursue a breach-of-contract claim in court. An employer has few rights when an employee terminates an employment agreement before the end of the term, because the courts will not force an employee to continue working against his or her will. Damages caused by the employee's departure also may be difficult to calculate.

For an employee who poses a competitive risk to the employer, *noncompetition and nonsolicitation clauses* may be the only way to protect the employer. An employee presented with an agreement that contains these clauses should consult an attorney before signing the documents, given that these clauses often significantly limit an employee's ability to work after termination of employment. Likewise, employers should seek legal counsel in preparing contracts with such clauses, given that these clauses may be unenforceable under state law. (See the language provided in the California Business and Professional Code § 16600, "Except as provided in this chapter, every contract by which anyone is restrained from engaging in a lawful profession, trade or business of any kind is to that extent void" or because they are unreasonable.) Furthermore, in the healthcare context, noncompete clauses may be against public policy for physicians in specialty practice areas, where there is limited availability to services in the restricted geographic region. See Figure 4.8 for an example of legal interpretation of a covenant not to compete.

Termination Procedures

Termination is rarely a happy event in an organization. Documentation of the circumstances surrounding the termination is as important as the reason for the termination itself. An employee, barring extreme circumstances in which the well-being of the organization is jeopardized, has the right to receive ample notice and explanation of the employer's dissatisfaction with the employee's attempts to remedy the problematic issues. Documentation of all incidents, requests for changes in conduct, employee evaluations, and employee responses to evaluations is the responsibility of the employer. Sufficient documentation of the choice to sever an employer-employee relationship is one of the best strategies to demonstrate the fair handling of a termination.

Although not required by law or otherwise, some employers will provide at-will employees an opportunity to correct a performance problem before termination. Under the concept of *progressive discipline*, an employee is made aware of the problems and what he or she must do to correct the problems. The employee sometimes has a reasonable amount of time to correct the problem and is made aware of the consequences of inaction. Many organizations implement a *termination at-will policy* that in theory permits the employer or the employee to sever employment relations at any time and for any reason. While these types of policies allow a heightened degree of employer discretion in termination matters, state and federal equal opportunity and discrimination standards supercede any private policies. A termination at-will policy does not permit an employer to terminate an employee-employer relationship on non-work-performance grounds. An employee has the right to contest a termination, even if a termination at-will policy exists, if the employee believes that he or she was fired for discriminatory reasons.

Furthermore, a prudent employer may regard termination at-will policies lightly for any termination circumstance. Organizational termination at-will policies have been likened to contract *termination without cause* clauses. Courts have pierced the veil of termination-without-cause policies even in cases when the termination was not of a discriminatory nature. In *Harper v. Healthsource New Hampshire, Inc.* (140 N.H. 770, 674 A.2d 962 [1996]), the termination of an employee without a specified reasonable

FIGURE 4.8

Case Example:
Covenant Not
to Compete
and Public
Policy

To be enforceable, most courts require that noncompetition clauses protect a legitimate business interest of the employer and are reasonable in terms of geography, time, and scope. For example, a hospital that prohibits a payroll clerk from working for any hospital in the United States for three years following termination probably is not protecting its legitimate business interest, and the court will find the clause unreasonable in terms of geography, time, and scope.

In *Medical Specialist, Inc. v Sleweon* (652 N.E.2d 517 [Ind. App. June 1995]), the plaintiff was an infectious disease specialist employed by a physician group practice. His employment agreement with the practice included a covenant not to compete. After resigning from his position, the defendant group practice sought to enforce the covenant not to compete. The plaintiff brought suit against his former employer, alleging the covenant was unenforceable based on public policy grounds. The court ruled against the doctor because there was no evidence of a shortage of such specialists in the restricted area.

cause was found to be against public policy. In this particular case, a physician was terminated without a cause or stated reason. Although this case stands alone in its findings, the ruling was intended to discourage bad-faith decisions that may endanger public welfare. Additionally, terminating without stating a cause was said to hamper the employee from properly responding to the termination. With these findings in mind, an employer may not retain much protection in termination at-will policies.

Once it is decided that termination of an employee is the proper course of action, several steps in the termination process must be considered, including the following (Mick 2004):

- *Analyze risk before termination.* Review carefully the personnel file and examine all facts and circumstances surrounding the termination. Ensure that human resources or management has investigated all valid complaints raised by the employee. Also examine the employee's personal situation or status (e.g., pregnancy, disability, age).
- *Avoid procrastination.* Do not delay an employee's termination after satisfying the risk analysis.
- *Strategically choose the termination date.* Employees who are fired on Friday have the weekend to think about the termination and about possible recourse against the employer. Therefore, termination

should be avoided on Fridays. Significant dates to the employee, such as a birthday, anniversary, or a holiday, should also be avoided.

- *Consult human resources personnel.* The HR department requires advance notification to consider the possibility of a severance agreement or the necessity of communicating the termination to other affected employees to avoid service disruption. Human resources also can process final paychecks and answer benefits questions.
- *Take action.* The individual who informs the employee of termination should be direct and to the point.

Separation Agreements

At the termination of employment, the employee and employer occasionally will enter into a separation or severance agreement. Such agreements often are required as a condition of receiving certain post-termination benefits such as severance, health benefit payments, or outplacement services. The separation or severance agreement will be enforceable in court only if supported by valid consideration. This means that each party to the agreement must receive some benefit in which he or she otherwise was not entitled to under a law, regulation, personnel policy, or employment agreement.

The benefits to an employer in obtaining a severance agreement are (1) a release of legal claims and (2) a covenant not to sue by the terminated employee. Because of the highly technical requirements of a release, the employer should consult experienced HR personnel or legal counsel. For example, in certain states, the severance agreement must specify state statutes to serve as a valid release of particular claims. Furthermore, to obtain a valid release for an age-discrimination claim, an employer must follow the Age Discrimination Employment Act (29 U.S.C. §§ 621–34) requirements: the employer must provide (1) a written agreement, (2) consideration, (3) advise in writing to seek counsel prior to signing, (4) 21 days to consider before signing, and (5) seven days to revoke after signing (29 U.S.C. § 626(f)[1]). Severance agreements also can require the employee to reaffirm or the employer to waive employment obligations, such as noncompetition and nonsolicitation provisions.

Dismissal for Cause

In the absence of an agreement or representation to the contrary, employers are not required to show cause to dismiss an employee. In many employment agreements, circumstances constituting a basis for "for-cause" termination are defined (see Figure 4.9).

FIGURE 4.9
Basis for
For-Cause
Termination

- Misconduct, including fraud, embezzlement, and commission of a criminal act
- Violation of corporate policy or practice
- Material failure to perform employment obligations
- For professionals, loss of license

Grievance Procedures

Public Employees' Right to Due Process

Despite the many exceptions described previously, at-will employment prevails for private employees. The same is not true, however, for public-sector employees, even in at-will states. Public employees enjoy certain due process rights and cannot be fired without a good reason or without notice and a hearing.

When considering the discharge of a public employee, an employer must remember that all public employees are protected by specific federal and state statutes and the federal and state constitutions. Both federal and most state governmental employees must be provided with written notice of the basis for any proposed disciplinary action. These employees also may be entitled to a hearing to allow them to defend against termination for cause. Because of these additional rights, management must seek professional assistance when terminating a public employee.

Alternative Dispute Resolution

Given the volume of employment litigation, some employers are attempting to control the escalating costs and media attention associated with litigation by including mandatory arbitration or *alternative dispute resolution* (ADR) clauses in employment contracts. These types of clauses mandate that any disagreement or claim that arises under the terms of employment will be subject to ADR. ADR agreements, however, do not preempt any rights that the EEOC or various state employment rights commissions may have to investigate claims of discrimination. ADR agreements also do not apply to unemployment or worker's compensation claims, nor do they relieve an employer of its obligation to conduct investigation of claims such as racial discrimination or sexual harassment.

There are two main types of ADR: mediation and arbitration. *Mediation* is generally a nonbinding process in which opposing parties conduct semi-formal settlement negotiations assisted by a neutral third-party mediator. *Arbitration*, much like a trial, is a more formal process in which both sides can present evidence and call witnesses; this form of ADR is typically binding on the parties and enforceable by the courts. Employers usually excempt from ADR clauses their right to seek injunctive relief for violation of noncompetition and nonsolicitation provisions.

Other Employment Issues

Employers, especially in the healthcare industry, cannot allow their employees to perform job duties while impaired or suffering from extreme stress. There are public health as well as liability problems associated with employers that do not take proactive measures in this regard. Employers should have confidential employee assistance programs available free of charge to all employees. Managers, with assistance from human resources or the legal department, also should discipline or terminate employees who work while impaired.

Job-Related Stress

Healthcare professionals and staff experience great levels of stress because of the nature of their work (Rowe 1998). Such stressful conditions can be exacerbated if employees suffer from depression or anxiety, as those who suffer from these disorders are less likely to have a person to confide in and have greater incidences of prior psychiatric disorders. Other work-related stress inducers include job insecurity, managers who are not supportive, and limited potential for job promotion.

Workplace Substance Abuse

Substance abuse is characterized as the unlawful, unauthorized, or improper use of alcohol, over-the-counter drugs, or products with mind-altering properties. Changes in the impaired individual's performance, appearance, and behavior are likely to be obvious. The impact these changes have on the employee's ability to carry out work-related duties without endangering their own safety or that of patients and coworkers is a substantial concern (McAndrew and McAndrew 2000).

Impaired Professionals

A unique and challenging set of circumstances faces healthcare professionals (e.g., doctors, nurses, other clinicians) who have substance abuse and dependence problems. Some of these issues are as follows:

1.   Fear of self-reporting because of the potential for loss of licensure
2.   Positions of accountability and high visibility (Consequences of addiction problems are both personal and isolating, which conflict

with public personas. Such problems also eventually affect their work and the care of their patients.)

3. Access to prescription medications that are highly addictive (Even when these professionals enter a treatment program and are highly motivated to change, their ongoing exposure and access to these medications put them at considerable risk for relapse.)

4. Tendency to self-treat and self-prescribe (Professionals view their illness as a weakness and failure, preventing them from accepting and complying with medical advice from other professionals.)

Summary

Many of the laws and regulations discussed in this chapter are complex, interdependent, and often conflicting. The legal environment surrounding HRM is under constant federal scrutiny and reform. Additionally, the legal requirements imposed on an organization often shift according to industry- and state-specific regulations. Blanket policies and regulations are imposed on all employers, but there are regulations that apply specifically to specific segments of employers.

To accommodate the complexity of the workplace, managers must learn as much as possible about work environment regulations and should not rely on instinct alone when faced with dilemmas in areas such as whistle-blowing, discrimination, or other types of highly sensitive situations. Because of the intricacy and specificity of workplace regulations, no single resource exists that managers can rely on. Instead, managers must acquire knowledge on specific and general areas of workplace laws. Table 4.3 lists resources available on the Internet.

Mishandling any situation can harm the employer's ability to attract and retain good employees and can lead to costly litigation and negative publicity. In general, a wise manager realizes the convoluted nature of his or her job and concedes to the necessity of ongoing education. An insightful manager executes thoughtful, deliberate choices. To make prudent law-abiding decisions, an employer must know the rights of both employer and employees. When dealing with employment issues, management should seek advice from experienced HR personnel, in-house legal counsel, or external legal advisors.

References

Allen, T. 2003. "Notes and Comments: The Foreseeability of Transference: Extending Employer Liability Under Washington Law for Therapist Sexual Exploitation of Patients." *Washington Law Review* 78: 525.

TABLE 4.3
Internet
Resources for
Employment
Law

Web Site	Content
www.dol.gov	General site for the U.S. Department of Labor; contains labor statistics, DOL online library, current news, listing of programs and services, and contacts
www.useeoc.gov	General site for the U.S. Equal Employment Opportunity Commission; contains information regarding filing of charges, enforcement and litigation, enforcement statistics, small business information, and the Freedom of Information Act
www.access.gpo.gov	General site for the Government Printing Office; allows access to any public document printed by the federal government
www.nlrb.gov	General site for the National Labor Relations Board, the organization charged with administering the National Labor Relations Act. Its main duties include (1) the facilitation of fair relations between unions and employers and (2) the prevention and remedies of unfair labor practices by both parties
www.business.gov	General site of the Office of the U.S. Business Advisor, the organization that provides guidance in all general business practices overseen by the government in some capacity
www.fmcs.gov	General site for the Federal Mediation and Conciliation Service, an independent agency created by Congress to facilitate strong and stable labor-management relations; contains information regarding dispute mediation, preventive mediation, alternative dispute resolution (litigation alternatives), arbitration services, and labor management grants

Anderson, P. 2001. "Study: U.S. Employees Put in Most Hours." [Online article; retrieved 2/25/04.] www.cnn.com/2001/CAREER/trends/08/30/ilo.study.

Becker, G. 1957. *The Economics of Discrimination*. Chicago: University of Chicago Press.

BNA. 1994. "Medical Center Employee Awarded $1 Million in Massachusetts Suit." *Employee Relations Weekly* 12 (January 31): 111–12.

Bouvier, C. 1996. "Why At-Will Employment Is Dying." *Personnel Journal* 75 (5): 123–28.

Castaneda, C. 1977. "Panel Backs FAA on Retire-at-60 Rule." *USA Today* (July 16): 11.

Cooter, R. 1994. "Market Affirmative Action." *San Diego Law Review* 31: 133–68.

Davis, E. 2002. "Comment: The Doctrine of Respondeat Superior: An Application to Employers' Liability for the Computer or Internet Crimes Committed by their Employees." *Albany Law Journal of Science & Technology* 12: 683–713.

Decker, P. J. 1997. "Sexual Harassment in Health Care: A Major Productivity Problem." *The Health Care Supervisor* 16 (1): 1–14.

Dobbin, F. 2004. "The Social Sciences: Do the Social Sciences Shape Corporate Anti-Discrimination Practice: The United States and France." *Comparative Labor Law and Policy Journal* 23 (3): 829–63.

Employment Law Update. 1991. "ADA: The Final Regulations (Title I): A Lawyer's Dream/An Employer's Nightmare." *Employment Law Update* 16 (9): 1.

England, P. 1994. "Neoclassical Economists' Theories of Discrimination." In *Equal Employment Opportunity: Labor Market Discrimination and Public Policy*, edited by P. Burstein. New York: Aldine de Gruyter.

Equal Employment Opportunity Commission, Civil Service Commission, Department of Labor, and Department of Justice. 1978. *Uniform Guidelines on Employee Selection Procedures. Federal Register* 43 (166): 38290–315.

Equal Employment Opportunity Commission. 2004. [Online information; retrieved 6/15/04.] www.eeoc.gov/types/sexual_harassment.

Fisher, A. B. 1994. "Businessmen Like to Hire by the Numbers." In *Equal Employment Opportunity: Labor Market Discrimination and Public Policy*, 269–73, edited by P. Burstein. New York: Aldine de Gruyter.

Furrow, B. R., T. L. Greaney, S. H. Johnson, T Jost, and R. L. Schwartz. 1997. *Health Law: Cases, Materials and Problems, 3rd Edition*, 237–307. St. Paul, MN: West Publishing Co.

Gabel, J., and N. Mansfield. 2003. "The Information Revolution and its Impact on the Employment Relationship: An Analysis of the Cyberspace Workplace." *American Business Law Journal* 40 (2): 301–53.

Greenberg, E. R. 2000. "Workplace Testing: Monitoring & Surveillance." [Online information; retrieved 6/15/04.] http://www.amanet.org/research/pdfs/monitr_surv.pdf.

Greenlaw, P. S., and J. P. Kohl. 1995. "The Equal Pay Act: Responsibilities and Rights." *Employee Rights and Responsibilities Journal* 8 (4): 295–307.

Kobata, M. 1992. "The Civil Rights Act of 1991." *Personnel Journal*, p. 48.

Kundu, K. 1999. "Hours of Work: A Matter of Choice for Most Working Americans." *Fact & Fallacy, Employment Policy Foundation.* [Online article; retrieved 6/15/04.] www.epf.org/ff/ff991014/htm.

Ledvinka, J., and V. G. Scarpello. 1991. *Federal Regulation of Personnel and Human Resource Management, 2nd Edition*. Boston: PWS-Kent.

Lee, R. D., and P. S. Greenlaw. 1995. "The Legal Evolution of Sexual Harassment." *Public Administration Review* 55 (4): 357–64.

McAndrew, K. G., and S. J. McAndrew. 2000. "Workplace Substance Abuse Impairment: The Occupational Health Care Provider's Role." *Journal of the American Association of Occupational Health Nurses* (January): 32–45.

Mick, G. 2004. "How to Fire Someone." [Online information; retrieved 6/10/04.] http://www.bsad.emba.uvm.edu/hrm/Discipline/article1.htm.

Mikulenak, M. 1992. "House Takes Stand Against Harassment, Discrimination." *The American Nurse* 1 (July–August): 13.

Modern Healthcare. 1999. "Healthcare Tattletales." *Modern Healthcare* 29 (47): 30–2, 37–8, 42.

Ramsey, R. 1999. "The 'Snoopervision' Debate: Employer Interest Vs. Employee Privacy." *Supervision* 60 (8): 40–45.

Reno, J., and D. Thornburgh. 1995. "ADA—Not a Disabling Mandate." *Wall Street Journal* (July 26): A12.

Rowe, M. M. 1998. "Hardiness as a Stress Mediating Factor of Burnout Among Healthcare Providers." *American Journal of Healthcare Studies* 14 (1): 16–20.

Segal, J. A. 1992. "Seven Ways to Reduce Harassment Claims." *HR Magazine* (January): 84–85.

Sherer, J. L. 1995. "Sexually Harassed." *Hospitals & Health Networks* 69 (2): 54–57.

U.S. Department of Labor. 2003. *Highlights of Women's Earnings in 2002,* Report 972. Washington, DC: U.S. Department of Labor.

Walsh, A., and S. C. Borowski. 1995. "Gender Differences in Factors Affecting Healthcare Administration Career Development." *Hospital & Health Services Administration* 40 (2): 263–77.

Yamada, D. C. 1998. "Voices from the Cubicle: Protecting and Encouraging Private Employee Speech in the Post Industrial Workplace." *Berkeley Journal of Employment and Labor Law* 19 (1): 1–51.

Discussion Questions

1. Is affirmative action still necessary to ensure equal employment opportunity? Given the diversity in the United States, should we begin to think about class-based rather than race-based affirmative action?

2. Has concern about sexual harassment gotten out of hand, and has political correctness replaced common sense?

3. Why is mental disability so difficult to define in the context of the Americans with Disabilities Act?

4. Should there be a uniform definition of reasonable accommodation in the Americans with Disabilities Act?

5. Why is sexual harassment so prevalent in the healthcare environment? What can be done to break this historical pattern?

6. Have federal antidiscrimination laws gone too far? Should public policy in the United States seek a return to employment at-will?

7. What does public policy exception to employment at-will mean?

8. Because employee handbooks may be used to contest a disciplinary procedure, what advice would you give to a work group that is assembling an employee handbook?

9. Under what circumstances would you use a progressive discipline process? When would you choose not to use such a procedure?

10. Given the great risks to the public that can result from the work of an impaired healthcare worker, should random drug testing be used in all healthcare organizations?

11. Consider the case of a physician who has been practicing for 15 years and is one of the few well-established physicians in a small community. How would you deal with information about this physician's abuse of alcohol or drugs?

Experiential Exercises

Case 1   Dr. Mind, a prominent psychiatrist at the Mensa Medical Center, a Department of Veterans Affairs (VA) Hospital, treated Ms. Puppet for anxiety and panic disorder. Dr. Mind used recognized techniques for treating Ms. Puppet, including medication, psychotherapy, and hypnosis. During the many hypnosis sessions, Dr. Mind began a sexual relationship with Ms. Puppet. She did not remember having relations with Dr. Mind, as Dr. Mind, during hypnosis, has instructed her to have no memory of her thoughts.

On one occasion, however, Ms. Puppet noticed that after she left Dr. Mind's office her undergarments were on backwards and that her skirt was not buttoned properly. She became suspicious of Dr. Mind, so she forced herself to not fall into a hypnotic state at her next session with Dr. Mind. At this session, when Dr. Mind believed Ms. Puppet was in a hypnotic state, he began undressing her. She then broke her silence, confronted him, and left his office.

Following the confrontation, Dr. Mind was placed on paid administrative leave pending an investigation, which resulted in his admission of guilt and termination. Ms. Puppet then sued the United States, because the actions occurred at a VA hospital, under the Federal Torts Claim Act (28 U.S.C. Section 2675[a]).

Ms. Puppet's attorney argued that Dr. Mind's acts took place during regularly scheduled therapy sessions, during working hours, and in an office provided to Dr. Mind by the VA hospital. Accordingly, under the doctrine of respondeat superior, the United States was liable for Dr. Mind's acts. The United States contented that it was not liable because Dr. Mind's motives were not intended to benefit the employee and that criminal and/or tortuous acts clearly fall outside the scope of employment.

Case Questions

1. Is the United States liable based on a theory that the wrongful acts of Dr. Mind took place within the scope of his employment?
2. What other theories may apply such as the foreseeability of transference?
3. What can employers do to prevent such wrongful acts?

For helpful information on this situation, see the basis for the hypothetical case—*Doe v. United States of America* (912 F. Supp. 193 [E.D. Va. 1995]). Also, for study of transference, see Allen 2003.

Case 2   Dr. Zhivago grew up in a small town in North Carolina. He was extremely intelligent and did well in college and medical school. After a fellowship in thoracic surgery, he was offered positions, with extremely good employment terms and conditions, in various reputable medical practices throughout the United States.

Feeling some duty to his hometown, however, Dr. Zhivago decided to return to his local community to practice medicine. He was offered and accepted employment with a multispecialty group practice. The practice paid his expenses to relocate back to his hometown and required him to sign an employment agreement that contained a non-competition provision. Being a trusting person, Dr. Zhivago did not seek an attorney's advice before signing the agreement. After several years of working at this practice, Dr. Zhivago fell in love with a patient who resided in another small town about 30 miles away. After this patient's recovery, Dr. Zhivago proposed marriage and agreed to move and work in his fiancé's hometown. He opened a private practice in this town.

After giving notice to his employer, however, Dr. Zhivago received a stern letter from the employer's counsel, reminding him of his employment agreement. The agreement's noncompetition provision prevented him from working as a thoracic surgeon within a 60-mile radius of his current employer for one year after leaving employment. Given the rural nature of the community, Dr. Zhivago was the only thoracic surgeon within a 90-mile radius of either practice. He would have to move to the big city to practice medicine, leaving all the residents of his hometown as well as those of his new wife's hometown without a practicing thoracic surgeon.

Case Questions

1. Given that such agreements restrict competition, under what circumstances should a court enforce a covenant not to compete?
2. In general, courts will enforce a covenant not to compete if it is (1) in writing, (2) entered into at the time of employment as part of the employment contract, (3) based on reasonable consideration, (4) reasonable with respect to time and territory, and (5) not against public policy. Using this as a guide, how should the court decide in this case?

For additional information, see *Iredell Digestive Disease Clinic, P.A., v. Petrozza*, 92 N.C.App. 21, 373 S.E.2d 449 (1988), aff'd per curiam, 324 N.C.327, 377 S.E.2d 750 (1989).

WORKFORCE DIVERSITY

Rupert M. Evans, Sr., FACHE

Learning Objectives

After completing this chapter, the reader should be able to

- understand how proactive use of diversity principles can transform the organization's culture;
- work toward creating an inclusive organizational culture;
- define the roles that healthcare providers, management, and governance play in building a business imperative for diversity within the organization; and
- discuss how healthcare leaders can develop a diversity program in their organizations.

Introduction

When you hear the term *diversity*, what comes to mind? To some, the word means the differences between human beings related to race or ethnicity. To others, it means the uniqueness of each individual. A few people still may jump up to argue that diversity is just a code word for affirmative action.

Healthcare organizations across the United States are beginning to make a commitment to move toward becoming institutions in which workforce diversity is embraced and fostered. This cultural change means adopting new values in terms of being inclusive and appropriately managing a diverse workforce. Diversity will drive the business practices of hospitals and other healthcare organizations and will require healthcare executives to provide strong leadership. This change will take time, but in the words of Reverend Jesse Jackson, "Time is neutral and does not change things. With courage and initiative, leaders change things."

In this chapter, we provide a definition of diversity and a framework for understanding how people view the term differently, highlight several studies and legal issues surrounding this topic, and enumerate methods for building a case for and establishing a diversity program.

A Definition of Diversity

People define diversity in many ways, depending on the way they live in and view society. In his book, *The 10 Lenses: Your Guide to Living and Working in a Multicultural World*, author Mark Williams (2001) discusses the framework that explains the way people see the world:

1. The *assimilationist* wants to conform and fit in with the group to which he or she belongs.
2. The *colorblind* ignores race, color, ethnicity, and other cultural factors.
3. The *cultural centrist* seeks to improve the welfare of his or her cultural group by accentuating its history and identity.
4. The *elitist* believes in the superiority of the upper class and embraces the importance of family roots, wealth, and social status.
5. The *integrationist* supports breaking down all barriers between racial groups by merging people of different cultures together in communities and in the workplace.
6. The *meritocratist* lives by the adage, "cream rises to the top"—the belief that hard work, personal merit, and winning a competition determine one's success.
7. The *multiculturist* celebrates the diversity of cultures, seeking to retain the native customs, languages, and ideas of people from other countries.
8. The *seclusionist* protects himself or herself from racial, cultural, and/or ethnic groups in fear that they may diminish the character and quality of his or her group's experiences within society.
9. The *transcendent* focuses on the human spirit and people's universal connection and shared humanity.
10. The *victim/caretaker* views liberation from societal barriers as a crucial goal and sees oppression as not only historical but also contemporary.

With this framework in mind, it is easier to understand why there are so many variations in the way diversity is defined.

For our purposes, we describe diversity in the context of three key dimensions: (1) human diversity, (2) cultural diversity, and (3) systems diversity. Each dimension needs to be understood and managed in the healthcare workplace.

Human diversity includes the attributes that make a human being who he or she is, such as race, ethnicity, age, gender, family status (single, married, divorced, widow, with or without children), sexual orientation, physical abilities, and so on. These traits are what frequently come to mind first when individuals consider the differences in people. Human diversity is a core dimension because it defines who we are as individuals. This dimension is with us throughout every stage of our lives, guiding how we define ourselves and how we are perceived by others. A workplace definition of diversity includes human diversity as a minimum.

Cultural diversity encompasses a person's beliefs, values, family structure practice (nuclear or extended family, independent living), and mindset as a result of his or her cultural, community, and environmental experiences. This dimension includes language, social class, learning style, and ethics or moral compass, religion, lifestyle, work style, global perspectives, and military views. Cultural diversity is a secondary dimension, but it can have a powerful impact on how a person behaves in the workplace. The cultural norms vary from one culture to another and influence how individuals interact with their work environments. For example, some religious groups are forbidden from working on the Sabbath, and this excemption has an impact on work scheduling and even hiring decisions.

Systems diversity relates to the differences among organizations in work structure and pursuits. This dimension includes teamwork reengineering, strategic alliances, employee empowerment, quality focus, educational development, corporate acquisitions, and innovation. Systems diversity deals with systems thinking and the ability to recognize how functions in the work environment are connected with diversity. In a multicultural, diverse, and inclusive workplace, organizational systems are integrated to enhance innovation, encourage teamwork, and improve productivity.

All of these dimensions are important and are present in the healthcare workplace, and all leaders should recognize them. The challenge is in seeing not only our differences but also our similarities as individuals, as professionals, and as members of a group. Leaders must develop effective strategies to manage the differences (and highlight similarities), and this will lead to building effective teams and a higher-performing organization (Guillory 2003).

Managing diversity is not an easy task, as a number of barriers often get in the way of achieving a harmonious working environment. Some of these barriers, which revolve around the diversity dimensions mentioned earlier, can be a great source of tension and conflict. For instance, a person's culture can be a barrier to a work team when other members of the group are not respectful of or misunderstand the person's values, beliefs, or even clothing, which that person gained through his or her cultural background. Examples of a cultural difference may be the person's hairstyle or affinity to wear religious artifacts. The education, race/ethnicity, work style, empowerment, and relationship/task orientation of an individual can also become barriers if they are not properly understood and managed.

Advancement Disparities Among Healthcare Administrators

The United States is becoming increasingly diverse. In 1900, one in eight Americans was non-white; today, this ratio is one in four. By 2050, it will be one in three (IOM 2004). The healthcare industry needs nurses and other healthcare providers, but it also needs to reflect the diversity of the population, who, in one point or another, become patients. Therefore, healthcare organizations need to employ caregivers and leaders who represent diverse backgrounds.

Healthcare managers and executives who are non-white are in the same situation when it comes to climbing the organizational ladder. In 1992, the American College of Healthcare Executives (ACHE) and the National Association of Health Services Executives (NAHSE) conducted a study that compares the career attainment of Caucasian and African-American healthcare executives. The study found that among executives with similar training and experience, African Americans were in lower-level positions, made less money, and had lower levels of job satisfaction (ACHE 2002). The results of this study made way for the creation of the Institute for Diversity in Health Management (IFD), the only organization in the industry committed exclusively to promoting managerial diversity within the healthcare field. In 1996, ACHE, with assistance and support from NAHSE, IFD, the Association of Hispanic Healthcare Executives, and the Executive Leadership Development Program of the Indian Health Services, conducted a follow-up survey using many of the items included in the first survey. This second survey, completed and published in 2003, revealed that 23 percent of the U.S. hospital workforce was made up of African Americans and Hispanics. Unfortunately, less than 2 percent of these minority groups held the positions of president, chief executive officer, and chief operating officer.

Following is a summary of the most important findings of the second study (ACHE 2003):

- More white administrators than minority administrators worked in hospital settings.
- White female administrators earned more than female minority administrators. When controlling for education and experience, compensation earned by white women remained higher than the compensation for male and female members of minority groups.
- White male administrators earned more than male minority administrators. When controlling for experience and education, the total compensation of male African-American and Hispanic administrators was approximately equal to that of their white counterparts.

- Minority administrators expressed lower levels of job satisfaction than did white administrators. The items with which low satisfaction was reported included the following:
  1. *Pay and fringe benefits* were not proportionate to the minority administrators' contribution to their organization.
  2. The *degree of respect and fair treatment* that minority administrators received from their leaders was inadequate.
  3. The *sanctions and treatment* that minority administrators faced when they made a mistake were more severe than their action called for.
- Fewer minority administrators than white administrators expressed that their organizations had great personal meaning to them.
- More minority administrators than white administrators stated that they experienced racial/ethnic discriminatory acts in the past five years, such as not being hired or being evaluated with inappropriate standards.
- Only about 15 percent of female minority administrators aspired to be chief executive officers. In contrast, more white male administrators had such aspirations than male minority administrators.
- The majority of minority administrators endorsed efforts to increase the percentage of racial/ethnic minorities in senior healthcare management positions. Nearly half of their white counterparts were neutral or opposed to such efforts.

Recommendations to address the disparities found between the white and minority groups are being developed. A third race/ethnic survey is expected to be conducted in 2007.

Prejudice in the Workplace

Prejudice is a set of views held by individuals about members of other groups. Prejudice is a pre-judgment and hence is not based on facts and/or experience. It affects the way people react toward and think of other people, and it can be as innocent as children choosing to not play with children they deem different from themselves or as harmful as adults not associating with certain people because English is not their native language.

Formally, prejudice can be defined as a set of institutionalized assumptions, attitudes, and practices that have an invisible-hand effect in systematically advantaging members of more powerful groups over members of less dominant groups. This type of prejudice occurs in many healthcare institutions. Some examples include culturally biased assessment and selection criteria, cultural norms that condone or permit racial or sexual harassment, lower performance expectations for certain groups, and collectively shared assumptions about a specific group that relegate members to certain positions. An example of the latter is the stereotypes assigned to certain groups. *Stereotypes* are generalizations about individuals based on their identity, group membership, or affiliations (Dreachslin 1996). A common stereotype in the healthcare management field is the assumption that black executives are not as qualified as their white counterparts. Thus, African-American executives are tested more often to prove their competence, while their white contemporaries are assumed to be competent from the start. This fact is substantiated in both the 1992 and 1997 race/ethnic surveys discussed earlier.

Comfort and risk refers to human being's natural need to feel comfortable and to avoid risk. People tend to prefer to work with others from similar racial or ethnic backgrounds because doing so provides them with a certain amount of comfort and shields them from a certain amount of risk. Although subordinate-superior relationships that involve people from different backgrounds work sufficiently to allow people to get the job done, they often fail to lead to the close bonds that form between a mentor and a protégé.

Given the systemic existence of prejudice and the way it influences people's mind-set and behavior, the fair and accurate assessment of the potential of employees of color remains an organizational dilemma rather than an established practice. For instance, there is evidence presented in the literature that managers systematically give higher performance ratings to subordinates who belong to the same racial group as they do, while high performers from minority groups remain comparatively invisible in the managerial/leadership selection process (Thomas and Gabarro 1999).

The Business Case for Diversity

Societal trends and a rapidly changing demographic picture in the United States require healthcare executives and their organizations to look for new insights, examples, and best practices to help them navigate through their diversity journey. A key challenge in establishing and implementing a diversity program is building a business case for having a diverse workforce.

The business case for diversity is unique for each organization. The circumstances, environment, and community demographics of one organization cannot be generalized to another institution. However, there are elements common in all organizations, which can be the basis of a diversity program. The healthcare marketplace, skills and talent of employees, and organizational effectiveness should be considered and will drive the institution's investment in and commitment to diversity. With a diversity focus in mind, an organization can achieve growth and profitability and sustain these results by doing the following:

- Expand market share by adding or enhancing services that target diverse populations.
- Link the marketplace with the workplace through recruiting, developing, and retaining employees with diverse racial/ethnic backgrounds.
- Create and implement workplace policies and management practices that maximize the talent and productivity of employees with diverse backgrounds.

The fact is that minority groups buy and consume healthcare services, many are educated and trained to provide either healthcare services or manage operations, and many already work within the field and know its complexities. Hospitals and other healthcare organizations cannot afford to miss such opportunities. They can seek, cultivate, and retain talent of minority candidates and current employees to compete in today's healthcare business environment that serves diverse people. Failure to do so will mean the difference between being a provider and employer of choice and losing ground to competitors.

Governance's Impact

The organization's governance can help in this regard. Trustees are the ultimate links to the communities served by a healthcare organization. They know the make-up of the population the organization serves and seeks to target, and they have insights into their communities' healthcare needs. Because trustees are part of the community, they have an interest in making sure that the healthcare organization that they represent is not only providing inclusive services but also is being a fair and equitable employer and neighbor. With this perspective in mind, governance should support a business strategy that promotes community goodwill, encourages growth, considers present social and demographic transformations and hence future needs, and emphasizes culturally competent and sensitive healthcare. The membership of a healthcare organization's governance or board of trustees should also reflect the multicultural mix of the communities.

Considering all of the challenges that any healthcare board is faced with today, why should they be concerned with diversity? One of the many reasons is protecting the organization's bottom line. The financial costs of problems stemming from racial discrimination and discriminatory practices can be substantial. Well-publicized cases of large organizations committing or turning their backs on such practices provide evidence of the extent of financial consequences. The Coca-Cola Company was directed by a court to pay $192 million to settle a race-bias lawsuit brought by its African-American workers. Similarly, Texaco, Denny's Restaurants, and Salomon Smith Barney have all been fined large sums for essentially not paying attention to this important issue (Jordan 2002).

Another reason to support diversity initiatives is to encourage and strengthen employee commitment to the organization. With such a workforce, the organization's competitive advantage in the marketplace is heightened, making the diverse workforce an asset and a difference from other organizations. Commitment by trustees to the principles of diversity may lead to shifts in the corporate culture as well, allowing all stakeholders to contribute to the overall success of the organization and its mission. Trustees should hold organizational leaders and management accountable for setting and following high diversity standards. This practice will lead to a healthier organization and to healthier communities as well.

Legal Issues Surrounding Diversity

The debate continues between those who think that the healthcare industry should be more diverse because it is the right thing to do and those who welcome diversity because it enhances shareholder/stakeholder value. The answer is diversity is both—not only is it the right thing to do, it also adds value to the organization. Women, people of color, and other professionals from minority groups who are trained and capable to serve in the healthcare field bring strategic, unique input and perspectives to their organizations; generate productive dialog; and challenge the status quo—all of which are essential to the practice and operations of a healthcare organization.

Another reason to pay attention to diversity matters is based on the law. The Civil Rights Act of 1964 was signed into law on July 2, 1964. This legislation was intended to ensure that the financial resources of the federal government would no longer subsidize racial discrimination (Smith 1999). This law bans discrimination in any activities, such as training, employment, or construction, funded by federal monies. Discrimination is also prohibited in entities that contract with organizations that receive federal funds. Every recipient of federal funds is required to provide written assurances that nondiscrimination is practiced throughout the entire institution. Among the first major tests of the Civil Rights Act was the decision of the U.S. Court of Appeals for the Fourth Circuit on the case of *Simkins v. Moses Cone Memorial Hospital.* The decision struck down the separate-but-equal provisions of the Hill-Burton Act and gave the federal government the necessary power to enforce the new law (Smith 1999).

The Civil Rights Act also provides protections for individuals who speak English as a second language. The U.S. Department of Justice has issued guidance to recipients of federal financial assistance regarding prohibitions against discrimination of people who have limited English-language proficiency. The law requires federally funded entities to ensure that people whose primary language is not English can access/understand programs and activities provided by these organizations. This issue is having a serious impact on the way healthcare organizations, especially those in areas with large numbers of individuals who speak English as a second language (ESL), are framing their service offerings. The National Council on Interpreting in Health Care has put together a glossary of terms intended to help healthcare leaders in developing programs for ESL patients; visit http://www.ncihc.org/mission.htm. See Chapter 4 for other laws that concern and address the issues of diversity.

The Impact of Diversity on Care Delivery

According to the National Institutes on Health, "the diversity of the American population is one of the nation's greatest assets; one of its greatest challenges is reducing the profound disparity in health status of America's racial and ethnic minorities" (Smedley and Stith 2002). The Institute of Medicine's landmark report in 2002, entitled *Unequal Treatment*, reveals the presence of significant disparities in the way white and minority patients receive healthcare services, especially in treatment for heart disease, cancer, and HIV (Smedley and Stith 2002).

Addressing such disparities in care, including the minority workforce in recruitment and selection, and ensuring cultural competence of caregivers are all interconnected. For care disparities to decrease, institutions and providers have to develop cultural competence. To develop cultural competence, embracing diversity and inclusion needs to be practiced in the workplace. *Cultural competence* may be defined as a set of complementary behaviors, practices, attitudes, and policies that enable a system, agency, or individuals to effectively work and serve pluralistic, multiethnic, and linguistically diverse communities.

An understanding of the factors that influence the disparities in healthcare is essential in developing effective strategies to combat these differences. Table 5.1 presents two sets of factors: patient-related factors and health-system-related factors.

Patient-related factors are cultural characteristics of individual patients that prevent them from getting fair and adequate treatment in an organization that is not culturally competent or sensitive. Health-system-related factors are organizational (including employee attributes and biases) dynamics that influence the methods they use to treat patients.

TABLE 5.1
Factors That
Influence
Disparities in
Healthcare

Patient-Related Factors	Health-System-Related Factors
Socioeconomic Low income and education	**Cultural competence** Insufficient knowledge of and sensitivity to cultural differences
Health education Lack of knowledge of health symptoms, conditions, and possible treatments	**Language** Inability to communicate sufficiently with patients and families whose native language is not English
Health behavior Patient willingness and ability to seek care, adhere to treatment protocols, and trust and work with healthcare providers	**Discrimination** Healthcare system and provider bias and stereotyping
	Workforce diversity Poor racial and ethnic match between healthcare professionals and the patients they serve
	Payment Insufficient reimbursement for treating Medicare, Medicaid, and uninsured patients

Source: Information from Smedley, B. D., and A. Y. Stith. 2002. *Unequal Treatment: Confronting Racial and Ethnic Disparities in Health Care.* Washington, DC: Institute of Medicine, National Academies Press.

Components of an Effective Diversity Program

Healthcare leaders can establish a diversity program that will lead to a more diverse and inclusive organization (see Figure 5.1). Some actions that leaders can take toward this goal include, but are not limited to, the following:

- Ensure that senior management and the board are committed to the development and implementation of a diversity program.
- Broaden the definition of diversity to include factors beyond race and ethnicity.
- Recognize the business case for bringing in diversity at the leadership level.
- Tie diversity goals to business objectives.
- Hold recruiting events that target racial and ethnic groups, women, people with disabilities, older but capable workers, and others who are considered minorities.

- Encourage senior executives to mentor minorities.
- Develop employee programs that emphasize and celebrate diversity and inclusivity.

The business imperatives and organizational necessities for aggressively creating a diversity program include, but are not limited to, the following:

1. *Reflection of the service population.* The healthcare organization's caregivers and support staff should mirror the diversity of the population that the institution serves. Toward this end, the organization should attract and take advantage of the talents, skills, and growth potential of minority professionals within the community.

2. *Workforce utilization.* Minority employees have a lot to contribute to the organization. Leaders should recognize this fact and should be open to, sensitive to, knowledgeable about, and understanding of the cultures, mind-set, and practices of the organization's diverse workforce. Doing so will not only enhance staff productivity and overall performance but will also boost staff morale.

3. *Work-life quality and balance.* Leaders should recognize that work and personal activities are interrelated, not separate preoccupations. Both are performed on the basis of necessity, practicality, efficiency, and spontaneity.

4. *Recruitment and retention.* Attracting and retaining a diverse workforce have a lot to do with the state of the workplace. Leaders should create an environment in which minorities feel included, professionally developed, and safe.

5. *Bridging generations.* Generational differences in expectations, education, and values exist between younger and older staff. Such gaps should be acknowledged, and attention should be paid to the physical, mental, and emotional well-being of all caregivers and staff at all ages regardless of backgrounds.

6. *Cultural competence.* This competence is an in-depth understanding of and sensitivity to the values and viewpoints of minority staff and patients and other customers. Leaders should master the skills necessary to work with and serve these groups and should provide training in this matter to all employees to ensure provision of culturally competent care.

7. *Organizationwide respect.* Leaders should create an environment in which the differences in title, role, position, and department are valued and respected but not held too lofty above everything else. Each employee, regardless of his or her level within the organization, should be viewed as integral to the overall success of the team.

FIGURE 5.1
How to
Create an
Inclusive
Culture

1. Study the culture, climate (i.e., what employees are thinking, feeling, or hearing about diversity issues), and demographics of the organization.

2. Select the diversity issues that allow the greatest breakthrough.

3. Create a diversity strategic plan.

4. Secure leadership's financial support for the plan.

5. Establish leadership and management accountabilities for the plan.

6. Implement the plan.

7. Provide continual training related to the new skills and competencies necessary to successfully achieve the plan goals.

8. Conduct a follow-up survey one or one-and-one-half years after implementing the plan.

Summary

Healthcare organizations in the United States are beginning to make a commitment to embracing and fostering workforce diversity. This cultural change means adopting new values in terms of being inclusive and attracting a diverse workforce. The business case for diversity is unique for each organization, as circumstances, the environment, and community demographics of one organization vary from those of another. However, there are elements common in all organizations, which can be the basis of a diversity program.

One of the many reasons that senior management and board should pay attention to diversity issues is to protect the organization's bottom line. The financial costs of problems stemming from racial discrimination and discriminatory practices can be substantial. Studies have found disparities in two areas: (1) minority healthcare administrators rise more slowly within their organizations than their white counterparts and (2) patients who belong to minority groups receive different medical treatments than patients who are white. Such disparities may be bridged with the development of a diversity program.

References

American College of Healthcare Executives. 2002. *A Race/Ethnic Comparison of Career Attainments in Healthcare Management*. Chicago: ACHE.

———. 2003. "Increasing and Sustaining Racial/Ethnic Diversity in Healthcare Management." *Healthcare Executive* 18 (6): 60–61.

Dreachslin, J. L. 1996. *Diversity Leadership*. Chicago: Health Administration Press.

Guillory, W. 2003. "The Business of Diversity: The Case for Action." *Health & Social Work* 28 (1): 3–7.

Institute of Medicine. 2004. "In the Nation's Compelling Interest: Ensuring Diversity in the Health Care Workforce." Washington, DC: National Academies Press.

Jordan, P. T. 2002. "Willie Gary vs. Coca-Cola: Angry Plaintiffs Protest Delays." [Online information; retrieved 6/1/04.] DiversityInc.com.

Smedley, B. D., and A. Y. Stith. 2002. *Unequal Treatment, Confronting Racial and Ethnic Disparities in Health Care*. Washington, DC: Institute of Medicine, National Academies Press.

Smith, D. B. 1999. *Health Care Divided: Race and Healing a Nation*. Ann Arbor, MI: The University of Michigan Press.

Thomas, D., and J. J. Gabarro. 1999. *Breaking Through: The Making of Minority Executives in Corporate America*. Boston: Harvard Business School Press.

Williams, M. 2001. *The 10 Lenses: Your Guide to Living and Working in a Multicultural World*. Sterling, VA: Capital Books.

Discussion Questions

1. What are the legal, moral, and ethical consequences that prohibit hospitals from turning away patients based on race?
2. Why are there are no such consequences to patients who demand doctors, nurses, or workers of a specific race to administer their healthcare?
3. Can hospitals that adhere to such patient demands face discrimination lawsuits from their employees?
4. When an employer denies an employee or group of employees their full employment opportunity based on the racial bias of customers, is the employer in violation of the employee's civil rights?

Experiential Exercises

Note: The following cases are included in "A Diversity and Cultural Proficiency Assessment Tool for Leaders." To access the complete tool, go to http://www.diversityconnection.org/userdocs/uploads/5_leadership_ifd.pdf.

Case 1   Hurley Medical Center is a publicly owned 463-bed teaching hospital that serves the five-county Flint,

Michigan, area. The hospital maintains clinical affiliations with the medical schools at Michigan State University and the University of Michigan as well as with the Henry Ford Health System, all of which are close by. Hurley's 300 physicians and 2,600 employees serve an area population of about 550,000. Hurley annually records 23,000 inpatient admissions, 318,000 outpatient visits, and 73,000 emergency room visits. The medical center's service area is 76 percent Caucasian and 21 percent African American. Minorities comprise approximately 40 percent of its workforce. Hurley and General Motors were each created in Flint in 1908, and local healthcare has been intertwined with the automotive industry since then. The departure of major segments of the area's automotive-manufacturing base in recent years hit Flint's economy and Hurley's patient base hard. Today, local unemployment wavers between 8 percent and nearly 11 percent; 16 percent of all residents and 14 percent of area families live under the poverty line. The hospital is the safety net healthcare provider in its service area.

Over the past decade, Hurley's leadership team and managers developed a two-tiered strategy to attract and advance women and racially/ethnically diverse individuals to senior management positions and roles throughout the workforce. In addition to maintaining a workforce that reflects the diversity of its community, Hurley's leadership team is minority led.

Executive succession planning at Hurley includes an extensive three-year management development program for high-potential candidates. This program is geared toward ensuring that Hurley's future management team has the skills and diversity needed to care for its communities. Recognizing the importance of diversity to the hospital's corporate culture, Hurley's board approved the creation of an executive HR position responsible for cultural diversity, equal-employment recruiting, and diversity training. Hospital managers are charged with increasing the number of women and minority employees by at least 0.5 percent per year. In 2003, 31 percent of all new hires were minorities; 42 percent of all promotions involved minorities; and 14 percent of all administrative professional/technical jobs were held by minorities. In the 1990s, Hurley's senior management retained an outside consultant to conduct a "cultural assessment" of the medical center and to help install a long-term cultural and racial-diversity training program. The first step was "train the trainer" sessions, which expanded to include the board, senior management, and all levels of the workforce. Today, all new hires receive diversity training as part of their orientation to the medical center. Managers also receive affirmative action training.

Hurley's leadership has asserted a highly visible role for the hospital as a steward of the community's health and as an organization that recognizes and celebrates diversity. A special board leadership task force directs the hospital's participation in key community health programs, such as the GM/UAW Health Initiative, Michigan's "Healthy Mother-Healthy Baby" program of immunizations, and care for indigent and underserved populations. Hurley also is a corporate leader and key participant in community efforts to showcase and celebrate cultural heritage and diversity. In addition to pursuing diversity initiatives as the right thing to do, Hurley also sees real benefits. The medical center is well recognized for its commitment to diversity, and its brand loyalty with the community and its reputation as a good corporate citizen are strengthened. This recognition also helps Hurley recruit and retain a high-quality workforce. Most importantly, this initiative provides a better healing environment for the people who entrust their care to Hurley.

CEO Action Steps

1. *Manage upward.* CEO vision and commitment to diversity can rally the board.
2. *Seek buy-in at all levels.* Top-to-bottom diversification can improve both the bottom line and community reputation.
3. *Take stock and mandate change.* Assess cultural and diversity needs, then tailor diversity training for everyone from the board to new hires.
4. *Make the hospital environment a haven.* A diverse, culturally proficient staff enhance quality-of-safety net care for diverse, stressed patients and families.

Case 2   Aventura Hospital and Medical Center is a 407-bed acute care medical/surgical facility that serves an unusually varied racial, ethnic, international, and socioeconomic patient population in the densely compressed South Florida neighborhoods of northeast Miami-Dade and southeast Broward counties. Mirroring the rapid growth of its bi-county service area, the hospital has undergone one geographic relocation and three name changes since its formation in 1965 by a group of local physicians. Aventura took its current name in 1993 from the 2.7-square-mile, high-rise condominium and shopping mall city (created by a realty company). The hospital's 725 physicians and 1,300 employees serve a patient base that includes retired Caucasians from the Northeast; Spanish- and Portuguese-speaking immigrants from Central and South America; émigrés from Russia; and European tourists from Italy, Germany, Poland, France, and the United Kingdom.

The hospital has developed an international patient services department to help provide healthcare services to patients from other countries or to patients whose first language is not English. Described by hospital administrators as a "commuter hospital," Aventura provides care for both high- and low-income families. In 2002, nearly 29 percent of all hospital expenditures were for charity and uncompensated care. Although Aventura, an HCA affiliate, does not follow a formal, structured plan to recruit and promote women and racially/ethnically diverse individuals, it has developed and sustains an impressively diverse management team through its own local and corporate national pipelines. Board diversity is widening through a long-term development program. A separate strategy for recruiting nurses is in place to address challenges that are peculiar to Aventura's location.

Aventura identifies, recruits, and mentors management talent through parallel talent pipeline streams. As a result, women and minorities make up more than half of the senior management team, including administrators originally from Cuba and Jamaica. Hospital executives monitor local healthcare students who are at the top of their graduate business and healthcare classes. An example of this practice is a London-born Jamaican woman who was enrolled in a hospital administration program at the University of Miami and was recruited by Aventura as an unpaid intern. She earned her degree and, through talent, drive, and a willingness to learn, rose through Aventura's management ranks. Today, she is a senior manager at one top hospital in the South Florida area.

Nationally, Aventura draws on HCA's corporatewide farm system of chief operating officer and controller/chief financial officer development programs for management talent. These programs train and develop high-potential managers before they are placed in hospitals like Aventura as "associate administrators" for two to five years. Advanced degrees in business or health administration are required. Importantly, candidates receive training in ethics along with finance and technology. Hospital bylaws require a 14-member board, supported by a 5-year diversity plan to ensure that the composition of the board reflects the changing racial and ethnic demographics of the community the hospital serves. Aventura's current trustees include three women from minority groups—an African American, a Cuban American, and two physicians from Colombia.

Aventura's immediate neighborhood is populated by high-income residents, and affordable housing for minority and other middle-class employees is scarce. Most staff commute to work, often passing other hospitals closer to home that offer more geographically desirable opportunities for employment, especially for trained nurses. To overcome this, Aventura bypasses nursing agencies and recruits directly from area nursing schools, offering permanent, full-time positions and registered-nurse training. The hospital also finds success recruiting minority nurses from overseas. HR managers take part in corporate-organized international recruiting tours, yielding English-speaking minority nurses from Singapore, the Philippines, Asia, India, southern Africa, Australia, and the United Kingdom. Surprisingly, nurses recruited from nearby Puerto Rico present a special challenge: Florida nursing licensing requirements include proficiency in English language skills.

CEO Action Steps

1. *Diversify the board.* Conform board membership to changing community demographics.
2. *Continue to recruit a diversified group of home-grown talent.* Draft raw, high-potential candidates from local education and healthcare entities and bring them in-house for development.
3. *Turn on the external pipeline.* Locate minority candidates through regional and national affiliates.
4. *Go global.* Recruit minority allied health professionals through cross-country and international searches. Relocate and retrain.

Case 3   Abington Memorial Hospital is a 508-bed hospital located in Abington, Pennsylvania. It services patients from Philadelphia and the surrounding white suburbs of Bucks and Montgomery counties. The hospital's mission "is to provide patients with the highest quality care possible, regardless of the health-care professionals' race. . . ."

The African-American workers at Abington were outraged when they were told not to enter the room of a white patient. Supervisors at the hospital told their African-American healthcare professionals, as well as food-service and housekeeping staff, not to enter the patient's room or interact with the family.

Abington administrators said they broke hospital policy to avoid a potentially "volatile situation" by adhering to the request of the patient's husband—only white employees could enter his wife's room on the maternity ward. "We were wrong," said Meg McGoldrick, a vice president at Abington Memorial Hospital. "We should have followed our policy. The whole incident has greatly upset many of our employees who perceived that we were acquiescing to the family's wishes."

Despite the hospital's policy that states, "care will be provided on a nondiscriminatory basis," the administrators' actions seemed as though patients are allowed to discriminate. Catholic Health Care West's medical ethicist, Carol Bayley, said that Abington failed in its responsibility to its employees and the community to accommodate a patient's racial preference: "This was a fundamental disrespect of these professionals' skills and their fundamental dignities . . . a hospital needs to stand against this undercurrent of racism in our society."

The Philadelphia office of the Anti-Defamation League (ADL) said that prohibiting African-American employees from carrying out the full scope of their duties is reprehensible: "I don't see why and how a hospital could justify accommodating a request that the professionals attending to a patient be of a particular background," said Barry Morrison, director of the Philadelphia chapter of the ADL. "Certainly, it's demoralizing for the people who work there." The American Hospital Association (AHA) acknowledged several similar instances that its staff knows about and that no hard-and-fast industry guidelines exist for hospitals to follow when such a request is made. With nearly 5,000 hospitals as members, the Chicago-based AHA is the largest hospital association in the United States. AHA does not offer hospitals a suggestion as to how to address this situation. "It's subjective," said Rick Wade, senior vice president at the AHA. "I'm sure the person who made the decision at Abington thought they were doing the right thing." Goldrick said supervisors at Abington were acting with good intentions and sought to deflect any confrontation between its African-American staff and the Caucasian family. No incident was reported during the patient's stay.

Since then, Abington president Richard L. Jones sent a letter to all its employees and volunteers apologizing for the situation, which he termed "morally reprehensible." In addition to creating a diversity task force at the 508-bed hospital, Abington has hired consultants and is revising its antidiscrimination policy.

The AHA bestowed on Abington the "Quest for Quality" award for raising awareness of the need for an organizational commitment to patient safety and quality. Wade said hospitals are constantly evaluating how to provide the best treatment for their patients, while protecting and maintaining the dignity of its employees. He said that a hospital's constant patient turnover sometimes subjected workers to society's underbelly. "Perhaps Abington could have been more protective of their employees," Wade said. "Patients come and go, [but] the most important thing at a hospital is the work-force," he said.

JOB ANALYSIS AND JOB DESIGN

Myron D. Fottler, Ph.D.

Learning Objectives

After completing this chapter, the reader should be able to

- distinguish between job analyses, job descriptions, and job specifications;
- describe the methods by which job analyses are typically accomplished;
- discuss the relationship of job requirements (as developed through job analyses, job descriptions, and job specifications) to other human resources management functions;
- enumerate the steps involved in a typical job analysis as well as the methods of job analysis;
- address the relationship between job analyses and strategic human resources management; and
- understand the changing nature of jobs and how jobs are being redesigned to enhance productivity.

Introduction

The interaction between an organization and its environment has important implications for the organization's internal organization and structure. For example, the environment affects how the institution organizes its human resources to achieve specific objectives and to perform different functions necessary in carrying out the organization's mission and goals. The organization formally groups the activities to be performed by its human resources (HR) into basic units referred to as jobs.

A *job* consists of a group of related activities and duties that entail natural units of work that are similar and related. Jobs should be clear and distinct from others to minimize misunderstandings and conflict among employees and to enable employees to recognize what is expected of them. Some jobs require to be performed by several employees, each of whom occupies a separate position. A *position* consists of different duties and responsibilities that are performed by only one employee. For example, in a hospital, 40 registered nurses fill 40 positions, but all of them perform only one job—that of a registered nurse. Different jobs that have similar duties and responsibilities may be grouped into a *job family* for purposes of recruitment, training, compensation, or advancement opportunities. For example, the nursing job family may consist of registered nurses, nursing supervisor, and director of nursing services.

Healthcare organizations are continually restructuring and reengineering themselves in an attempt to become more cost effective and customer focused. They have put emphasis on smaller scale, less hierarchy, fewer layers, and more decentralized work units. As these changes occur, more managers want their employees to operate more independently and flexibly to meet customer demands. To do this, they require that decisions be made by employees who are closest to the information and who are directly involved in the service delivery. The objective is to develop jobs and basic work units that are adaptable and can thrive in a world of high-velocity change.

In this chapter, we define the terms job analysis, job description, and job specification; indicate the processes that may be used to conduct job analyses; and identify the relevance of and relationship between the results of job analysis (i.e., job descriptions and job specifications) and other human resources management functions. In addition, we emphasize that these job processes provide the organization with a foundation for making objective and legally defensible decisions in managing human resources. We discuss how healthcare jobs have been redesigned to contribute to organizational objectives while simultaneously satisfying the needs of the employees, and we review several innovative job design and employee-contribution techniques to enhance job satisfaction and organizational performance.

Definitions

Job analyses are sometimes called the cornerstone of strategic human resources management because the information they collect serve so many HR functions. *Job analysis* is the process of obtaining information about jobs by determining the job's duties, tasks, and/or activities. The procedure involves undertaking a system investigation of jobs by following a number of predetermined steps specified in advance of the study (Ash 1988). When the analysis is completed, a written report is created that summarizes the information obtained from studying 20 or 30 individual job tasks or activities. HR managers use these data to develop job descriptions and job specifications.

A *job description* is a written explanation of a job and the types of duties the job involves. Because there is no standard format for job descriptions, these documents tend to vary in appearance and content from one organization to another. However, most job descriptions contain the job title, a job identification section, and a job duties section. They may also include a job specification section; sometimes a job specification is prepared as separate documents, but sometimes it is a part of the job description. A *specific job description* is a detailed summary of a job's tasks, duties, and responsibilities, emphasizing efficiency, control, and detailed work planning. This type of description fits best with a bureaucratic organizational structure, where there are well-defined boundaries that separate functions and different levels of management. A *general job description*, which is fairly new on the HR scene, emphasizes innovation, flexibility, and loose work planning. This type of job description fits best with an organization with flat boundaries, where few boundaries exist between functions and levels of management (Leonard 2000). Only the most generic duties, responsibilities, and skills for a position are documented in a general job description (Johnson 2001).

A *job specification* describes the personal qualifications an individual must possess to perform the duties and responsibilities contained in a job description. Typically, the job specification describes the skills required to perform the job and the physical demands the job places on the employee performing it. Skills relevant to a job include education and experience, specialized knowledge or training, licenses, personal abilities and traits, and manual dexterity. The physical demands of a job refer to the condition of the physical work environment; workplace hazards; and the amount of walking, standing, reaching, and lifting required by the job. Appendix A (end of chapter) provides an example of a combined job description/job specification document for the position of staff nurse in a hospital's labor and delivery department.

The Job Analysis Process

Figure 6.1 indicates how job analysis is performed, including the functions for which it is used. Analysis involves a systematic, step-by-step investigation of jobs. The end product of the analysis is a document that summarizes information about the various job tasks or activities examined. This information is then used by HR managers in developing job descriptions and job specifications, which in turn are used to guide performance and to enhance different HR functions such as development of performance appraisal criteria or the content of training classes (Clifford 1994). The ultimate purpose of a job analysis is to improve organizational performance and productivity.

Steps in Job Analysis

The process of conducting a job analysis involves a number of steps. Although healthcare organizations may perform their job analysis differently, they follow a general guide such as that listed below (Anthony, Perrewe, and Kacmar 1993):

1. *Determine the purpose of the job analysis.* As a result of rapid growth or downsizing, jobs may have changed in their content. Such changes may cause employee salaries to be inequitable. The purpose of conducting the job analysis should be explicit and tied to the organization's overall business strategy to increase the probability of a successful job analysis program.

2. *Identify the jobs to be analyzed.* All jobs are analyzed if no previous formal job analysis has been performed. If the organization has undergone changes that have affected only certain jobs or if new jobs have been added, then only those jobs are analyzed.

3. *Explain the process to employees, and determine their levels of involvement.* Employees should be informed of who will be conducting the analysis, why the analysis is needed, whom to contact to answer questions and concerns, when the analysis will take place, and what roles they are expected to play in the process. In addition to receiving good communication, employees may elect a committee to serve as a verification check and to reduce anxiety. Such a committee can also help answer employee questions and concerns.

4. *Collect the job analysis information.* Managers must decide which method or combination of methods will be used and how the information will be collected. Various alternatives are discussed in the next section of this chapter.

5. *Organize the job analysis information into a form that will be useful to managers and employees.* This form consists of job descriptions and job specifications. The job descriptions can vary from very broad to very specific and precise; the level of detail depends on the needs of the organization. The job specifications must be linked directly to the job description—that is, it must be relevant to the job.

6. *Review and update the job analysis information frequently.* Particularly in a dynamic environment such as healthcare, jobs seldom go unchanged for long periods of time. Even if no major changes have occurred within the organization, a complete review of all jobs should be performed every three years (Mathis and Jackson 1985). More frequent reviews are necessary when major organizational changes occur.

Data Sources and Data-Collection Methods

Conducting job analyses is usually the primary responsibility of the HR department or the individuals charged with this function. Although job analysts are typically responsible for the job analyses program, they usually enlist the cooperation of the employees and supervisors in the departments

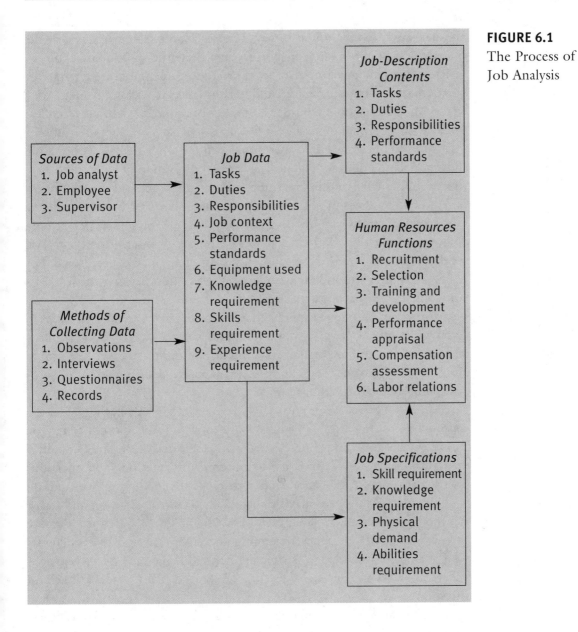

FIGURE 6.1

The Process of
Job Analysis

Sources of Data
1. Job analyst
2. Employee
3. Supervisor

*Methods of
Collecting Data*
1. Observations
2. Interviews
3. Questionnaires
4. Records

Job Data
1. Tasks
2. Duties
3. Responsibilities
4. Job context
5. Performance
   standards
6. Equipment used
7. Knowledge
   requirement
8. Skills
   requirement
9. Experience
   requirement

*Job-Description
Contents*
1. Tasks
2. Duties
3. Responsibilities
4. Performance
   standards

*Human Resources
Functions*
1. Recruitment
2. Selection
3. Training and
   development
4. Performance
   appraisal
5. Compensation
   assessment
6. Labor relations

Job Specifications
1. Skill requirement
2. Knowledge
   requirement
3. Physical
   demand
4. Abilities
   requirement

in which jobs are being analyzed. These supervisors and employees are the
sources of much of the job information generated through the process.

Job information is collected in several ways, depending on the purpose identified by the organization. Typically, the organizational chart is
reviewed to identify the jobs to be included in the analysis. Often, restructuring, downsizing, merger, or rapid growth initiates the job analysis. A
job may be selected because its content has undergone undocumented
changes. As new job demands arise and the nature of the work changes,

compensation for the job also may have to change. The employee or the manager may request a job analysis to determine the appropriate compensation. The manager may also be interested in documenting change for recruitment selection, training, and performance appraisal purposes.

Managers should consider a number of different methods to collect job analysis information because it is unlikely that any one method will provide all of the necessary information needed for a job analysis. Among the most popular methods of data collection are observation of tasks and behaviors of jobholders, conducting interviews, using structured questionnaires and checklists, assessing job performance, and reviewing critical incidents.

Observations require job analysts to observe jobholders performing their work. The observations may be continuous or intermittent based on work sampling—that is, observing only a sampling of tasks performed. For many jobs, observation may be of limited usefulness because the job does not consist of physically active tasks. For example, observing an accountant review an income statement may not provide valuable information. Even with more active jobs, observation does not always reveal vital information such as the importance or difficulty of the task. Given the limitations of observation, it is helpful to incorporate additional methods for obtaining job analysis information.

Employees who are knowledgeable about a particular job (i.e., the employee holding the job, supervisors, or former jobholders) may be interviewed concerning the specific work activities of the job. Usually a structured interview form is used to record information. The questions asked correspond to the data needed to prepare a job description and job specification. Employees may be suspicious of the interviewer and his or her motives, especially if the interviewer asks ambiguous questions. Because interviewing can be a time-consuming and costly method of data collection, managers and job analysts may prefer to use the interview as a means to get answers to specific questions generated from observations and questionnaires.

The use of structured questionnaires and checklists is most efficient because each method is a quick and inexpensive way to collect information about a job. If possible, it is desirable to have several knowledgeable employees complete the questionnaire for verification. Such survey data often can be quantified and processed by computer. Follow-up observations and interviews are not uncommon if a questionnaire or checklist is chosen as the primary means of collecting job analysis information. Although questionnaires and checklists provide the employer with a simplified method for obtaining job analysis information, the questionnaire must be extremely detailed and comprehensive so that valuable data are not missed. Compared to other methods, questionnaires are cheaper and easier to administer but are more time consuming and expensive to develop. Management must decide whether the benefits of a simplified method of data collection outweigh the costs of its construction.

Strategically, managers would favor methods of data collection that do not require a lot of work and up-front costs if the content of the job changes frequently. Another option may be to adopt an existing structured questionnaire. Among the more widely used structured questionnaires are the Position Analysis Questionnaire, the Management Position Description Questionnaire, and the Functional Job Analysis. Regardless of whether the questionnaire is developed in-house or purchased from a commercial source, rapport between analyst and respondent is not possible unless the analyst is available to explain items and to clarify misunderstandings. Without such rapport, such an impersonal approach may have adverse effects on the respondent's cooperation and motivation.

Finally, the analyst can actually perform the job in question. This approach allows exposure to the actual job tasks as well as the job's physical, environmental, and social demands. This method is appropriate for jobs that can be learned in a relatively short period of time. However, it is inappropriate for jobs that require extensive training and/or are hazardous to perform.

Relation to Other Human Resources Functions

Job analysis provides the basis for tying all the HR functional areas together and for developing a sound HR program. Not surprisingly, job requirements as documented in job descriptions and job specifications influence many of the HR functions that are performed as part of managing employees. When job requirements are modified, corresponding changes must be made in other HR activities. Job analysis is the foundation for forecasting future needs for human resources as well as plans for such activities as recruitment, selection, performance appraisal, compensation, training, transfer, or promotion. Job analysis information is often incorporated into the HR information systems.

Before attempting to recruit capable employees, recruiters need to know the job specifications for the positions needed to be filled, including the knowledge, skills, and abilities required for successful job performance. The information in the job specifications is used in job opening notices and provides a basis for attracting qualified applicants while discouraging unqualified applicants. A failure to update job specifications can result in a flood of applicants who are unqualified to perform one or more functions of the job.

Until 1971, job specifications used as a basis for employee selection decisions often bore little relation to the duties to be performed under the job description. In the case of *Griggs v. Duke Power Company* (401 U.S. 424) (1971), the Supreme Court ruled that employment practices must be job related. When discrimination charges arise, employers have the burden of proving that job requirements are job related or constitute a business necessity. Today, employers must be able to show that the job specifications used in selecting employees for a job relate specifically to that job's duties.

Any discrepancies between the knowledge, skills, and abilities demonstrated by the jobholders and the requirements contained in the job description and specification provide clues to training needs. Career development is concerned with preparing employees for advancement to jobs at which their capabilities can be used to the fullest extent possible. The formal qualifications set forth in the job specifications for higher-level jobs serve to indicate how much more training and development are needed for employees to advance to these jobs. The requirements contained in the job description provide the criteria for evaluating the performance of the jobholder. The appraisal may reveal, however, that certain performance criteria established for a particular job are not completely valid. These criteria must be specific and job related. If the criteria used to evaluate employee performance are overly broad, vague, and not job related, employers may be charged with unfair discrimination.

The relative worth of a job is one of the most important factors in determining the rate to be paid for performing a job. This worth is based on what the job demands of an employee in terms of skill, effort, and responsibility as well as the conditions and hazards under which the work is performed. Information derived from job analysis is also valuable in identifying safety and health considerations. If a job is hazardous (e.g., poses possibility of contracting AIDS), the job description and specification should reflect this condition. Employers need to provide specific information about such hazards to enable jobholders to perform their jobs safely.

Job analysis information is also important to the employee-relations and labor-relations functions. When employees are considered for promotion, transfer, or demotion, the job description provides a standard for comparison of talent. Regardless of whether the organization is unionized, information obtained through job analysis can often lead to more objective HR decisions. Job analysis can be used in employee selection to determine whether an applicant for a specific job should be required to take a particular kind of test. The performance standards used to judge employee performance for promotion, rewards, discipline, and loyalty should be job related and based on the job description. Job analysis information can also be used to compare the relative worth of each job's contribution to the organization's overall performance. Finally, job analysis can be used to determine training needs by comparing current employee skills to skills identified in the job analysis. Training programs can then be put in place to reduce employees' skill gaps.

Legal Aspects of Job Analysis

Although HR managers consider job descriptions a valuable tool for performing HR functions, they encounter several problems when using these documents (Grant 1988). First, they are often poorly written and provide little guidance for the jobholder. Second, they are generally not updated as job duties or specifications change. Third, they may violate the law by containing specifications not related to job performance. Fourth, the job duties they include are often written in vague, rather than specific, terms. Fifth, they can limit the scope of activities of the jobholder in a rapidly changing environment.

A major goal of job analysis is to help the organization establish the job relatedness of its selection and performance requirements. Job analysis helps employees to meet their legal duties under equal employment opportunity law. Section 14 C.2 of the *Uniform Guidelines for Employee Selection Procedures* states that "There shall be a job analysis which includes an analysis of the important work behaviors required for successful performance. . . . Any job analysis should focus on work behavior(s) and the task associated with them" (EEOC 1978).

Today's legal environment has created a need for higher levels of specificity in job analysis and job descriptions. Federal guidelines now require that the specific performance requirements of a job be based on valid job-related criteria (EEOC 1978). Employment decisions that involve either job applicants or employees and that are based on vague and non-job-related criteria are increasingly being challenged, and the challenges have mostly been successful. Managers of small healthcare organizations, where employees may perform many different job tasks, must be particularly concerned about writing specific job descriptions.

When writing job descriptions, employers must use statements that are terse, direct, and worded simply and must eliminate unnecessary phrases and terms. Typically, the sentences that describe job duties begin with verbs (see Appendix A). The term "may" is used for those duties performed only by some workers on the job. Excellent job descriptions are of value to both employee and employer. They can be used to help employees learn their job duties and to remind them of the results they are expected to achieve. For the employer, they can minimize the misunderstandings that occur between supervisors and their subordinates relative to job requirements. Good job descriptions also establish management's right to take corrective action in the events that the duties specified in the document are not performed at all or performed at an inadequate or inappropriate level.

Job analysis is surrounded by several legal constraints largely because it serves as a basis for selection decisions, compensation, performance appraisals, and training. These constraints have been articulated in the *Uniform Guidelines for Employee Selection Procedures* and several court decisions. Section 14.c.2 of the *Guidelines* states that "there shall be a job analysis of the important work behaviors required for successful performance. . . . Any job analysis should focus on work behavior(s) and the tasks associated with them." To determine this, organizations should assess job skills, knowledge, and abilities needed to perform the jobs. After this is known, selection procedures can be developed (Thompson and Thompson 1982).

Job analyses that were not performed in organizations have resulted in the successful challenge to the validity of the organizations' selection decisions; see *Albermarle Paper Company v. Moody* (422 U.S. 405) (1975). Numerous court decisions regarding promotion and job analysis also exist. In *Rowe v. General Motors* (32 5 U.S. 305) (1972), the court ruled that a company should have written objective standards for promotion to prevent discriminatory practices. In *U. S. v. City of Chicago* (573 F. 2nd 416 [7th Cir.]) (1978), the court ruled that the standards should describe the job for which the person is being considered for promotion. In both cases, these objective standards can be determined through job analysis (Nobile 1991).

Before the *Guidelines* and the associated court cases discussed earlier, labor contracts required consistent and equitable treatment of unionized employees. The information provided by job analysis is helpful to both management and unions in contract negotiations and in avoiding or resolving grievances, jurisdictional disputes, and other conflicts. For these reasons, unionized employers have found it advantageous to prepare written job descriptions and job specifications.

The passage of the Americans with Disabilities Act (ADA) also had a major impact on job analysis. Managers must now adhere to the legal mandates of the ADA when preparing job descriptions and job specifications (Mitchell, Alliger, and Morfopoalos 1997). The ADA requires that job duties and reasonability be essential functions for successful job performance. If the job requires the jobholder to perform certain essential physical and mental tasks, these requirements should be stated in the job description. Section 1630.2 (n) of the ADA provides three guidelines for rendering a job function essential (EEOC 1992):

1. The reason the position exists is to perform a function.
2. A limited number of employees are available among whom performance of the function may be distributed.

3. The function may be highly specialized, requiring needed expertise or abilities to complete the job.

Managers who write job descriptions in terms of essential functions reduce the risk of discriminating on the basis of disability. Once the essential functions of a job are defined, the organization is legally required to make a reasonable accommodation to the disability of the individual.

Job Analysis in a Changing Environment

The traditional approach to job analysis assumes a static job environment, where jobs remain relatively stable apart from incumbents who hold these jobs. It assumes jobs can be meaningfully defined in terms of tasks, duties, processes, and behaviors necessary for job success. Unfortunately, these assumptions discount technological advances that are often so accelerated that jobs that are defined today may be obsolete tomorrow. In a dynamic environment where job demands change rapidly, job analysis data can quickly become outdated and inaccurate. Obsolete job analysis information can hinder an organization's ability to adapt to change. Several approaches to job analysis may respond to the need for continuous change.

First, managers may adopt a future-oriented approach to job analysis. This "strategic" analysis of jobs requires managers to have a clear view of how duties and tasks can be restructured to meet organizational requirements in the future. One method to this approach is performed by researchers in one study. They asked experts on a particular job to identify aspects of the job, the organization, and the environment that might change in the next few years and how those changes might affect the nature of the job (Schneider and Konz 1989). The collected data were then used to describe the tasks, knowledge, skills, and abilities needed for doing the job in the future. By including future-oriented information in job descriptions, healthcare organizations can focus employee attention on new strategic directions. For example, one organization decided to change its strategic focus to increasing its "customer-consciousness" orientation (George 1990). Job descriptions were then amended to include tasks, knowledge, skills, and abilities related to customer contact and responsibilities. These new job descriptions focused more on what the organization wanted to be doing in the future.

Second, organizations may adopt a competency-based approach to job analysis that places emphasis on characteristics of successful performers rather than on standard job duties and tasks (Hunt 1996; Van Wart 2000). These competencies will match the organization's culture and strategy and will include such things as interpersonal communication skills, ability to work as part of a team, decision-making abilities, conflict resolution, adaptability, and self-motivation (Carson and Stewart 1996; Van Wart 2000). This technique enhances a culture of continuous improvement, as organizational improvement is a constant aim.

Both the first and second approaches to change-oriented job analysis have potential impracticalities, including the dependence on the ability of managers to accurately predict future job needs, the uncertainty that the analysis will comply with EEOC guidelines, and the ambiguity in job descriptions as a result of creating them based on estimates.

Third, conduct a generic job analysis. The traditional job analysis approach serves to constrain desired change and flexibility by compartmentalizing and specifically defining presumably static job characteristics. It impedes shifting decision making downward in the organization, cross-training employees, and getting employees involved in quality improvement efforts (Blayney 1992). Reducing the number of job titles and developing more generic job descriptions can provide needed flexibility to manage unanticipated change. For example, Nissan Motor Company has only one job description for hourly production employees. This description is generic and gives the organization the opportunity to use employees as needed. Cross-training and multiple job assignments are possible with this approach. However, employees may experience more conflict and ambiguity with generic job descriptions.

Undoubtedly, most jobs are getting bigger and more complex. The last item on a typical job description is often, "any other duty that may be assigned," and this is increasingly becoming *the* job description. This enlarged, flexible, complex job changes the way virtually every HR function is performed. For example, in recruitment and selection, individuals who possess the technical skills required to perform the job are not viewed as ideal candidates anymore. HR managers are also seeking for broader capabilities such as competencies, intelligence, adaptability, and an ability/willingness to work in teams.

The rapid pace of change in healthcare makes the need for accurate job analysis even more important now and in the future. Historically, job analysis was conducted and then set aside for a reasonable time. Today, however, job requirements are in such a constant state of flux that job descriptions and specifications must be constantly reviewed to keep them relevant. By one estimate, people may have to change their entire skill sets three or four times during their careers (Snyder 1996). If this projection is accurate, the need for accurate and timely job analysis is becoming even more important. Organizations that do not revise or review job descriptions and specifications may recruit new employees who do not possess the needed skills or may not provide necessary training to update employee skills.

Job Design

Job design is an outgrowth of job analysis and is a process of structuring jobs to help improve organizational efficiency and employee job satisfaction. The process involves changing, eliminating, modifying, and enriching duties and tasks to capture the talents of employees so that they can contribute to the fullest and develop professionally. Job design should simultaneously facilitate the achievement of organizational objectives and recognize the capabilities and needs of those who perform the job.

Job design encompasses the manner in which a given job is defined and how it will be conducted. This involves such decisions as will the job be handled by an individual or by a team of employees and such determination as how does the job fit into the overall organization. The organizing of tasks, duties, and responsibilities into a unit of work to achieve a certain objective requires a conscious effort. Each job design process must acknowledge any unique skills possessed by a number of employees of a given profession and must incorporate appropriate professional guidelines or task limitations. In healthcare, most professionals are constrained by which functions and tasks they may legally perform and under what type of supervision. For example, many technical functions require performance either by a physician or by another professional under the direct supervision of physicians. Such legal constraints obviously reduce the flexibility of healthcare executives in designing jobs.

Specialization in Healthcare

As a result of technological change, increased specialization, and the emergence of the hospital as the central focus of the healthcare system, there are approximately 700 different job categories in the healthcare industry. The most rapid growth in the supply of healthcare workforce has occurred in new categories: more than two-thirds of all healthcare employees work in nontraditional allied health or support service positions (U.S. Census Bureau 1998).

Researchers have concluded that specialization has inherent limitations and has been taken to extremes in healthcare (Fottler 1992). Because of the inherent disadvantages of specialization, new approaches to organizing work and job design are needed. The foremost criticism is that specialized workers may become bored and dissatisfied because their jobs may not offer enough challenge or stimulation. Boredom and monotony sets in and absenteeism rises, bringing in a possibility that the quality of work will suffer. To counter the problems of specialization and to enhance productivity and employee job satisfaction, healthcare executives have implemented a number of job-design and job-redesign options to achieve a better balance between organizational demands for efficiency and productivity and individual needs for creativity and autonomy. Four alternative redesign approaches are (1) job redesign (i.e., enlargement, enrichment, and rotation), (2) employee empowerment, (3) work-group redesign (e.g., employee involvement groups, employee teams), and (4) work-schedule redesign. Each of these approaches is explored below.

Job Redesign

Job enlargement involves changes in the scope of a job to provide greater variety to the employee. It is a horizontal expansion of duties with the same level of autonomy and responsibility. Alternatively, *job enrichment* adds additional autonomy and responsibility and is a vertical expansion of duties. One specific profession developed as a response to either job enlargement or job enrichment is the *multiskilled health practitioner* (MSHP). The MSHP is a "person cross-trained to provide more than one function, often in more than one discipline" (Vaughn et al. 1991). These combined functions can be found in a broad spectrum of healthcare-related jobs and ranges in complexity, from the nonprofessional to the professional level. The additional functions (skills) added to the original worker's job may be of a higher, lower, or parallel level.

Most theories of job enrichment stress that unless jobs are both horizontally and vertically enriched, little positive impact is made on motivation, productivity, and job satisfaction (Lawler 1986). Because the MSHP concept may involve horizontal, vertical, or both types of enrichment, whether it should be expected to enhance organizational outcomes is unclear. Research on the concept reveals that the outcomes have been positive in terms of enhanced productivity, job satisfaction, and patient satisfaction (Fottler 1996). However, those positive outcomes depend on many "contingencies" such as whether the "right" employees are chosen for the program (i.e., those with higher-order needs for personal growth), implementation processes, available training opportunities, legal constraints, and continuing top-management commitment.

Employee Empowerment

Various job enlargement/job enrichment approaches such as the MSHP are programs by which managers and supervisors formally change the job of employees. A less structured approach is to allow employees to initiate their own job changes through the concept of empowerment. Ann Howard of Development Dimensions International defines empowerment as "pushing down decision-making responsibility to those close to internal and external customers" (Simison 1999). To support empowerment, organizations must share information, knowledge, power to act, and rewards with the workforce. Empowerment encourages employees to become innovators and managers of their own work and gives them more control and autonomous decision-making capabilities (Ettore 1997).

Empowerment can involve employee control over the job content (i.e., functions and responsibilities), the job context (i.e., the environmental conditions under which the job is performed), or both (Ford and Fottler 1995). Most healthcare organizations are not ready for both and are advised to implement empowerment on an incremental basis. For empowerment to thrive and grow, organizations must encourage participation, innovation, access to information, accountability, and a culture that is open and receptive to change (Garcia 1997). Examples of organizations that have successfully implemented employee empowerment include Cigna Healthcare, the State of Illinois, Mesa (Arizona) Community College, and the State of Kentucky.

Work-Group Redesign

Table 6.1 outlines the six forms of work groups or teams currently being used in healthcare. Teams are groups of employees who assume a greater role in the service process. They provide a forum for employees to contribute to identifying and solving organizational problems. With work teams, managers accept the notion that the group is the logical work unit to resolve organizational problems and concerns.

Regardless of which team structure is employed, several team processes have been identified with successful teams. These include commitment to shared goals, motivated and energetic team members, consensus decision making, open and honest communication, shared leadership, a climate of trust and collaboration, valuing diversity, and acceptance of conflict and its positive resolution. A good team also requires that employee selection partially consider the potential employee's interpersonal skills and that extensive training for team members be provided (Bohlander and McCarthy 1996). The manager must also adapt to the role of the leader (rather than supervisor) and not be threatened by the growing power of the team.

Because many teams fail to operate at full potential, organizations must be aware of several obstacles to the effective functions of teams, including overly high expectations, inappropriate compensation, lack of training, and lack of power (Levy 2001). For example, new team members must be retrained to work outside their primary functional area, and compensation systems must be constructed to reward individuals for team achievements. New career paths to general management and/or higher clinical positions must be created from the team's experience. Finally, managers who feel threatened by the growing power of the team and reduced power of management may need further training or incentives to work with teams (Yandrick 2001). Complete training would enhance skills in team leadership, goal setting, conduct of meetings, team decision making, conflict resolution, effective communication, and diversity awareness (Bell and Smith 2003).

TABLE 6.1
Types of
Employee
Teams in
Healthcare

Type	Description
Cross-functional teams	A group staffed by a mix of specialists (i.e., nurses, physicians, and managers) and formed to accomplish a specific objective. Members usually are assigned rather than voluntary.
Project teams	A group formed specifically to design a new service. Members are assigned by management on the basis of their ability to contribute to success. The group normally dispatches after task completion.
Self-directed teams	Group of highly trained individuals who perform a set of interdependent job tasks within a natural work unit. Team members use consensus decision making to perform job duties, solve problems, or deal with internal or external customers.
Task force teams	A task force formed by management to resolve a major problem. The group is responsible for developing a long-term plan for problem resolution that may include a change for implementing the proposed solution.
Process improvement teams	A group made up of experienced employees from different departments or functions and charged with improving quality, decreasing waste, or enhancing productivity in processes that affect all departments. Team members are normally appointed by management.
Virtual teams	A group with any of the above purposes that uses advanced competitor and telecommunication technology to link geographically dispersed team members.

Work-Schedule Design

The goal of work-schedule design is to give employees greater control over their time. Various types of adjustments in work schedules alter the normal workweek of five eight-hour days in which everyone begins and ends their workday at the same time. Such adjustments are made to improve organizational productivity and morale by giving employees increased control over their work schedules.

Under the *compressed workweek*, the number of days in the workweek is shortened by lengthening the number of hours worked per day. The 4-day 40-hour week (4/40) is the most common form of compressed work-weeks, and the 3-day 39-hour week (3/39) schedule is less common. The compressed schedule accommodates the leisure-time activities and personal appointments of employees. Potential barriers to this schedule design are the stringent rules under the Fair Labor Standards Act that require the payment of overtime to nonsupervisory employees who work more than 40 hours a week. Long workdays may also increase the amount of exhaustion and stress for employees and managers.

Flextime, or flexible working hours, allows employees to choose daily starting and quitting times, provided they work a certain number of hours per day or week. There is typically a "core period" during the morning and afternoon when all employees on a given shift are required to be on the job. In healthcare, flextime is most common in clerical or management functions such as claims processing, health insurance, and human resources. By allowing employees greater flexibility in work scheduling, employers can reduce some of the most common causes of tardiness and absenteeism—that is, the time pressures of life. Employees can adjust their work schedules to accommodate their lifestyles, reduce pressure to meet a rigid schedule, and gain greater satisfaction. Employers can enhance their attractiveness when recruiting and retaining personnel while they improve customer service (poor service is a direct result of low levels of employee satisfaction). Productivity and quality may also be enhanced. However, flextime is not appropriate for patient care positions, because these functions must be staffed at all times, while communication and coordination are a continuing challenge in other positions.

Job sharing is an arrangement whereby two part-time employees share a job that otherwise is held by a full-time employee. Job sharers sometimes work three days a week to create an overlap day for face-to-face conferencing. Job sharing can be scheduled to conform to peaks in the daily or weekly workload. However, more time may be needed to orient, train, and develop two employees who share one role. The key to successful job sharing is good communication between partners through phone calls, e-mails, and voice mails. Among notable healthcare organizations that have developed a job-sharing program is HMO Kaiser Permanente in northern California. This program allows physicians to job share. Job sharing is best suited for employees who wish to work part time and older workers who wish to phase into retirement. Job sharing can reduce absenteeism because it allows employees to have time to accommodate their personal needs even when employed.

One of the most significant work-schedule innovations is telecommuting (Conklin 1999). *Telecommuting* is the system of performing work away from the office with the use of computers, networks, and fax machines. In 2000, an estimated 25 percent of the workforce were telecommuting either full time or part-time. The number of telecommuting employees increased from an estimated 19 million in 2000 to 31.5 million in 2002 (Garvey 2001). The most important reasons employers use telecommuting are to reduce costs (33 percent), improve productivity (16 percent), increase employee retention (16 percent), improve employee morale (15 percent), and improve customer service (11 percent) (Reilly 1997). It also reduces overhead costs by eliminating or reducing office space. The two most important advantages of telecommuting are increased flexibility for employees and the ability to attract workers who may not otherwise be available (Wells 2001).

Drawbacks of telecommuting include the potential loss of employee creativity because of lower levels of face-to-face interaction, the difficulty of developing appropriate performance standards and evaluation systems, and the challenge of formulating an appropriate technology system for telecommuting (Capowski 1998). Telecommuting may also negatively affect employee-supervisor relationships (Wells 2001). In addition, if some employees are denied the opportunity to work from home, they may pursue legal action and/or become dissatisfied employees. Telecommuting is obviously more appropriate for employers who are not engaged in direct patient care.

In sum, the healthcare industry can and does use all four work-schedule design approaches discussed here for positions that do not involve clinical care of patients. Positions that involve direct patient care must be staffed 24 hours a day, 7 days a week. A compressed workweek or job sharing are the most appropriate work-schedule adjustments for employees in such positions.

Summary

Job analysis is the collection of information relevant to the preparation of job description and job specifications. An overall written summary of the task requirements for a particular job is called a job description, and an overall written summary of the personal requirements an individual must possess to successfully perform the job is called a job specification. Job analysis information developed in the form of job descriptions and job specifications provides the basic foundation for all human resources management functions.

Some combination of available job analysis methods (i.e., observation, interviews, questionnaires, job performance, critical incidents) should be used because all have advantages and disadvantages. Key considerations regarding the choice of methods should be the fit between the method and the purpose, cost, practicality, and an overall judgment on the appropriateness of the methods for the situation in question. The primary purpose of conducting a job analysis should be described clearly to ensure that all relevant information is collected. In addition, time and cost constraints should be specified before choosing one or more of the available data-collection methods.

Healthcare executives should follow these steps when conducting a job analysis: (1) determine purpose, (2) identify jobs to be analyzed, (3) explain the process to employees, (4) collect job analysis information, (5) organize the information into job descriptions and job specifications, and (6) review and update the documents frequently. Job descriptions and job specifications, as derived from job analyses, must be done and their processes must be valid, accurate, and job related. Otherwise, the healthcare organization may face legal repercussions, particularly in the areas of employee selection, promotions, and compensation. The *Uniform Guidelines* and associated court cases provide standards to help executives avoid charges of discrimination when developing job analysis data. In today's rapidly changing healthcare environment, healthcare executives should consider the potential advantage of future-oriented job analyses when change is more predictable and generic job analyses when change is less predictable. Both are relatively new concepts that may have legal or practical limitations that must be considered before they are fully adopted.

Various new approaches to job design are required as healthcare organizations strive to overcome the effects of excessive specialization. Among the most significant of these are job redesign approaches such as the multiskilled health practitioners, employee empowerment, various team concepts, and work-schedule redesign.

References

Anthony, W. P., P. L. Perrewe, and K. M. Kacmar. 1993. *Strategic Human Resource Management*. Fort Worth, TX: Dryden Press.

Ash, R. A. 1988. "Job Analysis in the World of Work." In *The Job Analysis Handbook for Business*, edited by S. Grael, 3–23. New York: Wiley.

Bell, A. H., and D. M. Smith. 2003. *Learning Team Skills*. Upper Saddle River, NJ: Prentice-Hall.

Blayney, K. D. (ed.). 1992. *Healing Hands: Customizing Your Health Team for Institutional Survival*. Battle Creek, MI: W. K. Kellogg Foundation.

Bohlander, G. W., and K. M. McCarthy. 1996. "How to Get the Most from Team Training." *National Productivity Review* 20 (3): 25–35.

Capowski, G. 1998. "Telecommuting: The New Frontier." *HR Focus* 75 (4): 2.

Carson, K. P., and G. L. Stewart. 1996. "Job Analysis and the Sociotechnical Approach to Quality: A Critical Explanation." *Journal of Quality Management* 1 (1): 49–56.

Clifford, J. P. 1994. "Job Analysis: Why Do It and How Should It Be Done?" *Public Personnel Management* 23 (3): 321–40.

Conklin, M. 1999. "9 to 5 Isn't Working Anymore." *Business Week* (September 20): 94–98.

Equal Employment Opportunity Commission, Civil Service Commission, Department of Labor, and Department of Justice. 1978. *Uniform Guidelines for Employee Selection Procedures. Federal Register* 43 (166): 38290–315.

Equal Employment Opportunity Commission. 1992. *A Technical Assistance Manual on the Employment Provisions (Title 1) of the Americans with Disabilities Act.* Washington, DC: EEOC.

Ettore, B. 1997. "The Empowerment Gap: Hope vs. Reality." *HR Focus* 74 (7): 1–6.

Ford, R. L., and M. D. Fottler. 1995. "Empowerment: A Matter of Degree." *Academy of Management Executive* 4 (31): 21–29.

Fottler, M. D. 1992. "The Evolution of Health Manpower Utilization Pattern in Health Services and American Industry: Implications for Implementing the Multiskilled Concept." In *Healthy Hands: Customizing Your Health Team for Industrial Survival*, edited by K. D. Blayney, 1–23. Battle Creek, MI: W. K. Kellogg Foundation.

———. 1996. "The Role and Impact of Multiskilled Health Practitioners in the Health Services Industry." *Hospital & Health Services Administration* 41 (1): 55–75.

Garcia, J. 1997. "How's Your Organizational Commitment?" *HR Focus* 74 (1): 22–34.

Garvey, C. 2001. "Teleworking HR." *HR Magazine* 46 (8): 56–60.

George, W. 1990. "Internal Marketing and Organizational Behavior: A Partnership in Developing Customer-Conscious Employees at Every Level." *Journal of Business Research* 20 (1): 63–70.

Grant, P. C. 1988. "Why Job Descriptions Don't Work." *Personnel Journal* 67 (1): 53–59.

Hunt, S. T. 1996. "Generic Work Behavior: An Investigation into the Dimensions of Entry-level Hourly Job Performance." *Personnel Psychology* 49 (1): 51–83.

Johnson, C. 2001. "Refocusing Job Descriptions." *HR Magazine* 48 (8): 66–72.

Lawler, E. E. 1986. *High Involvement Management.* San Francisco: Jossey-Bass.

Leonard, S. 2000. "The Demise of the Job Description." *HR Magazine* 45 (1): 184.

Levy, P. F. 2001. "When Teams Go Wrong." *Harvard Business Review* 79 (3): 51–67.

Mathis, R. L., and J. H. Jackson. 1985. *Personnel/Human Resources Management.* St. Paul, MN: West Publishing.

Mitchell, K. E., G. M. Alliger, and R. Morfopoalos. 1997. "Toward an ADA-

Appropriate Job Analysis." *Human Resource Management Review* 7 (1):
5–26.

Nobile, R. J. 1991. "The Law of Performance Appraisals." *Personnel* 35 (1): 1.

Reilly, E. M. 1997. "Telecommuting: Putting Policy into Practice." *HR Focus*
74 (9): 5–6.

Schneider, B., and A. M. Konz. 1989. "Strategic Job Analysis." *Human
Resource Management* 28 (1): 51–63.

Simison, R. L. 1999. "Ford Rolls Out New Model of Corporate Culture." *Wall
Street Journal* (January 13): A-1.

Snyder, D. 1996. "The Revolution in the Workplace: What's Happening to Our
Jobs?" *Futurist* 30: 8.

Thompson, D. E., and T. A. Thompson. 1982. "Court Standards for Job
Analysis in Test Validation." *Personnel Psychology* 35: 865–74.

U.S. Census Bureau. 1998. *Statistical Abstract of the United States*. Washington,
DC: U.S. Government Printing Office.

Van Wart, M. 2000. "The Return to Simpler Strategies in Job Analysis." *Review
of Public Personnel Administration* 20 (3): 5–23.

Vaughan, D. G., M. D. Fottler, R. W. Bamberg, and K. D. Blayney. 1991.
"Utilization of Multiskilled Health Practitioners in U. S. Hospitals."
Hospital & Health Services Administration 36 (3): 397–419.

Wells, S. J. 2001. "Making Telecommuting Work." *HR Magazine* 46 (10):
34–45.

Yandrick, R. M. 2001. "A Team Effort." *HR Magazine* 46 (6): 136–41.

Discussion Questions

1. Why should healthcare executives conduct a job analysis? What pur-
    pose does it serve?
2. What are job descriptions and job specifications? What is their rela-
    tionship to job analysis? What will happen if a healthcare organiza-
    tion decides not to use any job descriptions at all?
3. Consider the position of the registered nurse in a large hospital.
    Which of the five methods of job analysis will you use to collect data
    on this position, and why?
4. Describe the steps involved in the job analysis process.
5. How can the existence of a high-quality job analysis make a particu-
    lar human resources function, such as employee selection, less
    legally vulnerable?
6. Are healthcare jobs static, or do they change over time? What may
    cause a job to change over time? What implications does this change
    have for job analysis?
7. Describe and discuss future-oriented job analysis and generic job
    analysis. How may each be used to help healthcare executives cope

with a rapidly changing and competitive environment? What are some potential pitfalls of each approach?

8. What are the advantages and disadvantages of using multiskilled health practitioners?

9. Access information on work teams at www.workteams.unt.edu. What types of work teams are most appropriate for achieving which objectives in the healthcare industry? Cite at least one successful team effort in healthcare.

10. Select one healthcare position with which you are familiar. What work schedule innovations make the most sense for this position? Why?

Experiential Exercises

Case 1   Assume that your professor required you to form a team with four of your fellow students and assigned you to make a 30-minute presentation to the entire class on this topic: The Future of Job Analysis in the Healthcare of Industry. The professor requires that all the work on this challenging project be done by the team; however, your group cannot have any face-to-face meetings.

Case Assignment

Your virtual team must come up with ways to deal with the following issues:

1. How will you organize the virtual team? Would you select a team leader? If so, based on what criteria?

2. On what bases would you select team members?

3. Without face-to-face encounters, how will you ensure that every member on the team does his or her assigned tasks so that a high-quality presentation is produced?

Case 2   Your professor divides the class into small groups of four or five members. Each group is asked to select one healthcare job (e.g., registered nurse, physical therapist, receptionist) with which the group members have some familiarity. Based solely on the group members' understanding of the selected job, outline the methods for conducting an analysis of the job. Draft a job description and a job specification that you believe represent the job. What future changes to the job do you think may affect your job description and job specification?

ST. VINCENT'S HOSPITAL
Birmingham, Alabama

JOB TITLE   Staff Nurse
DEPARTMENT   Nursing-Labor and Delivery

DATE   8/17192   JOB CODE   2339   FLSA STATUS   Nonexempt

DEPARTMENT APPROVAL:_____

PERSONNEL APPROVAL:_____

ADMINISTRATIVE APPROVAL:_____

JOB SUMMARY

Assesses, prescribes, delegates, coordinates, and evaluates the nursing care provided. Ensures provision of quality care for selected groups of patients through utilization of nursing process, established standards of care, and policies and procedures.

SUPERVISION

A. SUPERVISED BY: Unit Manager, indirectly by Charge Nurse

B. SUPERVISES: No one

C. LEADS/GUIDES: Unit Associates/Ancillary Associates in the delivery of direct patient care

JOB SPECIFICATIONS

A. EDUCATION
    — Required: Graduate of an accredited school of professional nursing
    — Desired:

B. EXPERIENCE
    — Required: None
    — Desired: Previous clinical experience

C. LICENSES, CERTIFICATIONS, AND/OR REGISTRATIONS: Current R.N. license in the State of Alabama; BCLS and certifications specific to areas of clinical specialty preferred.

D. EQUIPMENT/TOOLS/WORK AIDS: POA infusors, infusion pumps and other medical equipment, computer terminal and printer, facsimile machine, photocopier, and patient charts

E. SPECIALIZED KNOWLEDGE AND SKILLS: Ability to work with female patients of child-bearing age and new-born patients in all specialty and subspecialty categories, both urgent and nonurgent in nature.

APPENDIX A
An Example
of a
Combined Job
Description/
Job
Specification
Document

APPENDIX A
(continued)

F. PERSONAL TRAITS, QUALITIES, AND APTITUDES: Must be able to: 1) perform a variety of duties often changing from one task to another of a different nature without loss of efficiency or composure; 2) accept responsibility for the direction, control, and planning of an activity; 3) make evaluations and decisions based on measurable or verifiable criteria; 4) work independently; 5) recognize the rights and responsibilities of patient confidentiality; 6) convey empathy and compassion to those experiencing pain or grief; 7) relate to others in a manner that creates a sense of teamwork and cooperation; and 8) communicate effectively with people from every socioeconomic background.

G. WORKING CONDITIONS: Inside environment, protected from the weather but not necessarily temperature changes. Subject to frequent exposure to infection, contagious disease, combative patients, and potentially hazardous materials and equipment. Variable noise levels. Also subject to rapid pace, multiple stimuli, unpredictable environment, and critical situations.

H. PHYSICAL DEMANDS/TRAITS: Must be able to: 1) perceive the nature of sounds by the ear; 2) express or exchange ideas by means of the spoken word; 3) perceive characteristics of objects through the eyes; 4) extend arms and hands in any direction; 5) seize, hold, grasp, turn, or otherwise work with hands; 6) pick, pinch, or otherwise work with the fingers; 7) perceive such attributes of objects or materials as size, shape, temperature, or texture; and 8) stoop, kneel, crouch, and crawl. Must be able to lift 50 pounds maximum with frequent lifting, carrying, pushing, and pulling of objects weighing up to 25 pounds. Continuous walking and standing. Must be able to identify, match, and distinguish colors. Rare lifting of greater than 100 pounds.

JOB RESPONSIBILITIES AND PERFORMANCE STANDARDS

Assigned
Weight

10% 1. UTILIZES THE NURSING PROCESS (i.e., ASSESSMENT, PLANNING, IMPLEMENTATION, AND EVALUATION) IN THE PROVISION OF PATIENT CARE IN ACCORDANCE WITH THE STANDARDS OF CARE AND POLICIES AS WRITTEN

Assessment
— Admission assessment includes at least the following:
• Patient identification
• Current medical history
• Current obstetrical history
• Reason for admission
• Relevant physical, psychological, and sociological status
Allergies
Drug use

Disabilities Impairment
Surgical Consent Form Medical Consent Form
Pediatrician's Consent Form
— Assessments performed in accordance with the patient care standard, S-2-7010-VI:
• Admission physical assessment
• Affected system each shift
• Labor patients:
Maternal temperature q 4 hours Maternal pulse q 4 hours
Maternal blood pressure q 1 hour
Pitocin order
Vaginal exam prior to Pitocin
Epidural level of anesthesia hourly
FHR q 30 minutes during 1st stage
FHR q 15 minutes during 2nd stage
— Plan of care
• Conceptualized plan of care is developed for each patient:
Identify one nursing diagnosis pertinent to this patient's care.
Identify one nursing intervention related to this diagnosis.
Identify to whom this plan of care should be communicated.
• Nursing intervention(s) relative to the identified nursing diagnosis is documented.
• Written plan of care is initiated on patients whose stay in Labor and Delivery exceeds 24 hours (Exception: patients in labor).
• Plan of care mutually developed with patient and/or SO.
• Written plan of care updated in response to changes in patient care needs.
• Plan of care consistent with medical plan of care.
• All components of the written plan of care are included:
Date
Problem number
Nursing diagnosis
Nursing orders
Patient goal(s)
Projected resolution date
• Patient goals stated are:
Realistic
Measurable
• Patient's response to care given is documented.
• Changes in patient's condition are documented.
10% 2. DETERMINES CONDITION OF PATIENTS AND CLASSIFIES APPROPRIATELY

— Appropriate acuity level is determined based on care provided to the patient/So.

— All asterisk (*) items have narrative documentation.

APPENDIX A
(continued)

5%   3. DEMONSTRATES KNOWLEDGE OF DISCHARGE PLANNING REHABILITA-
TIVE MEASURES AND COMMUNITY RESOURCES BY MAKING APPRO-
PRIATE AND TIMELY REFERRALS

— Initial assessment of discharge needs is accomplished through a
complete patient/family history on admission.

5%   4. DEMONSTRATES KNOWLEDGE AND UNDERSTANDING OF TEACHING/
LEARNING PROCESS AND IMPLEMENTS PATIENT TEACHING TO MEET
LEARNING NEEDS OF PATIENT AND/OR SIGNIFICANT OTHERS

— Patient and/or significant other are involved in the identification
of learning needs for short-term teaching/counseling during labor.
— Patient teaching during labor is evidenced by anticipatory guidance
relative to all procedures and events.

5%   5. ASSUMES RESPONSIBILITY FOR ASSIGNING, DIRECTING, AND
PROVIDING CARE FOR GROUPS OF PATIENTS

— Demonstrates necessary skills and knowledge to make appropri-
ate assignments and considers the following factors when making
patient care assignments:
  — The patient's status
  — The environment in which nursing care is provided
  — The competence of the nursing staff members who are to pro-
  vide the care
  — The degree of supervision required by and available to the
  associates
  — The complexity of the assessment required by the patient
  — The type of technology employed in providing nursing care
  — Relevant infection control and safety issues
— Demonstrates the necessary skills and knowledge to provide care
for patients in accordance with the Nursing Department and unit
specific required skills and competencies
— Compassionately gives personal patient care to provide comfort
and well-being to the patient, acknowledging psychological needs
— Delegates aspects of care to other nursing staff members as
appropriate
— Appropriately documents and communicates pertinent observations and care provided

10% 6. ADMINISTERS MEDICATIONS, INTRAVASCULAR FLUIDS, AND TREAT-
MENTS IN ACCORDANCE WITH HOSPITAL STANDARDS AND FEDERAL
REGULATIONS

— Demonstrates or obtains knowledge of drugs and fluids to be
administered
— Accurately administers medications and intravascular fluids as
ordered and scheduled
— Accurately and completely documents administration and
patient's response to drugs and intravascular fluids

— Demonstrates ability and appropriate technical skills and procedures in accordance with physician's orders and nursing policies and procedures:
— Procedures and treatments performed in a timely manner
— Makes adequate preparation for performance of procedures and/or treatments
— Completes appropriate documentation

10% 7. MAINTAINS EFFECTIVE COMMUNICATION WITH SUPERVISORS, HOSPITAL ASSOCIATES, MEDICAL STAFF, PATIENTS, FAMILIES, AND VISITORS

— Enhances cohesiveness of unit staff group through effective interpersonal communication
— Communicates with all persons involved in a patient's care in a manner that facilitates timely meeting of stated goals
— Utilizes approved lines of authority and channels of communication in sharing concerns
— Actively participates in a minimum of four (4) interdepartmental meetings annually
— Interacts effectively with patients, families, and/or significant others
— Supports problem-solving approach to both unit and patient needs
— Follows through on problems that may compromise patient care by using the appropriate chain-of-command
— Gives a thorough concise change of shift report

5% 8. RESPONDS APPROPRIATELY TO ENVIRONMENTAL AND SAFETY HAZARDS AND FUNCTIONS EFFECTIVELY IN EMERGENCY SITUATIONS

— Recognizes, takes action, and reports unsafe acts or situations involving patients, visitors, or staff
— Responds promptly and appropriately to environmental and safety hazards
— Promptly removes unsafe equipment from patient care areas and notifies the appropriate department
— Functions promptly and effectively in codes, emergencies, or other stressful patient situations
— Identifies high-risk patients and monitors accordingly
— Complies with hospital and departmental policies and procedures concerning infection control
— Demonstrates correct and safe technique in the use of equipment according to specific product information and policy and procedure manuals
— Maintains a clean, neat, and safe environment for patients, visitors, and staff according to hospital and unit policies

5%   9. UTILIZES HOSPITAL SYSTEMS EFFECTIVELY TO ENSURE ECONOMICAL USE OF EQUIPMENT AND SUPPLIES
   — Effectively utilizes unit dose, classification, pneumatic tube, beepers, emergency checks, and services of other hospital departments
   — Demonstrates appropriate economical use of supplies and equipment
   — Ensures appropriate handling of charges
   — Accurately utilizes the computer system
   — Correctly initiates and discontinues daily charges when indicated
   — Ensures that supplies and equipment necessary for patient care are stored in an organized and efficient manner
   — Follows appropriate procedure for obtaining and returning or cleaning and/or disposing of equipment and supplies

5%   10. DEMONSTRATES THROUGH ACTIONS THE ACCEPTANCE OF LEGAL AND ETHICAL RESPONSIBILITIES OF THE PROFESSIONAL NURSE

   — Documents effectively, accurately, and in a timely manner, on the patient's medical record according to hospital and department standards and policies
   — Adheres to drug handling regulations
   — Exhibits knowledge of reportable incidents, appropriate documentation, and follow-up
   — Maintains current State R.N. license
   — Protects patients' rights to privacy and confidentiality
   — Demonstrates professional responsibility for nonprofessional group members
   — Accurately transcribes or verifies accuracy of physician orders

5%   11. ASSUMES RESPONSIBILITY FOR KEEPING SKILLS CURRENT AND KNOWLEDGE UPDATED THROUGH STAFF DEVELOPMENT AND CONTINUING EDUCATION PROGRAMS

   — Actively seeks learning experiences
   — Appropriately verbalizes learning needs
   — Attends a minimum of eight (8) hours or eight classes of relevant continuing education/staff development programs annually
   — Maintains current Educational Profile

10% 12. COMPLETES A VOLUME OF WORK THAT ENSURES OPTIMUM PRODUCTIVITY WHILE MAINTAINING QUALITY PATIENT CARE

   — Completes care of assigned patients in a timely manner

   — Assists other associates in completing their assignments in a timely manner. Supports cost-effective methods for improving patient care

- Willingly accepts adjustment of posted schedule to meet unit emergencies and patient care needs as requested
- Demonstrates an ongoing awareness of, and participation in, the Quality Review (QR) program
- Is alert to potential OR problems and actively participates in solving such problems. Responds with improved performance to results obtained from OR monitors. Does not incur excessive unscheduled overtime

5% 13. PARTICIPATES IN ASSIGNED COMMITTEES, CONFERENCES, PROJECTS, STAFF DEVELOPMENT PROGRAMS, AND STAFF MEETINGS

- Attends and actively contributes to assigned committees, projects, and so forth
- Assists immediate supervisor in the orientation and performance evaluation of associates
- Actively supports departmental projects
- Effectively implements approved departmental changes
- Adapts to changes in a positive, professional manner
- Attends staff meeting or reads and signs all minutes of staff meetings not attended

The associate is expected to perform this job in a manner consistent with the values, mission, and philosophy of St. Vincent's Hospital and the Daughters of Charity National Health System.

Reviewed/Revised By:

_____ Date_____

_____ Date_____

_____

_____

This job description is meant to be only a representative summary of the major duties and responsibilities performed by incumbents of this job. The incumbents may be requested to perform job-related tasks other than those stated in this description.

_____

Source: Reprinted with permission from St. Vincent's Hospital, Birmingham, Alabama.

RECRUITMENT, SELECTION, AND RETENTION

Bruce J. Fried, Ph.D.

Learning Objectives

After completing this chapter, the reader should be able to

- understand the major decisions involved in designing and implementing a recruitment effort,
- discuss the factors associated with an individual choosing to accept a job offer,
- describe the relationship of job requirements (as developed through job analyses, job descriptions, and job specifications) to other human resources management functions,
- design a recruitment effort for a particular job,
- address the advantages and disadvantages of internal and external recruitment,
- explain the concept of organizational fit and its relevance to recruitment and selection,
- discuss alternative selection tools and how they should be used in the selection process,
- define the concept of validity in the use of selection tools, and
- identify the most important factors related to turnover and retention and related to strategies that can improve retention.

Introduction

In this chapter, attention turns to the processes of recruitment, selection, and retention. We explore these three topics together because they are integrally related not only with each other but also with other human resources management (HRM) functions. For example, the development and stringency of criteria for selecting job applicants depend, to a large degree, on the success of the recruitment effort. An organization can be more selective when a relatively large supply of qualified applicants exists. Similarly, developing a recruitment plan for a particular position depends on the availability of an accurate, current, and comprehensive job description. If our concern is with retaining valued employees, then we may include in our selection process the criteria that increase the probability that employees will stay with the organization. As with all HRM functions, organizations must be cognizant of legal considerations when developing recruitment and selection procedures. Each of these functions must be addressed from both strategic and operational perspectives.

Recruitment and selection are key to employee retention. An important measure of the effectiveness of these functions is the extent to which the organization is able to attract committed employees who remain with the organization. Many factors affect retention, and as discussed later, recruitment and selection processes can have an impact on retention. Further, we know that employee retention is tied to the effectiveness of orientation and "on-boarding" procedures; therefore, we should focus on these practices in our efforts to improve retention.

These three functions are highly interdependent, but we address them separately and sequentially in this chapter. Related concepts discussed in this chapter include the following:

- Recruitment steps
- Internal and external recruitment
- Organizational fit, and its role in the selection process
- Reliability and validity of selection decisions
- Selection instruments, and the positive and negative aspects of each
- Types of selection interviews, and ways to make them valid and reliable
- Factors related to employee retention and turnover

Recruitment

The goal of recruitment is to generate a pool of qualified job applicants. Specifically, *recruitment* refers to the various processes an organization implements to attract qualified individuals on a timely basis and in sufficient numbers and to encourage them to apply for jobs in the organization. When we think of recruitment strategies, attention usually focuses on what the organization needs to do to recruit candidates. A number of decisions need to be made by the organization in developing recruitment strategies, including the following:

- Should the organization recruit and promote from within, or should it focus on recruiting external applicants?
- Should the organization consider alternative approaches to filling jobs with full-time employees, such as outsourcing, flexible staffing, and hiring contingent workers?
- Should the organization find applicants with precisely the right technical qualifications or applicants who best fit the culture of the organization but need training to improve their technical skills?

The success of recruitment is dependent on many factors, including the attractiveness of the organization, the community in which the organization is located, the work climate and culture of the organization, managerial and supervisory attitudes and behavior, and workload and other job-related considerations. Before we explore these aspects, first we should address recruitment from the perspective of potential employees. What factors influence an individual's decision to apply for and accept employment with a particular organization? If we consider applicants and employees as customers, then an understanding of their needs and expectations is central to the development and implementation of effective recruitment strategies.

Factors That Influence Job Choice

What do potential employees look for in a job? Once an individual is offered a position, how does that person make the decision to accept or reject the offer? People consider a number of factors related to the attractiveness of the position and the organization, and other factors are personal. Applicants consider their own competitiveness in the job market and whether alternative positions that provide better opportunities are available. They are also sensitive to the attitudes and behaviors of the recruiter, or whoever the first contact with the organization is. First impressions are very potent because the issue of "fitting in" with the organization is decided at this stage, and early negative first impressions may be difficult to reverse. Questions foremost in the applicants' mind are, "Is this the kind of place I can see myself spending 40 or more hours a week?" and "Will I fit in?" As discussed later, employers go through a similar process when making selection decisions, determining if the applicant will fit into the organizational culture and ways of working. Applicants are more likely to accept positions in organizations that share their values and style. Organizations engage in a "signaling" process, in which they send out messages about their values in an attempt to attract candidates with similar beliefs (Barber 1998). Consider, for example, the recruitment potential of the following mottoes:

- *The power to heal. A passion for care* (WakeMed Health & Hospitals 2005).
- *Every life deserves world class care* (The Cleveland Clinic 2005).

Consider the values statement of the world-renowned Mayo Clinic (2005) (spoken by Dr. Charles W. Mayo) in Rochester, Minnesota: "There are no inferior jobs in any organization. No matter what the assigned task, if it is done well and with dignity, it contributes to the function of everything around it and should be valued accordingly by all." Seeking to attract members of minority groups to its workforce, Kaiser Permanente (2005) devotes a substantial portion of its web-based recruitment efforts to promoting its National Diversity Program and its emphasis on culturally competent care.

With these examples in mind, we can see that people consider a variety of factors when choosing to accept employment with an organization. Considerable research has been done on job choice factors (Schwab, Rynes, and Aldag 1987); however, it is difficult to make a generalization about which factors are most important in employment decisions. The relative importance of these factors varies, depending on the individual, the job, and environmental factors such as the level of unemployment. The factors considered by a family physician to accept employment with a rural health center are quite different from the factors that drive a nurse's decision to accept employment with an urban teaching hospital. One's life stage may also affect the salience of these decision factors. Such personal factors make up *individual characteristics*.

Understanding these factors is important in developing recruitment strategies. A convenient way to think about the reasons for a job choice is to distinguish between vacancy characteristics and individual characteristics. *Vacancy characteristics* are those associated with the job, such as compensation, challenge and responsibility, advancement opportunities, job security, geographic location, and employee benefits; each of these factors are explained below.

The level of compensation and benefits is often considered, on face value, as a key element in an individual's decision to accept a position with an organization. For many positions in healthcare, we have seen the area of compensation further complicated by differential pay rates, hiring (or signing) bonuses, and relocation assistance. *Hot-skill premiums*, or temporary pay premiums added to base pay to account for temporary market escalations in pay (Heneman and Judge 2003, 588–89), have become particularly common in healthcare, although it is not uncommon for premiums to remain in place even after market pressures cease. The role of compensation, however, should not be overemphasized. Even a relatively generous level of compensation can be outweighed by the presence or absence of other important factors.

The amount of challenge and responsibility inherent in a particular job is frequently cited as an important job choice factor, and it is likely even more salient in healthcare organizations where individuals with professional training seek out positions that maximize use of their professional knowledge and skills. Similarly, applicants may seek out jobs with substantial advancement opportunities, which are likely to be particularly important choice determinants for professionally trained individuals and those in management roles (London and Stumpf 1982). Advancement opportunities in healthcare are traditionally difficult for clinically or technically trained individuals, because often in healthcare the only avenue to advancement is through promotion to supervisory or management responsibilities. For many clinicians, taking on these new responsibilities may lead to a feeling of loss of at least part of their professional identity. In healthcare (and other industries as well), dual career-path systems have been established to enable highly talented clinicians to "move up" while not forcing them to abandon their clinical interests and expertise. Such systems provide specialists who are interested in pursuing a technical career with alternative career paths while maintaining an adequate pool of talent in clinical and technical areas within the organization (Roth 1982).

Job security is clearly an important determinant of job choice. The current healthcare and general business environment is characterized by an unprecedented number of mergers and acquisitions, which lead to frequent downsizing and worker displacement. This phenomenon was once limited largely to blue-collar workers, but professionals and employees in middle and senior management are clearly at risk in the current environment. An illustrative manifestation of the importance of job security is evident in union organizing and collective bargaining. Not too long ago, compensation and benefits were the most highly valued issues in labor relations. Today, however, job security and restrictions on outsourcing have gained increasing importance in employees' decision to unionize (Caudron 1995). In fact, in many situations, unionized employees have made wage concessions in return for higher levels of job security (Henderson 1986).

Geographic location, along with other lifestyle concerns, is becoming increasingly important in job-choice decisions, especially for individuals in dual-income families, in which the employment of a spouse may be a significant determinant of the other partner's job acceptance. In healthcare, location is a particularly acute issue because organizations can establish business in less-than-desirable locales that are not attractive to applicants. The level and type of employee benefits continue to grow as an important determinant of job acceptance. Particularly in highly competitive industries, many companies have moved beyond traditional benefits, such as health insurance and vacation pay, into more innovative offers, including membership in country/health clubs, onsite day care, and financial counseling. SAS, Inc., in Cary, North Carolina, is known worldwide for its extensive and innovative benefits.

Table 7.1 exemplifies how individual job applicants assess the relative importance of different features of a job. Although the depiction in the table oversimplifies the job choice process, it illustrates how different individuals value different aspects of the job depending on personal preferences and life circumstances. The first column briefly describes each applicant. The second column states each applicant's minimum standards for job acceptance along four dimensions: pay, benefits, advancement opportunities, and travel requirements. These four dimensions are sometimes categorized as *noncompensatory standards*—that is, nothing about the job can compensate for any one of these factors being below the applicant's required standard. Thus, for Person 3, who does not like to travel, she will not take a job that requires substantial travel, regardless of anything else. Similarly, for Person 2, health insurance coverage is an absolute requirement for job acceptance. The third column showcases each of the three jobs according to the four noncompensatory standards.

This type of analysis is useful for applicants because it provides a way of narrowing down job choices. Assuming a job applicant is weighing in on several job possibilities that meet minimum requirements, she can engage in a more refined job-choice process that allows for compensatory relationships among other job factors (Barber et al. 1994). Using less important job-choice factors, an individual can trade-off one job dimension for another.

The Recruitment Process

The recruitment process uses the organization's HR plan as a foundation. An HR plan includes specific information about the organization's strategies, the types of individuals required to achieve organizational goals, the recruitment and hiring approaches, and a clear statement of how HR practices support organizational goals.

Those involved in recruitment and selection must have a thorough understanding of the position that needs to be filled. This clear knowledge makes the recruitment process easier. The recruitment process begins with a job analysis, which addresses the following questions, at a minimum: What are the tasks required for the job? What skills and knowledge are required? What qualifications are required of job applicants?

The process then assesses information about past recruitment efforts for this and similar positions: Is this a job that will require an international

TABLE 7.1
Three
Hypothetical
Job Applicants

Job Applicant	Minimum Standards for Job Acceptance	Job Description
Person 1: 23 years old, single	*Pay:* at least $40,000 *Benefits:* Health insurance coverage of at least 25 percent *Advancement opportunities:* Very important *Travel requirements:* Unimportant	*Job:* Insurance company provider relations coordinator *Pay:* $45,000 *Benefits:* Health insurance covered at 50 percent *Advancement opportunities:* Recruitment done internally and externally *Travel requirements:* Average 25 percent travel
Person 2: Sole wage earner for large family	*Pay:* at least $50,000 *Benefits:* Health insurance coverage of at least 50 percent *Advancement opportunities:* Very important *Travel requirements:* Cannot travel more than 25 percent of the time	*Job:* Healthcare consultant *Pay:* $55,000 *Benefits:* Health insurance covered at 50 percent *Advancement opportunities:* Strong history of promotions within one year *Travel requirements:* Average 50 percent travel
Person 3: Spouse of high-wage earner	*Pay:* at least $35,000 *Benefits:* Unimportant *Advancement opportunities:* Unimportant *Travel requirements:* Cannot travel more than one week per year	*Job:* Research assistant in academic medical center *Pay:* $37,000 *Benefits:* Health insurance covered at 50 percent *Advancement opportunities:* Generally hires externally for higher-level positions *Travel requirements:* Little or none

search, or will the applicants in the local labor market suffice? Optimally, an HR information system (HRIS) will provide useful information in the recruitment process. While the sophistication of an HRIS varies from organization to organization, many such systems include some or all of the information described in Table 7.2.

A *skills inventory* database maintains information on every employee's skills, educational background, work history, and other important job-related factors. This inventory can be very useful in identifying internal employees who have attributes needed for a particular job. To be effective, however, skills inventories need to be kept current, which is often not a high-priority task for organizations. In contrast, an *upgraded skills inventory* database maintains current information on employees, such as latest skills acquired or recent seminar attended; this inventory may also include data on applicants for positions who were not hired. This database provides a broader base of possible applicants from which to draw (Heneman and Judge 2003).

Recruitment, and subsequent hiring, can be a very costly process, and information on this cost is essential. Table 7.3 illustrates the variety of measures that may be used to assess the effectiveness and efficiency of the recruitment process. Each of these factors varies depending on the job, but overall it is important to use cost-effective recruitment methods. Again, a good HRIS and cost accounting system can help the organization to understand the major costs associated with recruitment and selection.

The early stages of the recruitment process involve an examination of the external environment, in particular the supply of potential job applicants and the relative competitiveness for a certain position. This analysis should also look into the compensation and benefits given to individuals who hold similar jobs in competing organizations. It may also entail an evaluation of external recruitment sources, such as colleges, other organizations, and professional associations, to determine if these were successful avenues. Other aspects to consider in this assessment are the logistics and timing for hiring a particular professional group or groups. For example, certain positions may be easier to recruit for at particular times of year.

Internal and External Recruitment

An initial question in the recruitment process is whether one should recruit from within the organization through promotion or transfer or seek applicants from outside the organization. Table 7.4 provides a summary of the advantages and disadvantages of internal and external recruitment. On the positive side of internal recruitment, candidates are generally already known—the organization is familiar with their past performance and future potential and is aware of what to expect from them. Internal candidates

HRIS Data	Uses in Recruitment
Skills and knowledge inventory	Identifies potential internal job candidates
Previous applicants	Identifies potential external job candidates
Recruitment source information • Yield ratios • Cost • Cost per applicant • Cost per hire	Helps in the analysis of cost effectiveness of recruitment sources
Employee performance and retention information	Provides information on the success of recruitment sources used in the past

TABLE 7.2

Human Resources Information System Recruitment Data

also tend to know the specific processes and procedures of the organization and may not require as much training and start-up time. Internal recruitment also encourages highly valued and ambitious employees to stay with the organization because of the possibility of promotion. This also provides employees with a sense of job security because it sends a message to employees that the organization looks to them first before venturing out to fill a position.

On the negative side of internal recruitment, however, is the manifestation of the *Peter Principle*, which suggests that people are typically promoted one position above their level of competence (Peter and Hull 1969) regardless of their aptitude for the new position. This is a particular problem in healthcare, where individuals with clinical skills are frequently promoted into supervisory and management roles without the requisite skills and training. Internal recruitment may at times create a ripple effect in an organization: one individual moves into a different position and leaves a vacancy, and this vacancy has to be filled by someone else in the organization, and so forth.

An advantage to external recruiting is that the candidate may bring new ideas into the organization. In addition, the organization may be able to more specifically target the skills it is looking for rather than settle for an internal candidate who may know the organization but lack specific job-related skills and knowledge. External candidates are also easier to bring into difficult political environments, as they have no dysfunctional alliances and conflict with existing employees. An external candidate typically is unencumbered by these political problems.

Traditional selection processes are based on matching the individual with the job. Research and practice reveal that a match between the person and the organization is important for individual performance and

TABLE 7.3
Measures of
Recruitment
Effectiveness
and Efficiency

Type of Cost	Expenses
Cost per hire	• Advertising, agency fees, employee referral bonuses, recruitment fairs and travel, and sign-on bonuses • Staff time: salary; benefits; and overhead costs for employees to review applications, set up interviews, conduct interviews, check references, and make and confirm an offer • Processing costs: opening a new file, medical examination, drug screening, and credential checking • Travel and lodging for applicants, relocation costs • Orientation and training
Application rate	• Ratio-referral factor: number of candidates to number of openings • Applicants per posting • Qualified applicants per posting • Protected class applicants per posting • Number of internal candidates, number of qualified internal candidates • Number of external candidates, number of qualified external candidates *The measures above can be calculated for all referral sources or by individual referral source.*
Time to hire	• Time between job requisition and first interview • Time between job requisition and offer • Time between job offer and offer acceptance • Time between job requisition and starting work
Recruitment source effectiveness	• Offers by recruitment source • Hires by recruitment source • Employee performance (using performance evaluation information and promotion rates) • Employee retention by recruitment source • Offer acceptance rate (overall and by recruitment source)
Recruiter effectiveness	• Response time, time to fill, cost per hire, acceptance rate, employee performance, and retention
Miscellaneous	• Materials and other special or unplanned expenses, new employee orientation, reference checking, and drug screening

Source: Adapted from Fitz-enz, J., and B. Davison. 2002. *How to Measure Human Resources Management.* New York: McGraw-Hill.

Advantages	Disadvantages
Recruiting Internal Candidates	
• May improve employee morale, and encourage valued employees to stay with the organization	• Possible morale problems among those not selected
• Permits greater assessment of applicant abilities; candidate is a known entity	• May lead to inbreeding
	• May lead to conflict among internal job applicants
• May be faster, and may involve lower cost for certain jobs	• May require strong training and management development activities
• Good motivator for employee performance	• May manifest the Peter Principle
• Applicants have a good understanding of the organization	• May cause ripple effect in vacancies, which need to be filled
• May reinforce employees' sense of job security	
Recruiting External Candidates	
• Brings new ideas into the organization	• May identify candidate who has technical skills but does not fit the culture of the organization
• May be less expensive than training internal candidates	
• External candidates come without dysfunctional relationships with others and without being involved in organizational politics	• May cause morale problems for internal candidates who were not selected
	• May require longer adjustment and socialization
• May bring new ideas to the organization	• Uncertainty about candidate skills and abilities, and difficulty obtaining reliable information about applicant

TABLE 7.4
Advantages and Disadvantages of Internal and External Recruitment

retention (Kristoff-Brown 2000). In the past, the question of fit often had a negative discriminatory connotation. For example, at one time (and perhaps even today) some recruiters believed that a woman in a management role is not a good fit because she would be out of place in a male-dominated corporate culture. However, organizational fit refers to the alignment between an applicant's values and those of the organization, which is an important ingredient in the employee-organization relationship. Fit between the applicant and the culture of the organization affects not only the willingness of the employer to make a job offer but also the willingness of the applicant to accept a job with the organization (Bretz and Judge 1994). Measuring potential fit is a challenge, but organizations should pay more attention to hiring individuals who fit the characteristics of the organization, not just the requirements of the job (Bowen, Ledford, and Nathan 1991). Generally, organizations know more about the potential fit of internal candidates than the potential fit of external candidates. Considering an applicant's fit is critical when the organization is trying to change its culture. In this instance, the organization may seek change-oriented candidates who do not fit the current dysfunctional organizational culture.

More often, however, organizations use fit to select people with attitudes that match the mission of the organization. For example, Women & Infants Hospital of Rhode Island made an explicit effort to select employees on the basis of their fit with the culture, believing that a "person must be qualified to do the job, but they also require the right personality." After starting a hiring program using behavior-based interviews and in-depth analysis of candidates, the hospital saw patient satisfaction rise from the 71st percentile to the 89th percentile nationally, while its turnover was reduced to 8.5 percent. Labor disputes also decreased, while productivity increased (Greengard 2003).

The choice between seeking internal or external candidates is not often clear, and it is not at all unusual for organizations to pursue simultaneously both internal and external candidates.

Internal and External Recruitment Sources

As a general rule, it is a good idea to obtain as many qualified job applicants as possible in a particular recruiting effort. From the organization's perspective, a large number of applicants permits choice and sometimes may even stimulate a rethinking of the design of the job, such as when applicants appear who have additional skill sets that are useful to the organization; successful organizations are flexible enough to take advantage of these opportunities. Note also that it is important to design recruitment efforts in such a way that they yield job applicants who have at least the minimum job qualifications. Processing unqualified applicants can be expensive as well as a waste of time for both the organization and the candidate.

The most common sources of internal candidate are as follows:

- *Current employees.* Many organizations have a policy of informing current employees about job openings. *Job posting* is such a notification system. Internal job postings may increase morale, motivation, and retention by highlighting the career ladders possible for current employees. A skills inventory of current employees may help the organization to identify internal candidates. Current employees typically move into new positions through either a promotion or transfer. In some organizations and for certain positions, internal job posting is done prior to initiating external recruitment efforts.

- *Employee referrals.* Many organizations rely on current employees to refer other individuals to work for the organization. The value of this approach is that current employees, who tend to have a good understanding of organizational needs and culture, act as the initial screen for applicants. Employee referral can be a powerful recruitment strategy, yielding employees who typically stay with the organization longer and who exhibit higher levels of loyalty and job satisfaction than employees recruited through other mechanisms (Rynes 1991; Taylor 1994). Interestingly, an increasing number of organizations are using web-based systems to encourage employee referrals for internal as well as external recruitment (Calandra 2001).
- *Former employees.* Employees who are no longer with the organization are sometimes an excellent source of job applicants or even can be applicants themselves. Employees may have left for a number of reasons, including other employment opportunities, organizational downsizing and restructuring, relocation, and personal factors. Sometimes such employees may seek or be available for reemployment with the organization. As with current employees, their capabilities and potential are well known to the organization.
- *Former applicants.* An organization can identify candidates from its database of previous job applicants. These individuals may already be employees of other organizations or may still be seeking employment.
- *Skills inventory.* An updated and user-friendly skills inventory is a useful resource. As noted earlier, these systems must be managed and updated to ensure that knowledge and skills sets for employees are current.
- *In-house temporary pools.* Temporary pools are typically used to provide a ready source of employees. Because individuals in these pools are already known in and by the organization, evaluation of these persons for permanent positions is easier.

External recruitment tends to be more costly than internal recruitment because of costs associated with advertising, applicant travel, and commissions paid to employment agencies. The particular recruitment sources listed below are highly dependent on the job that is being filled.

- *Professional and trade associations.* Use of national, regional, and state professional associations is particularly common in healthcare organizations. Recruitment of this type is often done through academic and trade journals and at professional meetings.
- *Employment agencies and executive search firms.* These include both state-sponsored as well as private employment agencies and executive search firms. Private agencies specialize in different types of searches and work either on a commission or on a flat-fee basis.
- *Media.* This is a very common recruitment source and involves a range of newspapers, magazines, television, radio, billboards, and the Internet. Because of the wide circulation possible through use of the media, targeting the advertisement to the appropriate media outlet and specificity in advertisement are particularly important.
- *High schools, colleges, and universities.* Recruitment through educational institutions is common for virtually all levels of work.
- *Competitor organizations.* In many instances, the right candidate for a job may be found in a competing organization. In an era when commitment to one's current organization is on the decline, "raiding" other organizations is not at all unusual.

Content of the Recruiting Message

An important objective of recruitment is to maximize the possibility that the right candidate will select the organization after a job offer has been made. What are the appropriate messages to include in recruitment messages? At its core, four types of information should be made available to applicants:

1. *Applicant qualifications:* education, experience, required credentials, and any other preferences that the employer has within legal constraints
2. *Job basics:* title, responsibilities, pay, benefits, location of the job, and other pertinent working conditions (e.g., night work, travel, promotion potential)
3. *Application process:* deadlines, inclusion of resumes, cover letters, transcripts, application, references, and where and to whom applications should be submitted
4. *Organization and department basics:* name and type of organization, an equal-employer statement, and other relevant information

Realistic Recruitment Message and Realistic Job Preview

An innovative tool for recruitment is the use of a *realistic recruitment message*—a direct statement to the applicant that includes facts about the organization and the job rather than a public relations pitch that the employer thinks the applicant wishes to hear (Heneman and Judge 2003). So far, there is limited research on the effectiveness of this technique.

There is considerable research on the effectiveness of the realistic job preview, however. The goal of a *realistic job preview* is to present practical information about job requirements, organizational expectations, and the actual work environment. This preview includes negative as well as positive information about the job and the organization, and it may be presented to new hires before they start work. The use of realistic job previews is related to higher performance and lower attrition from the recruitment process, lower initial expectations, lower voluntary turnover, and lower turnover overall (Phillips 1998). A realistic job preview can be presented in a number of ways: verbally, in writing, or through media (Wanous 1992). Certainly the most straightforward approach is for the prospective or new employee to hold frank discussions with coworkers and supervisors. In addition, the new employee may observe the work setting and perhaps shadow an employee who is doing a similar job.

Regardless of the approach used, preventing surprises and providing the employee with an honest assessment of the job and work environment are key.

Evaluating the Recruitment Function

Assessing the effectiveness of recruitment efforts is critical. Such an evaluation process is dependent on the existence of reliable and comprehensive data on applicants, the quality of applicants, the applicants' disposition, and recruitment costs. Common measures of the success of a recruitment process include the following:

- *Quantity of applicants.* The proper use of recruitment methods and sources should yield a substantial number of candidates (depending on the market supply) who meet at least minimum job requirements. Having a big pool of potential employees allows the organization a better chance at coming up with the most qualified people.
- *Diverse mix of applicants.* Assuming one of the goals of a recruitment program is to identify and hire qualified candidates who represent the diversity of the population, the organization can consider its recruitment goal met if it can show that candidates from diverse

cultural and demographic backgrounds have been considered for and/or are holding positions for which they are qualified.

• *Quality of applicants.* A recruitment effort should bring in employees who have the appropriate education, qualifications, skills, and attitudes.

• *Overall recruitment cost and cost per applicant.* A recruitment effort's costs are often unacceptable to the organization. In addition to looking at overall costs per applicant, the costs associated with the recruiting methods and sources used should also be examined. This analysis provides the opportunity to examine the cost effectiveness of alternative recruitment methods. The financial impact of using part-time or temporary help while looking for the right applicant should also be considered as these costs are likely substantial.

• *Recruitment time.* The more time spent on proper recruitment, the greater the chance that the ideal candidate will emerge. However, a lengthy recruitment process also results in greater costs, disruption of service or work, and potential dissatisfaction of current staff who end up filling in for the missing jobholder.

Selection

Employee selection is the process of collecting and evaluating information about job applicants to allow the employer to extend an employment offer. The selection process is to a great extent a matter of predicting which person, among a set of applicants, is likely to achieve success in the job being filled. Of course, the definition of success is not always straightforward. Job performance may be defined in terms of technical proficiency, but the goals of a selection process may also include longevity in the position or fit with the culture and goals of the organization. Thus, evaluating the effectiveness of selection processes may include not only the time taken to fill the position but also the hired individual's performance, length of service in the organization, and other factors.

It is important to distinguish selection from simple hiring (Gatewood and Feild 1998). In selection, a careful analysis is performed of an applicant's knowledge, skills, and abilities (KSAs) as well as attitudes and other relevant factors. The applicant who scores highest on these factors is then extended an offer of employment. Sometimes, however, offers are made with little or no systematic collection and analysis of job-related information. A common example is hiring an individual based on political considerations or on the applicant's relationship with owners or managers in the organization (e.g., family). In such instances, these non-job-related factors take precedence over objective measures of job suitability. In circumstances where a position has to be filled in a short period of time, or when there are labor shortages in a particular area, an organization may simply hire whoever is available, assuming the individual possesses the minimum level of qualifications. This is a frequent occurrence in staffing health centers in remote or otherwise undesirable locations. Applicant availability, rather than the comparative competence of the applicant, is key in such situations.

Job Requirements and Selection Tools

If the goal of selection is to identify among a group of applicants the person to whom a job offer should be made, then the organization needs to use tools to evaluate each applicant's KSAs. *Selection tools* refer to any procedures or systems used to obtain job-related information or KSAs on job applicants. A great many selection tools are available, including the job application form, standardized tests, personal interviews, simulations, and references. However, having a clear understanding of job requirements should come before choosing selection tools. While this may seem obvious, it is not uncommon for a selection process to move forward without adequate information about job requirements.

The design and utilization of selection tools should be based on the knowledge of the technical and qualification requirements of the job, such as education, credentials, and experience. The informal and less technical aspects of job performance, such as the jobholder's interpersonal skills, attitude, judgment, values, fit, ability to work in teams, and management abilities, should also be specified first. Without this determination, an organization may hire someone who has the technical skills but lacks the ability to perform effectively. The job requirements in essence direct the design of selection tools, allowing the tools to properly assess the applicants' KSAs related to the requirements.

Among the most common methods for understanding job requirements are as follows:

* Conducting a job analysis
* Seeking out the views of individuals currently in the position or in similar positions
* Obtaining the perspectives of supervisors and coworkers
* Conducting a critical incidents analysis

A *critical incidents analysis* is very useful for discovering the hidden or less formal aspects of job performance. This process is designed to generate a list of good and poor examples of job performance by current or potential jobholders. Once these examples of behaviors are collected, they are grouped into job dimensions. Measures are then developed for each of these job dimensions. This approach involves the following steps:

1. *Identify job experts, and select methods for collecting critical incidents.* Incidents can be obtained from the job incumbent, coworkers, subordinates, customers, and supervisors. Collection of critical incidents can be done in a group setting, with individual interviews, or through administration of a questionnaire. Note that different job experts may view the job differently and hence may identify different aspects of job performance. This in fact is the strength of this method.
2. *Generate critical incidents.* Job experts should be asked to reflect on the job and identify examples of good and poor performance. According to Bowns and Bernardin (1998), each critical incident should be structured such that
    *   it is specific and pertains to a specific behavior;
    *   it focuses on observable behaviors that have been, or can be, exhibited on the job;
    *   it briefly describes the context in which the behavior occurred; and
    *   it indicates the positive or negative consequences of the behavior.
3. *Define job dimensions.* Job dimensions are defined by analyzing the critical incidents and extracting common themes that arise.

Table 7.5 provides examples of three critical incidents and the job dimensions in which each incident is grouped. This exercise yields a thorough understanding of the job's technical requirements, formal qualifications (e.g., training, credentials), and the informal but critical aspects of successful job performance. Not only does a critical incidents analysis provide a solid foundation for selection, it also provides strong protection against charges of unfair hiring practices as it specifically identifies aspects of the job related to performance.

Reliability and Validity of Selection Tools

As noted earlier, selection tools comprise any method used to assess job applicants' KSAs along job requirements and qualifications. At the most fundamental level, selection tools should elicit information that is predictive of job performance. Applicants who "score" better on selection instruments should exhibit higher levels of job performance than individuals who score at lower levels. To be useful, selection tools should be both reliable and valid.

Reliability is defined as the degree of dependability, consistency, or stability of the measure used. A reliable selection procedure is one that

TABLE 7.5
Critical
Incidents
Approach to
Understanding
Job
Requirements

Job	Critical Incident	Job Dimensions
Physician, Public Health Department	In an administrative staff meeting to review plans for the coming year, this physician exhibited strongly condescending and rude behaviors toward other team members.	• Ability to work in teams • Respect for other professionals
Nurse, Emergency Room	After a school bus accident, the emergency department was overwhelmed with children and frightened parents. This nurse effectively and appropriately managed communication with parents and successfully obtained further assistance from elsewhere in the hospital.	• Creativity and resourcefulness • Leadership • Ability to work effectively under crisis conditions • Strong interpersonal skills
Medical director, local Public Health Department	The local media reported an outbreak of salmonella that resulted in one child being hospitalized with the effects of this serious condition. The outbreak was traced to a fast-food restaurant that was inspected by health department personnel less than one week ago. The health department was blamed for not preventing the outbreak. This medical director conducted a thorough internal investigation and found that this was an isolated incident caused by mishandling of food on a single occasion. She communicated effectively at a press conference, defending the health department and assuring the public of the safety of local eating establishments.	• Effective crisis manager • Strong communication and media skills • Strong sense of public accountability

yields the same findings regardless of who administers the tool and the context (e.g., time of day, version of the tool) in which the tool is used. Consider the employment interview, a notoriously unreliable selection tool. A job applicant may be evaluated very differently by different interviewers. One interviewer may be particularly struck by an applicant's impressive management skills, which may be unrelated to job performance. Similarly, if an interviewer has just interviewed several strong candidates, he or she may find an applicant who seems soft spoken mediocre by comparison; the reverse may also hold. Time pressures may also constrain an interviewer's ability to obtain information from an applicant. The reliability of interviews can be increased with, for example, the use of multiple interviewers.

A word processing test is among the more reliable selection tools. Assuming the same computer and word processing program is used, and the physical environment of the test is roughly the same, it is likely that an individual's score will not vary significantly between different administrations of the test. In general, physical and observable traits and skills, such as height and weight, ability to lift a given weight, and ability to compute manually, are more reliably measured than psychological or behavioral traits. Table 7.6 provides an interesting perspective on the relative reliability of measuring different human attributes.

Validity of selection tools refers to the extent to which a selection tool actually corresponds to job performance—that is, does a particular predictor of future job performance actually foretell the quality of performance? Three types of validity are commonly considered with selection tools: criterion-related validity, content validity, and construct validity.

Criterion-related validity is the extent to which a selection tool is associated with job performance, and this validity can be demonstrated through two strategies. First is concurrent validity, whereby a selection tool is administered to a current group of employees. These employees' scores are then correlated with actual job performance. For the selection tool to be deemed valid, there needs to be a correlation between scores on the selection tool and actual job performance. Second is *predictive validity*, whereby the selection tool is administered to a group of job applicants. Because the selection tool has not yet been validated, actual selection decisions are made on the basis of other measures and criteria. Over time, data are obtained on actual job performance, and the two sets of scores—those from the selection tool under study and those from actual performance measures—are correlated and examined for possible relationships.

Content validity is the extent to which a selection tool representatively samples the content of the job for which the measure will be used. Using this strategy, if a selection tool includes a sufficient amount of actual job-related content, it is considered valid. Expert judgment, rather than

TABLE 7.6
Relative
Reliability of
Human
Attributes

Level of Reliability	Human Attributes
High	*Personal*
	Height
	Weight
	Vision
	Hearing
Medium	*Attitudes and Skills*
	Dexterity
	Mathematical skills
	Verbal ability
	Intelligence
	Clerical skills
	Mechanical skills
Medium to low	*Interests*
	Economic
	Scientific
	Mechanical
	Cultural
Low	*Personality*
	Sociability
	Dominance
	Cooperativeness
	Tolerance

Sources: Adapted from Albright, L. E., J. R. Glennon, and W. J. Smith. 1963. *The Use of Psychological Tests in Industry.* Cleveland, OH: Howard Allen; Gatewood, R. D., and H. S. Feild. 1998. *Human Resource Selection, 4th Edition.* Fort Worth, TX: Dryden.

statistical analysis, is typically used to assess content validity. One may look to content validity in designing a knowledge-based selection tool for laboratory technicians. An exercise that requires applicants to describe procedures associated with the most common laboratory tests is likely to be judged to have content validity.

Construct validity refers to the extent to which a selection tool actually measures the construct it is intended to measure. Assume that a selection committee has determined that a particular job requires the employee to exhibit strong time-management skills. The selection committee has designed a simulation exercise that is expected to assess this construct of time management. To determine if this selection tool actually predicts an individual's time-management skills, the exercise may be evaluated on the basis of a criterion-related validation study between the time-management simulation and actual measures of the individual's time-management skills exhibited on the job. Construct validity studies are most useful for determining whether selection tools actually measure the constructs they are expected to measure.

Most organizations employ a range of selection tools but pay little or no attention to issues of reliability and validity. In the section below, we examine the reliability and validity of some of the more common selection tools.

Reference Checks

A study of about 700 HR directors reveals that 87 percent of them used reference checks, 69 percent conducted background employment checks, 61 percent checked criminal records, 56 percent checked driving records, and 35 percent did credit checks (BNA 2001). Few studies, however, assess the reliability of using reference checks to gauge performance in previous jobs. In those studies that have been conducted, researchers have sought to determine the level of agreement (interrater reliability) between different individuals who provide a reference for the same prospective employee. Reliability estimates are typically poor, at a level of .40 or less. This may be explained by a number of factors, including the reluctance of many referees to provide negative feedback and the real possibility that different raters may be evaluating different aspects of job performance. Studies of the validity of reference checks have found that this tool has low-to-moderate predictive validity (Hunter and Hunter 1984). Several explanations have been suggested for the poor predictive power of reference checks:

- Many measures used in reference checks have low reliability; where reliability is low, validity must be low as well.
- Individuals who provide references frequently only use a restricted range of scores—typically in the high range—in evaluating job applicants. If virtually all reference checks are positive, they are still unlikely predictors of performance success for all individuals.
- In many instances, job applicants preselect the individuals who will provide the reference, and applicants are highly likely to select only those who will provide a positive reference.

How can the validity of reference checks be improved? Research in this area concludes the following (Gatewood and Feild 1998):

- The most recent employer tends to provide the most accurate evaluation of an individual's work.
- Prediction improves when the reference giver has had adequate time to observe the applicant and when the applicant is the same gender, ethnicity, and nationality as the reference giver.
- The old and new jobs are similar in content.

Reference checks have an intuitive appeal and are well institutional-ized in virtually all selection processes. The usefulness of references, how-ever, is decreasing as many organizations advise their employees to provide only skeletal information on former employees, such as job title and dates of employment. This is being done to reduce the liability of the referring organization to lawsuits from both the hiring organization (through charges of negligent hiring) and the prospective employee (through claims of defama-tion of character). Figure 7.1 provides some basic guidelines for the appro-priate use of references.

The job interview is used for virtually all positions largely because those involved in hiring simply wish to find out more about applicants than can be obtained from the application, references, and other documen-tation. The result of the interview is often given the greatest weight in hiring decisions. Job interviews, however, typically have low reliability and validity, are often unfair to applicants, and may be at least partially illegal. They are not reliable in that the questions vary from interviewer to interviewer, and two applicants vying for the same position are some-times asked different questions. Similarly, the manner in which answers to interview questions are interpreted and scored by interviewers may vary substantially as well.

Interviews

Validity of the job interview—that is, does a positive interview actu-ally predict job success?—has also been questioned. Questions asked in an interview are often not planned in advance and may bear little relationship with future job success. This factor makes interviews unfair to job appli-cants, as candidates are not given the opportunity to prepare for such unplanned questions and hence prevent them from showcasing their abil-ities; this also results in inequitable treatment of job applicants. Untrained interviewers also have a tendency to pose questions that violate the law or compromise ethical principles, such as inquiries about plans for starting a family or for maternity leaves.

Notwithstanding these problems, the job interview can be a very effective and efficient method of obtaining job-related information and of assessing the applicant's suitability for a position and his or her fit within the organization. Furthermore, the interview itself can be used as an effec-tive recruitment tool, giving the interviewer an opportunity to highlight the positive features of the organization as a whole and the department in particular.

Those involved in selection can choose between unstructured and structured interview techniques. *Unstructured interviews* present few con-straints in how interviewers go about gathering information and evaluat-ing applicants. As a result, unstructured interviews may be very subjective and thus tend to be less reliable than structured interviews. However,

FIGURE 7.1
Guidelines
for the
Appropriate
Use of
Reference
Checks

1. Ask for and obtain only job-related information.

2. Do not ask for information in an application or personal interview that may be deemed illegal.

3. Applicants should provide written permission to contact references; this may be included in the application form.

4. Individuals who check references should be trained in how to interview references, probe for additional information, and accurately record reference information.

5. Reference information should be recorded in writing.

6. Use the reference-checking process to confirm information provided by the applicant and to identify gaps in the employment record.

7. Use the reference-checking method appropriate to the job.

8. Be aware if the individual who provides a reference is trying to damage a prospective employee by giving a negative reference.

9. Use the references provided by the applicant as a source for additional references or information.

10. Consider using preemployment information services, particularly for sensitive positions.

because of the free reign frequently given to interviewers, unstructured interviews may be more effective than the structured type in screening out unsuitable candidates.

The basic premise of a *structured interview* is that the questions are clearly job related in that they are based on the result of a thorough job analysis. In highly structured interviews, the "correctness" of answers are predetermined and scores are allocated to different answers prior to the interview. Ideally, interviewers are not given ancillary information about applicants that may have a positive or negative impact on their evaluation of the information provided in a job interview. The most common types of questions in a structured interview are situational questions, experience-based questions, job-knowledge questions, and worker-requirements questions.

Situational questions relate to how applicants may handle a hypothetical work situation, while *experience-based questions* ask how applicants previously handled a situation similar to the type of situation they may encounter on the new job. Following are examples of a situational question and an experience-based question for the position of office manager in a pediatric group practice. The constructs being assessed in this case are handling stressful situations, dealing with the public, and professionalism.

Scenario: Seven pediatricians work in a busy medical practice, and Monday morning is the busiest time of the week. The waiting room is overcrowded, and two of the pediatricians unexpectedly are called away from the office—one for a personal situation and the other to attend to a patient in the hospital. Children and their parents now have to wait up to two hours to see the remaining doctors, and their level of anger and frustration increases as they wait. They are taking out their anger on you.

Situational questions: How would you handle this situation? What and how would you communicate with the remaining physicians about this situation?

Experience-based questions: Think about a situation on your last job in which you were faced with angry and upset patients or customers. What was the situation? What did you do? What was the outcome?

With situational questions, the question designers should decide a priori how alternative responses will be evaluated or scored. If an interview panel is used in which two or more interviewers are in the same room as the applicant, the interviewers can confirm answers and their meaning.

Job-knowledge questions assess whether job applicants have the knowledge to do the job. These questions and follow-up probes are predetermined and are based on the job description. Similarly, *worker-requirements questions* seek to determine if the candidate is able and willing to work under the conditions of the job. For example, applicants for a consulting position may be asked if they are able and willing to travel for a designated portion of their work.

Whatever form is used, job interviews must be conducted with the following guidelines in mind:

1. Prepare yourself. For an unstructured interview, learn the KSAs required for the job. For a structured interview, become familiar with the questions to be asked. Review materials or information about the candidate as well.
2. Tidy up the physical environment in which the interview will take place.
3. Describe the job, and invite questions about the job.
4. Put the applicant at ease, and convey an interest in him or her. The idea of a purposefully stressful interview is rarely desirable, as there are other reliable and ethical ways to assess an applicant's ability to handle stress. Furthermore, a stressful interview reflects the organization poorly.

5. Do not come to premature conclusions (positive or negative) about a candidate. This is particularly important for unstructured interviews.
6. Listen carefully, and ask for clarity if an applicant's responses are vague.
7. Observe the candidate, and take notes on relevant aspects of dress, mannerisms, and affect.
8. Provide an opportunity for the applicant to ask questions.
9. Do not talk excessively. Remember that this is an opportunity to hear from the applicant.
10. Do not ask questions that are unethical or that put the organization in a legally vulnerable position (see Figure 7.2).
11. Explain the selection process that comes after the interview.
12. Evaluate the candidate as soon as possible after the interview.

Application Forms and Resumes

Application forms and resumes usually contain useful information about job applicants. The major drawback to these information-gathering tools is that they may be inaccurate or may exaggerate an applicant's qualifications. Several methods can be used to improve the usefulness of application forms. First, create an addendum to the application that asks candidates to provide information specific to the job for which they are applying. This way, specific KSAs can be targeted for different jobs. Second, include a statement on the application form that allows the applicant to indicate that all information he or she reported is accurate; the applicant should then be required to sign or initial this statement. Third, ensure that illegal inquiries about personal information (e.g., marital status, height, weight) are *not* included on the form.

Ability and Aptitude Tests

A variety of ability and aptitude tests are available, many of which demonstrate reliability and validity. The list of tests is massive and includes tests on personality, honesty, integrity, cognitive reasoning, and fine motor coordination. A number of firms specialize in the production and assessment of tests; see, for example, the web site for Walden Personnel Testing and Consulting: http://www. waldentesting.com/booklet/booklet.htm. Debate is currently brewing about the issue of *situational validity*—the notion that the nature of job performance differs across work settings and that the validity of tests may vary according to the setting. In general, studies tend to conclude that in fact most basic abilities are generalizable across work settings, assuming that the test itself is valid and reliable. The key is to ensure that such tests are actually representative of the work involved in a particular job.

FIGURE 7.2

Inappropriate and Appropriate Job Interview Questions

Personal and Marital Status

Inappropriate: How tall are you?

How much do you weigh? (acceptable if these are safety requirements)

What is your maiden name?

Are you married?

Is this your maiden or married name?

With whom do you live?

Do you smoke?

Appropriate: After hiring, inquire about marital status for tax and insurance forms purposes

Are you able to lift 50 pounds and carry it 20 yards? (acceptable if this is part of the job)

Parental Status and Family Responsibilities

Inappropriate: How many kids do you have?

Do you plan to have children?

What are your childcare arrangements?

Are you pregnant?

Appropriate: Would you be willing to relocate if necessary?

Travel is an important part of this job. Would you be willing to travel as needed by the job?

This job requires overtime occasionally. Would you be able and willing to work overtime as necessary?

After hiring, inquire about dependent information for tax and insurance forms purposes

Age

Inappropriate: How old are you?

What year were you born?

When did you graduate from high school and college?

Appropriate: Before hiring, asking if the applicant is above the legal minimum age for the hours or working conditions is appropriate, as this is in compliance with state or federal labor laws. After hiring, verifying legal minimum age with a birth certificate or other ID and asking for age on insurance forms are permissible.

National Origin

Inappropriate: Where were you born?

Where are your parents from?

What is your heritage?

What is your native tongue?

What languages do you read, speak, or write fluently? (Acceptable if this is relevant to the job)

Appropriate: Are you authorized to work in the United States?

May we verify that you are a legal U.S. resident, or may we have a copy of your work visa status?

FIGURE 7.2
(continued)

Race or Skin Color
Inappropriate: What is your racial background?
Are you a member of a minority group?
Appropriate: This organization is an equal opportunity employer. Race is required information only for affirmative-action programs.

Religion or Creed
Inappropriate: What religion do you follow?
Which religious holidays will you be taking off from work?
Do you attend church regularly?
Appropriate: May we contact religious or other organizations related to your beliefs to provide us with references, per your list of employers and references?

Criminal Record
Inappropriate: Have you ever been arrested?
Have you ever spent a night in jail?
Appropriate: Questions about convictions by civil or military courts are appropriate if accompanied by a disclaimer that the answers will not necessarily cause loss of job opportunity. Generally, employers can ask only about convictions and not arrests (except for jobs in law-enforcement and security-clearance agencies) when the answers are relevant to the job performance.

Disability
Inappropriate: Do you have any disabilities?
What is your medical history?
How does your condition affect your abilities?
Please fill out this medical history document.
Have you had recent illnesses or hospitalizations?
When was your last physical exam?
Are you HIV positive?
Appropriate: Can you perform specific physical tasks? (such as lifting heavy objects, bending, kneeling that are required for the job)
After hiring, asking about the person's medical history on insurance forms is appropriate.
Are you able to perform the essential functions of this job with or without reasonable accommodations?

Affiliations
Inappropriate: To what clubs or association do you belong?
Appropriate: Do you belong to any professional or trade groups or other organizations that you consider relevant to your ability to perform this job?

Note: Questions listed here are not necessarily illegal. For example, it is not illegal to ask an applicant's date of birth, but it is illegal to deny employment to an applicant solely because he or she is 40 years of age or older. In this case, the question is not illegal, but a discriminatory motive for asking is illegal. Unknown or ambiguous motive is what makes any question with discriminatory implications inappropriate. If an individual is denied employment, having asked this and similar questions can lead to the applicant claiming that the selection decision was made on the basis of age, gender, or other characteristic for which it is illegal to discriminate.

The use of assessment centers is an increasingly popular method of evalu- **Assessment**
ating applicants. Assessment centers may be an actual physical location **Centers**
where testing is done, but they may also refer to a series of assessment procedures that are administered, professionally scored, and reported to hiring personnel. Assessment centers have traditionally been used to test
applicants' management skills, but they are now employed for a variety of
hiring situations. Typical assessment formats include paper-and-pencil tests,
intelligence tests, personality tests, interest measures, work-task simulations, in-basket exercises, interviews, and situational exercises. Evidence
indicates positive statistical relationships between use of assessment centers and high-level of job performance (Gaugler et al. 1997).

Retention

Ranking among the most important healthcare workforce challenges is staff
shortages, and related to this issue are employee retention and turnover.
Shortages of healthcare personnel are related to turnover and retention,
but larger pressures contribute to the chronic shortages the industry is
experiencing and will likely see in the foreseeable future. Although employee
turnover is not appreciably increasing in healthcare, its rates are higher in
healthcare than in other industries. A number of factors are associated
with increased demand for healthcare workers: population growth, the
aging of the population, improved diagnostic techniques that enable earlier detection of disease and increase patient loads, and heightened consumer demand for a full range of diagnostic and therapeutic technologies
(HCAB 2001). About 60 percent of the registered nurse (RN) workforce
is older than 40, and the percentage of RNs under 30 has fallen by nearly
40 percent since 1980 (Buerhaus, Staiger, and Auerbach 2000).
Approximately half of the RN workforce will reach retirement age in the
next 10 to 15 years (Maes 2000). Increases in demand, together with
decreasing supply and changing demographic patterns in the nursing workforce, have created a chronic shortage that is unlike past shortages (Ponte
2004; Mee and Robinson 2003).

    These broad societal factors are largely out of the control of health-
care organizations and contribute substantially to increasing worker vacancy
rates in hospitals. These vacancy rates in turn highlight the need for organizations to do a better job at recruiting, selecting, and retaining staff. In this
section, we explain our concern with turnover, enumerate the costs associated with turnover, discuss the factors that contribute to turnover, and explore
the methods proven to improve retention. Although we use the nursing
shortage as a basis to explore the retention issue, we are aware also of the
shortages in other healthcare professions—for example, radiological techni-

cians and pharmacists. The reasons for turnover and strategies for improving retention for nursing can be applied as well to other professions.

Studies on Turnover and Retention

The demand for healthcare workers is increasing, while the quality of their work life is decreasing. The average annual turnover rate for hospital workers is about 20 percent, with substantially higher percentages for particular professional groups. At any one time, approximately 126,000 nursing positions in U.S. hospitals are unfilled (JCAHO 2004). Nurse turnover in hospitals ranges generally between 10 percent and 25 percent. In certain sectors, vacancy rates are even higher. Ninety percent of nursing homes lack nursing staff sufficient to provide even basic care (CMS 2002). Recently, the turnover rate in nursing homes for RNs, LPNs, and directors of nursing was a staggering 50 percent (American Health Care Association 2003).

Nurse dissatisfaction has been cited as a key reason for turnover and for nurses leaving the profession entirely. In a worldwide study of nurses, those surveyed in the United States had the highest rate of job dissatisfaction at 41 percent, which is four times that of the professional workforce in general (Albaugh 2003; Aiken et al. 2001). A multitude of studies have examined reasons for nurse dissatisfaction and the consequences of dissatisfaction. McFarland, Leonard, and Morris (1984) cite lack of involvement in decision making, problems with supervisors, poor working conditions, inadequate compensation, and lack of job security. Swansburg (1990) identifies compensation, poor recognition, lack of flexible scheduling, and increased stress as dissatisfiers. The Maryland Nurses Association (2000) articulates the top five reasons for poor nurse retention: (1) absence of advancement opportunities, (2) stress and burnout related to mandatory overtime, (3) unrealistic workloads, (4) increased paperwork, and (5) nurses' perception of lack of respect and recognition from the workplace. The Joint Commission on Accreditation of Healthcare Organizations (2004) finds that overtime requirements are major sources of dissatisfaction.

Turnover has an adverse effect on the performance of organizations, with data increasingly pointing to the impact of turnover and shortages on healthcare quality. A survey conducted by the American Nurses Association (ANA 2001) reveals that 75 percent of nurses felt that the quality of nursing care has declined in the past two years. Among those respondents who claimed that quality has declined, over 92 percent cited inadequate staffing as the reason, while 80 percent indicated nurse dissatisfaction. The ANA survey also reports that over 54 percent of nurse respondents would not recommend their profession to their children or friends.

A study conducted by the Voluntary Hospitals Association of America finds a correlation between nurse retention and quality measures. Hospitals with nurse turnover rates under 12 percent had lower risk-adjusted mortality scores and lower severity-adjusted lengths of stay than hospitals whose nurse turnover was above 22 percent. Confirming evidence from earlier studies, Aiken and colleagues (2002) argue that nurse-patient ratios are strongly related to higher levels of dissatisfaction and emotional exhaustion. These studies present the connection that exists among nurse dissatisfaction, turnover, and quality of care.

In addition to the effect on quality, nurse shortages and turnover also have very significant financial implications for healthcare organizations. The costs associated with employee termination, recruitment, selection, hiring, and training represent a very substantial non-value-adding element in the organizational budget. A 2004 study of turnover estimates various costs associated with turnover in an academic medical center in the southwest (Waldman et al. 2004). Depending on assumptions made in the analysis, the total cost of turnover decreased somewhere between $7 million and 19 million, or between 3.4 percent and 5.8 percent, of the annual operating budget. This research indicates that over one-fourth of the total turnover costs were attributable to nurse turnover.

Several studies have focused specifically on the cost of nursing turnover. While difficult to measure, Jones (1990) estimates that the cost of a single nurse leaving is somewhere between $10,000 and $15,000. The Healthcare Advisory Board estimates that 21 percent of these costs are direct hiring costs, while 79 percent are hidden costs of reduced productivity (i.e., predeparture, vacancy, and new employee on-boarding). Assuming a turnover rate of 20 percent and the cost of nurse turnover at 100 percent of a nurse's annual salary, the Voluntary Hospitals Association of America estimates that a hospital that employs 600 nurses will spend $5.5 million in staff replacement costs each year (Kosel and Olivo 2002).

Turnover can be viewed as costly in terms of patient care, financial stability, and staff morale. Nurse turnover affects communication among nurses and between nurses and other healthcare professionals. It affects quality of care and the care continuity, which are crucial in healthcare provision. The work of teams is affected as well, as team composition changes when staff come and go. Those left behind often feel low morale and a sense of rejection.

Retention Strategies

Many of the factors associated with effective recruitment are also applicable to retention. People come to work in an organization for a number of professional and personal reasons, including compensation, the quality of work life (e.g., relationships with peers, supervisors, and members of other professional groups), and opportunities for professional growth. Retention strategies are a necessary follow-up to recruitment. With the opportunities available to nurses in other organizations and professions, the organization needs to view retention as an essential function, not unlike compensation and training.

One study examined the strategies used by nurse managers who had succeeded in achieving low turnover rates and high satisfaction among patients, employees, and providers; good patient outcomes; and positive working relationships (Manion 2004). The study finds that these nurse managers were able to develop a "culture of retention." Through their daily work, these managers created an environment where people want to stay because they enjoy their work and where staff contribute to this sense of attachment. These managers emphasized sincere caring for the welfare of their staff, forging authentic connections with each staff member, and focusing on results and problem solving. In the discussion below of retention strategies, keep in mind that these strategies are not likely to succeed without a culture of retention.

In today's healthcare environment, much of the turnover that occurs is beyond the control of a single organization. We have seen the virtual evaporation of employee commitment to their employers. Except in rare instances, the market profoundly affects the movement of employees. Organizations can still control turnover, but their influence is becoming limited. Retention strategies have simply not achieved the type of consistent success once anticipated. Furthermore, each organization needs to develop its own retention strategies and tailor them to the particular circumstances of the institution (Cappelli 2000).

Several generic retention strategies have shown success in particular circumstances. Compensation is a primary strategy and comes in many forms. Signing bonuses, premium and differential pay, forgivable loans, bonuses, and extensive benefits are all included under the umbrella of compensation. Job design and job customization are based on the premise that job satisfaction is a determinant of retention. We may improve retention if we can structure jobs so that they are more appealing and satisfying. This can be done by careful assignment and grouping of tasks and by providing employees with sufficient autonomy. It may also include being flexible with work hours and scheduling, enhancing the collegiality of the work environment, and instituting work policies that are respectful of individual needs. In the nursing environment, job design encompasses such strategies as nurse-patient staffing ratios and the existence of mandatory overtime. Based on the idea that people leave supervisors, not jobs, the quality of supervision is extremely important. This is clearly true in nursing; nurses sometimes leave because of poor working relationships with other healthcare professionals as well as poor relationships with colleagues and supervisors. Career-growth potential is a retention factor for many employees and, in particular, those in professional roles. Providing career ladders is increasingly difficult as organizations become flatter and have wider spans of control. Alternatives to promotion to managerial positions need to be developed and implemented.

The Magnet Nursing Service Recognition Program was developed to acknowledge and reward hospitals that have exhibited excellent nursing care. Designated magnet hospitals are characterized by fewer hierarchical organizational structures, decentralized decision making, flexibility in scheduling, positive nurse-physician relationships, and nursing leadership that supports and invests in nurses' career development (Cameron et al. 2004). Magnet hospitals have been found to have better patient outcomes and higher levels of patient satisfaction (Scott, Sochalski, and Aiken 1999). Compared to nonmagnet hospitals, magnet hospitals have lower turnover and higher job satisfaction among nurses (Huerta 2003; Upenieks 2002).

The Healthcare Advisory Board (HCAB 2002) conducted an extensive review of recruitment and retention strategies and identified each strategy's relative effectiveness. Much of the discussion in the literature about retention focuses on improving job satisfaction. The HCAB, however, distinguishes between strategies that boost morale and those that improve retention. The HCAB categorizes retention strategies into four types:

1. *Strategies that neither increase morale nor improve retention.* These well-intentioned strategies fail to have an impact on morale or retention. They include individualized benefits, concierge services, and employee lounge areas.
2. *Strategies that increase morale but do not improve retention.* These strategies include morale committees, on-site childcare, recognition programs, and educational benefits.
3. *Strategies that do not increase morale but improve retention.* Such strategies as improving screening of applicants, monitoring turnover in key areas, and tracking turnover of key employees are effective in reducing turnover.
4. *Strategies that increase morale and improve retention.* Improved staffing ratios, career ladders, buddy programs, and flexible scheduling are strategies that improve both morale and retention.

The HCAB's review yields five key strategies that are found to be effective in improving retention: (1) selecting the right employees; (2) improving orientation and on-boarding through such practices as creating buddy programs and providing opportunities for new employees to establish professional and personal relationships; (3) tracking turnover to identify specific root causes, including identifying managers whose departments have high turnover rates; (4) identifying and implementing retention strategies for employees who are particularly valued; and (5) although marginal in its effectiveness, systematically attempting to reverse turnover decisions.

Every organization faces different challenges in its efforts to retain valued employees. Successful retention is dependent on the ability of organizations to correctly identify the most important causes of turnover (and retention) and to implement strategies that appropriately target these factors. The effectiveness of strategies differs in each organization, but organizations must recognize the current evidence on the advantages and usefulness of alternative retention strategies. This provides a basis for thinking about alternative approaches.

Summary

Hiring and retaining employees continue to be important as healthcare organizations struggle to be competitive and operate under pressures for effectiveness, efficiency, and consumer responsiveness. The challenges that face recruiters are enormous. Organizations need to seek employees who (1) have specialized skills yet are flexible to fill in for other positions, (2) bring in new expertise yet are able to work in groups whose members are not experts, (3) are strongly motivated yet are comfortable with relatively flat organizational structures in which traditional upward mobility may be difficult, and (4) represent diversity yet also fit into the organizational culture. With strong HRM practices and positive organizational cultures, recruiting and retaining employees with dual traits may be possible.

References

Aiken, L. H., S. P. Clarke, D. M. Sloane, J. A. Sochalski, R. Busse, H. Clarke, P. Giovannetti, J. Hunt, A. M. Rafferty, and J. Shamian. 2001. "Nurses' Report on Hospital Care in Five Countries." *Health Affairs* 20 (3): 43–53.

Albaugh, J. 2003. "Keeping Nurses in Nursing: The Profession's Challenge for Today." *Urologic Nursing* 23 (3): 193–99.

Albright, L. E., J. R. Glennon, and W. J. Smith. 1963. *The Use of Psychological Tests in Industry*. Cleveland, OH: Howard Allen.

American Health Care Association. 2003. *Results of the 2002 AHCA Survey of Nursing Staff Vacancy and Turnover in Nursing Homes*. Chesterfield, MO: Health Services Research and Evaluation, American Health Care Association.

American Nurses Association. 2001. *Analysis of American Nurses Association Staffing Survey*. Silver Spring, MD: American Nurses Association.

Barber, A. 1998. *Recruiting Employees: Individual and Organizational Perspectives.* Thousand Oaks, CA: Sage Publishing.

Barber, A. E., C. L. Daly, C. M. Giannantonio, and J. M. Phillips. 1994. "Job Search Activities: An Examination of Changes Over Time." *Personnel Psychology* 47 (4): 739–65.

BNA. 2001. "Internet, E-mail Monitoring Common at Most Workplaces." *BNA Bulletin to Management*, February 1.

Bowen, D. E., G. E. Ledford, and B. R. Nathan. 1991. "Hiring for the Organization, Not the Job." *Academy of Management Executive* 5 (4): 35–51.

Bowns, D. A., and H. J. Bernardin. 1988. "Critical Incident Technique." In *The Job Analysis Handbook for Business, Industry, and Government*, edited by S. Gael, 1120–37. New York: Wiley.

Bretz, R. D., and T. A. Judge. 1994. "The Role of Human-Resource Systems in Job Applicant Decision-Processes." *Journal of Management* 20 (3): 531–51.

Buerhaus, P. I., D. Staiger, and D. I. Auerbach. 2000. "Implications of an Aging Registered Nurse Workforce." *Journal of the American Medical Association* 283 (22): 2948–954.

Calandra, B. 2001. "You've Got Friends." *HR Magazine* 46 (8): 49–55.

Cameron, S., M. Armstrong-Stassen, S. Bergeron, and J. Out. 2004. "Recruitment and Retention of Nurses: Challenges Facing Hospital and Community Employers." *Nursing Leadership* 17 (3): 79–92.

Cappelli, P. 2000. "A Market-Driven Approach to Retaining Talent." *Harvard Business Review* (January–February): 103–11.

Caudron, S. 1995. "The Changing Union Agenda." *Personnel Journal* 74 (3): 42–49.

Centers for Medicaid & Medicare Services. 2002. *Minimum Nurse Staffing Ratios in Nursing Homes.* Washington, DC: CMS.

The Cleveland Clinic. 2005. [Online information; retrieved 6/04.] http://www.clevelandclinic.org.

Fitz-enz, J., and B. Davison. 2002. *How to Measure Human Resources Management.* New York: McGraw-Hill.

Gatewood, R. D., and H. S. Feild. 1998. *Human Resource Selection, 4th Edition.* Fort Worth, TX: Dryden.

Gaugler, B. B., D. B. Rosenthal, G. C. Thornton, and C. Bentson. 1997. "Meta-Analysis of Assessment Center Validity." *Journal of Applied Psychology* 72 (3): 493–511.

Greengard, S. 2003. "Gimme Attitude." *Workforce Management* 81 (7): 56–60.

The Healthcare Advisory Board. 2001. *Competing for Talent: Recovering America's Hospital Workforce.* Washington, DC: The Advisory Board Company.

———. 2002. *Hardwiring for Right Retention: Best Practices for Retaining a High Performance Workforce.* Washington, DC: The Advisory Board Company.

Henderson, R. I. 1986. "Contract Concessions: Is the Past Prologue?" *Compensation and Benefits Review* 18 (5): 17–30.

Heneman, H. G., and T. A. Judge. 2003. *Staffing Organizations*. Middleton, WI: Mendota House.

Huerta, S. 2003. "Recruitment and Retention: The Magnet Perspective." Chart. *Journal of Illinois Nursing* 100 (4): 4–6.

Hunter, J., and R. Hunter. 1984. "The Validity and Utility of Alternative Predictors of Job Performance." *Psychological Bulletin* 96 (1): 72–98.

Joint Commission on Accreditation of Healthcare Organizations. 2004. "Healthcare at the Crossroads: Strategies for Addressing the Evolving Nursing Crisis." [Online information; retrieved 11/7/0404.] http://www.jcaho.org.

Jones, C. B. 1990. "Staff Nurse Turnover Costs: Part II, Measurement and Results." *Journal of Nursing Administration* 20 (5): 27–32.

Kaiser Permanente. 2005. [Online information; retrieved 6/04.] http://www.kaiserpermanentejobs.org/workinghere/diversity.asp#care.

Kosel, K. C., and T. Olivo. 2002. *The Business Case for Work Force Stability*. VHA's 2002 Research Series. Irving, TX: Voluntary Hospitals of America, Inc.

Kristof-Brown, A. L. 2000. "Perceived Applicant Fit: Distinguishing Between Recruiters' Perceptions of Person-Job and Person-Organization Fit." *Personnel Psychology* 53 (3): 643–71.

London, M., and S. A. Stumpf. 1982. *Managing Careers*. Reading, MA: Addison-Wesley.

Maes, S. 2000. "Where Have All the Nurses Gone?" *Oncology Nursing Society News* 15 (5): 1, 4–5.

Manion, J. 2004. "Nurture a Culture of Retention." *Nursing Management* 35 (4): 28–39.

Maryland Nurses Association. 2000. "Commission on the Crisis in Nursing Summit 2000." *Maryland Nurse* 3 (2): 1–10.

Mayo Clinic. 2005. [Online information; retrieved 6/04.] http://www.mayoclinic.org/jobs.

McFarland, G. K., H. S. Leonard, and M. M. Morris. 1984. *Nursing Leadership and Management: Contemporary Strategies*. New York: John Wiley & Sons.

Mee, C. L., and E. Robinson. 2003. "Nursing: What's Different About This Nursing Shortage?" *Nursing* 33 (1): 51–55.

Peter, L. J., and R. Hull. 1969. *The Peter Principle*. New York: William Morrow.

Phillips, J. M. 1998. "Effects of Realistic Job Previews on Multiple Organizational Outcomes." *Academy of Management Journal* 41 (6): 673–90.

Ponte, R. P. 2004. "The American Healthcare System at a Crossroads: An Overview of the American Organization of Nurse Executives Monograph." *Online Journal of Issues in Nursing* 9 (2). www.nursingworld.org/ojin/topic24/tpc24_2.htm.

Roth, L. M. 1982. *A Critical Examination of the Dual Ladder Approach to Career Advancement*. New York: Center for Research in Career Development, Columbia University Graduate School of Business.

Rynes, S. L. 1991. "Recruitment, Job Choice, and Post-Hire Consequences: A Call for New Research Directions." In *Handbook of Industrial and Organizational Psychology, 2nd Edition*, edited by M. D. Dunnette and L. M. Hough, 399–444. Palo Alto, CA: Consulting Psychologists Press, Inc.

Schwab, D. P., S. L. Rynes, and R. J. Aldag. 1987. "Theories and Research on Job Search and Choice." In *Research in Personnel and Human Resources Management*, edited by G. Ferris and T. R. Mitchell. Greenwich, CT: JAI Press.

Scott, J. G., J. Sochalski, and L. Aiken. 1999. "Review of Magnet Hospital Research: Findings and Implications for Professional Nursing." *Journal of Nursing Administration* 29 (1): 9–19.

Swansburg, R. C. 1990. *Management and Leadership for Nurse Managers.* Boston: Jones & Bartlett.

Taylor, G. S. 1994. "The Relationship Between Sources of New Employees and Attitudes Toward the Job." *Journal of Social Psychology* 134 (1): 99–110.

Upenieks, V. 2002. "Assessing Differences in Job Satisfaction of Nurses in Magnet and Nonmagnet Hospitals." *Journal of Nursing Administration* 32 (11): 564–76.

WakeMed Health & Hospitals. 2005. [Online information; retrieved 6/04.] http://wakemed.com.

Waldman, J. D., F. Kelly, S. Arora, and H. L. Smith. 2004. "The Shocking Cost of Turnover in Healthcare." *Healthcare Management Review* 29 (1): 2–7.

Wanous, J. P. 1992. *Recruitment, Selection, Orientation, and Socialization of Newcomers, 2nd Edition.* Reading, MA: Addison-Wesley.

Discussion Questions

1. Given two apparently equally qualified job applicants—one from inside and one from outside the organization—how would you go about deciding which one to hire?

2. For a variety of reasons, some healthcare organizations are unable to pay market rates for certain positions. What advice would you give such an organization about possible recruitment and retention strategies?

3. The use of references is increasingly viewed as unreliable. How can employers legally and ethically obtain information about an applicant's past performance? What measures can be taken to verify information contained in a job application or resume?

4. What are the advantages and disadvantages of recruiting through the Internet? What advice would you give to a hospital that is considering spending resources on using the Internet for recruitment?

Experiential Exercises

This case was developed in collaboration with Caroline LeGarde.

Grayson County Regional Health Center is a private, not-for-profit, 225-bed acute care hospital located in a rural community in a southeastern state. The hospital provides a broad range of inpatient and outpatient services, including cardiology, obstetrics, gynecology, general surgery, internal medicine, urology, family medicine, dermatology, pediatrics, psychiatry, radiology, nephrology, ophthalmology, occupational medicine, and rehabilitation services. The Center offers 24-hour emergency care.

The Center covers 310,000 square feet built on an approximately 96-acre site. Its service area includes Grayson County as well as parts of three neighboring rural counties. Grayson County's population is 60,879, with African Americans making up 53 percent of the population, Caucasian making up 42 percent, and Hispanics and other groups making up 5 percent.

Agriculture is the main industry in the area, with cotton as the major crop. Fifteen percent of the labor force works in manufacturing, which includes molded plastics, metal fabrication, paper and wood products, textiles, rubber materials, and clothing. In the last 20 years, the region has suffered severe economic setbacks. Most of the textile industry has moved out of the region because of outsourcing, and the town itself has fallen into disrepair. An increasing proportion of the population lives in poverty. The county has a civilian labor force of 27,568 and currently has an unemployment rate of 13 percent.

Between 2003 and 2004, private non-farm employment decreased by 7 percent. Younger, educated people have tended to leave the region, particularly to relocate in a well-established and economically developed region of the state only 90 miles away. Between 2000 and 2003, Grayson County's population has decreased by 2 percent. Grayson County has an overall poverty rate of 25 percent. Thirty-three percent of children and 22 percent of the elderly live below the poverty line. Per capita income is $12,000, down from $13,000 three years earlier. Over one-third of the adults do not have a high school diploma. The county's infant mortality rate is 12 percent, and 24 percent of the population does not have health insurance.

The Center has approximately 85 physicians on its active staff, representing 29 subspecialties. It has affiliation relationships with two academic health centers—one is located about 90 miles away and the other is located 100 miles from Grayson. The Center currently employs over 800 employees, is fully certified by JCAHO, and is certified to participate in the Medicare and Medicaid programs. The Center is governed by an 18-member board of trustees, which includes the chief of the medical staff, the immediate past chief of the medical staff, the chief executive officer, and 13 members selected by the board from the community at large. Criteria for board election, as specified in the corporation's charter, include an interest in healthcare, aptitude in business, and evidence of a strong moral and ethical background. The board is required by the corporation's charter to reflect the economic, racial, and ethnic diversity of the service area.

The Center has strong community ties and is active in the community. Its staff participate in such activities as community health screenings, health education programs, and health fairs. It serves as the meeting place for many support groups. Although it has been under financial stress for the last five years, it continues to have strong support in the community.

The turnover rate for all employees is 40 percent. Over the last few years, the turnover rate for nurses has ranged from 15 percent to 50 percent. Physician recruitment and retention is also a major concern. There is currently only one radiologist in Grayson County, and rumor has it that she is planning to move out of the area, and there is a shortage of physicians in all specialties.

The Center relies heavily on Medicaid and Medicare revenue, leaving the hospital in a difficult financial condition. It is unable to pay market rates for nurses and other professionals. As a result, nursing units are understaffed, and nurses have expressed concerns about being overworked and underpaid. There is evidence that this has resulted in concerns about the quality of care for patients. A recent newspaper article reported that patients were often left on stretchers in the hallway for long periods of time, that staff were unresponsive to patient and family concerns, and that it was not unusual to hear crying in the hallways.

Nurses and other professional groups report poor communication between senior management and employees. Poor relationships between middle managers and frontline staff are also a problem in some departments. This situation became particularly difficult two years ago when the Center embarked on a large building project. Employees could not understand how the Center could afford to build new facilities but was unable to pay market rates to its staff.

The nursing turnover problem at the Center has reached crisis proportions. Recent exit interview surveys indicate that financial concerns are the major reason for leaving. The Center has tried numerous strategies, including improving the work environment by adding amenities (such as lowering prices in the cafeteria) and training middle managers. For a short time 18 months ago, nurse salaries matched market rates, but the Center fell behind again shortly thereafter. The RN vacancy rate currently is 18 percent.

Case Exercise

As a consultant to the Center, you are expected to make recommendations to address the nursing shortage. Specifically, you have been asked to develop short-term strategies to cope with the current crisis as well as long-term strategies to improve the overall recruitment and retention picture.

1. How will you go about identifying the most important reasons for the current shortage?
2. How will you proceed with developing short-term and long-term strategies?

Project   Chronic and worsening healthcare workforce shortages are likely in the foreseeable future. The objective of this project is for readers to learn about how hospitals and other healthcare organizations are coping with healthcare workforce shortages. Specifically, how do they perceive the causes of turnover, and what strategies have they found successful in improving both their recruitment and retention.

1. Identify one professional group that has been cited as having recruitment and retention problems, such as nurses, laboratory technicians, radiologic technicians, and certain information technology personnel.
2. Choose two organizations that employ this professional group.
3. Locate the individual or individuals most directly accountable for recruitment and retention of professionals in this group. This may

be an individual or individuals within the HR department, a nurse recruiter, or other staff responsible for recruitment and retention.

4. Find the approximate number of professionals in this group that are needed by the organization.

5. Obtain information on the following:
   a. Current vacancy rate
   b. Turnover and retention rates for the last five years

6. Discuss with the appropriate individuals their perception of the causes of recruitment challenges and of turnover and the reasons people choose to stay with their organizations. If possible, interview frontline staff in this professional group to obtain their perceptions on these issues.

7. In your discussions, explore the strategies the organization has used to increase the success rate of recruitment and retention efforts. Does the organization know which strategies have been successful and unsuccessful? If so, which strategies have proven successful? Which strategies have not been effective? What strategies may be effective but are difficult to implement?

8. Summarize your findings in a four-page paper.

ORGANIZATIONAL DEVELOPMENT, TRAINING, AND KNOWLEDGE MANAGEMENT

James A. Johnson, Ph.D.; Gerald R. Ledlow, Ph.D., CHE; and Bernard J. Kerr, Jr.,

Ed.D., FACHE

Learning Objectives

After completing this chapter, readers should be able to

- articulate training and organizational-development methods,
- better understand the organization as a learning system,
- distinguish training from longer-range organizational development, and
- view training and development as central to organizational performance.

Introduction

As discussed by Kilpatrick and Johnson (1999), we work in an era of major social and cultural changes that present us with many challenges and compel us to manage our healthcare organizations with greater efficiency, effectiveness, and value. Many healthcare insiders even believe that we are engaged in refining the best healthcare system in the world. If this is so, then we need new knowledge, tools, skills, and particularly new perspectives. With exponential increases in information, technological breakthroughs, and scientific discovery, a solid commitment to lifelong learning is critical.

Healthcare organizations are fundamentally dependent on people who have to fill an extensive range of roles to accomplish the institution's tasks and goals. Leading and managing complex institutions, considering the scope and scale of tasks in healthcare delivery, are a complicated undertaking and also entail *organizational development*—a system for providing to employees learning and training that are closely tied to the purpose, mission, vision, culture, and strategy of the organization. To operationalize organizational strategies, development plans must be created and employed to enhance employees' knowledge, skills, and abilities (KSAs).

Organizational development involves assessment of training and learning needs across the organization. Once identified, needs are then used as a basis for developing programs and projects that are given appropriate resources so that skill and knowledge deficiencies in the organization can be overcome through training and learning. It is important to identify development, training, and knowledge management needs for all staff throughout the organization. Many times, however, individual or groups of employees are left out of this analysis. For example, receptionists and other entry-level staff are not heavily involved in the development-analysis process and do not receive development and training. This is an unfortunate practice in that these staff members are the first and most interactive contacts for patients. In the competitive healthcare industry, such oversights can lead to decreased patient and employee satisfaction. Needs analysis is discussed further in this chapter.

Additionally, healthcare organizations need to manage their knowledge appropriately and create a culture that enables everyone to learn continuously. Organizational purpose, mission, vision, culture, and strategies dictate, in most circumstances, the need for organizational development plans, and these plans drive group and individual training and learning needs to enhance as well as acquire KSAs. Managing organizational knowledge and fostering organizational learning are a necessity in the fast-paced, information- and bio-information-heavy world of healthcare. Figure 8.1 presents a model that illustrates the sequence and progression of these concepts.

In this chapter, we explore the unique aspects of organizational development that lead to training and learning needs and to management of knowledge in healthcare organizations. The distinction between organizational development, training and education, and knowledge management is provided, and the role of learning theory and principles is discussed. Also, techniques for development design, evaluation, and implementation are described.

Organizational Development

Organizational development (OD) is a preferred approach to dealing with change. The processes of OD are designed to improve the ability of an organization to effectively manage changes in its environment while also meeting the needs of its members. OD uses planned interventions (Bennis 1969; Johnson 1996), including force field analysis, survey feedback, confrontation meetings, and coaching. These are approaches that tend to be diagnostic in nature but offer solution-oriented interventions.

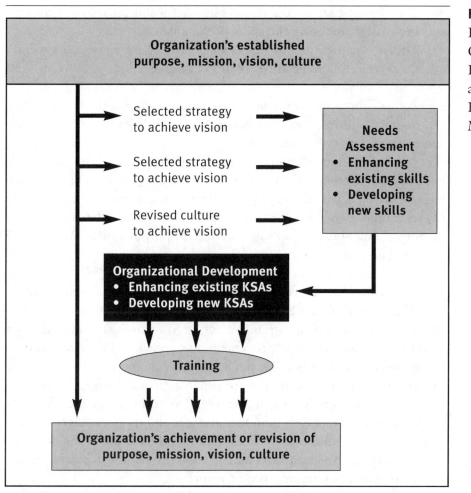

FIGURE 8.1

Process of Organizational Development and Knowledge Management

OD has been demonstrated to be successful in working through people's natural resistance to change. This is in part a result of the way OD empowers participants in the change process, encouraging understanding of and a commitment to the desired change. OD embraces a philosophy of participation, mutuality, and the value of knowledge at all levels of the organization. At the core of any OD effort is the involvement of employees in developing a commitment to change, which occurs for the following reasons (Blanchard and Thacker 1999):

- They are intimately familiar with the current system and can make valuable contributions to the change effort, increasing its chances of success.

- They become knowledgeable about what will happen as a result of the change, reducing their fear of the unknown.
- They are acting in a way that is supportive of the change, allowing them to feel more positive about the change.

An excellent resource for further information on OD is the Organization Development Institute, with its international network of OD practitioners and its information dissemination.[1]

Based on organizational needs and assessment of those needs, OD encompasses two major areas: (1) enhancement, improvement, or updating of existing KSAs of employees, affiliates, and other stakeholders and (2) creation of new KSAs for employees, affiliates, and other stakeholders to support the organization's new or revised purpose, mission, vision, or culture. These ideas and concepts are explained below.

The leadership and management teams, preferably using a predetermined and defined process of leadership and management (Ledlow, Cwiek, and Johnson 2002), determine the purpose, mission, and vision of the organization and the strategies required to move the organization toward its aspirations of improvement and enhancement. According to Kent, Johnson, and Graber (1996, 28), "Leaders go beyond a narrow focus on power and control in periods of organizational change. They create commitment and energy among stakeholders to make the change work. They create a sense of direction, then nurture and support others who can make the new organization a success." Often, the culture of the organization must change or must be recreated to best meet the expectations of a revised or new purpose, mission, or vision.

Purpose is the organization's reason for existing. It is what the organization provides in a competitive, effective, efficacious, and efficient way to meet the needs and demands of the external environment (e.g., customers, patients, community). Mission is closely tied to purpose. It is a statement of purpose that discloses why, where, and for whom the organization exists. Vision is a statement of aspiration. It is a future state of an improved, enhanced, or different organization. Healthcare organizations should have purpose, mission, and vision statements. The leadership and management teams create goals, resource needs, and monitor progress toward achievement of the improved organization in relation to its purpose, mission, and vision. Challenging yet achievable goals (Locke 1968; Locke et al. 1981; Locke and Latham 1984; Locke 1986; Locke, Gist, and Taylor 1987) and objectives and monitoring and reporting of progress (Ledlow, Bradshaw, and Shockley 2000) are critical in the attainment and evaluation of strategies that are used to achieve organizational success. OD programs and projects, as a strategy of organizational renewal and improvement, are also monitored and evaluated for effectiveness and efficiency. In essence, did the OD program or project make a positive impact on the organization's learning to meet a higher or new standard of performance? This becomes the salient issue in OD evaluation.

Healthcare organizations have an internal culture. The unique and important function of leadership is the conceptualization, creation, and management of this culture (Schein 1999). Organizational culture is a learned system of knowledge, behavior, attitudes, beliefs, values, and norms that is shared by a group of people (Schein 1999). Culture is a complex concept, but it can be evaluated through assessment of organizational climate, artifacts, traditions, and decisions made within the organization. Culture in one healthcare organization is unique from the culture of another, but the strong beliefs, values, attitudes, and assumptions about caring for other people are shared by those who work within the healthcare industry as a whole.

Organizational strategies are developed and used to create a roadmap or step-by-step sequence of goals, objectives, and action plans to reach the improved future state, or vision, of the organization. In essence, strategy is a systematic set of decisions, tasks, and events that are focused on and related to achieving an ideal state in the coming years. Revising, changing, or recreating organizational culture can be a strategy to move an organization toward its desired goals or vision.

Managing knowledge and creating a learning organization are strategies that fit today's evolving, demanding, and information-reliant age of healthcare. Considering the scope and depth of work involved in patient care activities, considering only the development of upper-level employees or functions is inappropriate. OD should involve training all people in the organization and learning together as a whole.

Fried (1999) defines healthcare personnel as both those with little formal training and education who provide support as well as those who are highly skilled and educated and are engaged in very complex tasks and decision making. Healthcare work has led to a point where ensuring employee competencies has become a critical strategic value (Friesen and Johnson 1996), dramatically increasing the pace and intensity of staff training and development (Blanchard and Thacker 1999). Training and development is essential to continuous quality improvement (Johnson and Omachanu 1999) and to strategic management (McIlwain and Johnson 1999). It is also the bedrock for creating a capacity for change and organizational learning (Senge 1990; Friesen and Johnson 1996; Tobin 1998). Lastly, one of the most salient approaches to improving our healthcare systems, according to the Robert Wood Johnson Foundation, is to "invest in people" (Isaacs and Knickman 2001). Healthcare at its most fundamental level is about people caring for people. Knowledge and skill, coupled with compassion and a commitment to continuous learning, will lead to an even better system of care.

Training

Training is typically a function of the human resources department and is the main vehicle for human resources development (HRD). Blanchard and Thacker (1999) describe the role of the HRD function as "improving the organization's effectiveness by providing employees with the learning needed to improve their current or future job performance." Training in organizations primarily focuses on the acquisition of KSAs. Focusing on areas that do not meet the needs of the organization will not be effective, and neither will training that fails to be seen by employees as relevant and important. The most effective approaches to training will simultaneously meet the needs of the organization and the individual employee.

KSAs required from and used by healthcare professionals and workers are extremely varied. For example, a nurse needs to be skilled in giving an injection with a syringe, while a radiological technician has to know how to work imaging technology. Even administrative tasks require KSAs from their performers. For example, an administrator needs to know how to use computers, to understand compliance issues, and to generate a flowchart.

There are distinctions between knowledge, skills, and abilities, although each requires learning and warrants different approaches to the learning process. *Knowledge* is the result of acquiring information and placing it in memory. When doing so, humans organize the information in a meaningful or useful way. Knowledge is often a byproduct of both remembering and understanding. *Skills* are defined as general capacities to perform a task or set of tasks. This capacity results from training or experience. *Abilities* are capabilities to perform based on experience, social and physical conditioning, or heredity. Many methods used in training have been demonstrated to be effective in improving KSAs.

Training is different from education. Training focuses on learning that is targeted at the enhancement of a given job or role, while education tends to be more global in its purpose. *Education* is viewed as the development of general knowledge related to a person's career or life but is not necessarily designed for a specific position. Examples of education include acquiring a master's in health administration, which allows the degree holder to fill different roles within a healthcare organization, or earning a doctor of medicine degree, which can lead to many different areas of medical specialization through further training and education.

Training Cycle

Training typically follows a systematic design, from an analysis of training need through the training design, implementation, and evaluation phase. This process helps to ensure control over the training process so that organizational goals can be accomplished. Without a systematic design, training has been shown to be only moderately effective and often a time and resources waste. A basic flow of the training cycle is shown in Figure 8.2.

The identification of training needs and evaluation of training (see Figure 8.1) are discussed later in this chapter. Other steps in the training cycle are important as well. Following are techniques to keep in mind when setting training objectives:

- Make sure that objectives are closely aligned with the organization's performance goals. Individual learning should be linked to the strategic direction of the organization.
- Always write the objectives clearly in terms that are easy to understand. Each objective should have a behavioral component that describes a desired outcome.

The selection of training methods is based on the learning objectives and the resources available. Training material and human resources needs have to be reviewed. Being aware of the context and the audience of the training is important when designing a training program. Once the objectives are established and the method of training is identified, then the training can be delivered. Methods of delivery can range from computer-assisted learning programs to formal lectures, which are discussed later in this chapter along with ways to implement the training program. Once training is presented and evaluated, a feedback loop should start, reporting to the original sponsors and designers the outcomes of the effort. This feedback helps to inform the need for future training and development in the organization.

Needs Analysis

The primary purpose of training is to improve the performance of both the individual and the organization. Thus, it is important to do a *needs analysis* before developing a training program. This assessment may encompass organizational analysis, operational analysis, and person analysis and should be done in a systematic manner to determine ways to bring performance up to an expected level. Sometimes the analysis reveals that the employee or group of employees lacks the necessary KSAs to perform the job effectively and hence requires training. Other times the analysis identifies the barriers within the organization or its culture that warrant OD interven-

FIGURE 8.2
Training Cycle

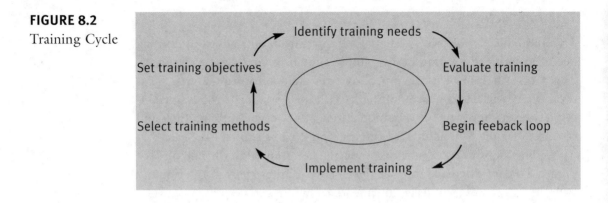

tion to tear down. A needs analysis may also disclose elements of a given job or task that have to be redesigned or altered accordingly. Most importantly, a needs analysis ensures that the right training and development are provided to the right people in the organization.

Organizational analysis is an evaluation of the strategic objectives, resources, and internal environment of the institution. These data are taken from the strategic plan, labor and skill inventories, interviews with leaders and workers, organizational climate surveys, and customer service records. *Operational analysis* examines the tasks and levels of, and the KSAs needed to effectively perform, a specific job or closely aligned set of jobs. This analysis often uncovers barriers that impede performance. Data sources for this assessment include job descriptions, task specifications, performance standards, performance appraisals, observation of the job itself, literature on the job, interviews with jobholder and supervisor, and quality control data. *Person analysis* is done once the organizational and operational analyses are complete. This type of evaluation identifies individuals who are not meeting the desired performance requirements or goals. Here, expected performance is compared to actual performance, resulting in an understanding of the gaps or discrepancies, which then become the basis for the design of the training intervention. Data sources for this analysis include supervisor ratings, performance appraisals, observation, interviews, questionnaires, tests, attitude surveys, checklists, rating scales, in-basket exercises and simulations, self-ratings, and assessment centers.

The design of a training program follows these three types of needs analysis, taking into account all of the findings from the assessment so that the effort targets the appropriate performance challenges and demands. Development of the training effort involves the identification of desired outcomes or program objectives, the conditions for goal accomplishment, and the standards by which achievements can be measured. The importance of a thorough needs analysis and clear learning objectives cannot be overstated. Objectives that are based on actual performance needs help the trainee to know what is expected and the trainer to design and implement a program that is applicable and relevant.

Training Methods

Several methods can be used to facilitate learning, and new techniques are being developed constantly. The American Society of Training and Development and other training-related organizations monitor and distribute available training tools and technologies as well as offer continuing education for trainers. The most popular methods are lectures and discussions, which are most useful in the dissemination of information and can be done live or face to face, through videotaped presentations, and via video conferencing. Other commonly used methods are computer-based training, programmed instruction, games and simulations, in-basket exercises, case studies, role playing, and on-the-job training. Each of these methods has its strengths and weaknesses, and depending on the desired learning objective and job tasks involved, each technique may be used independently or in combination.

Gordon, Morgan, and Ponticell (1995) and Blanchard and Thacker (1999) advise the trainer or training department to consider nine principles before undertaking or during any training initiative:

1. Identify the types of individual learning strengths and problems, and tailor the training around these factors.
2. Align learning objectives to organizational goals.
3. Clearly define program goals and objectives at the start.
4. Actively engage the trainee to maximize his or her attention, expectations, and memory.
5. Use a systematic, logical sequencing of learning activities so that trainees are able to master lower levels of learning before they can move on to higher levels.
6. Use a variety of training methods.
7. Use realistic and job- or life-relevant training material.
8. Allow trainees to work together and to share experiences with each other.
9. Provide constant feedback and reinforcement while encouraging self-assessment.

An important point to emphasize is this: Training evolves to learning, learning evolves to knowledge, and knowledge is then used in the workplace. To best improve the effectiveness of training, and achieve the progression to knowledge, trainers need to understand and evaluate the preferred learning styles of those who are being trained. There are four basic learning styles:

1. Auditory: listening and hearing
2. Visual-verbal: reading and then explaining
3. Visual-nonverbal: using pictures, graphs, and charts
4. Kinesthetic: learning by doing an activity

A good approach is to use multiple modes of learning media. In this instance, auditory, visual–verbal, visual–nonverbal, and kinesthetic learning styles can be used in coordination with and as a complement to each other. Not only does the use of multiple styles reinforce the strength of each style, it also increases the likelihood that trainees can grasp and remember concepts better as they learn according to their preferred style. Computer technology enables the use of multiple forms of media.

The Learning Environment

For training, or any other effort to improve organizational performance, to be effective a positive *learning environment* is critical. Ideally the organization has a culture in which continuous learning is central to the institution's definition of itself. Tobin (1998) asserts that the key to developing knowledge and skills that support organizational goals is the establishment of a positive learning environment where the following occur:

*   All employees recognize the need for continuous learning to improve their own performance and that of the organization as well.
*   Open sharing of knowledge and ideas is encouraged.
*   Opportunities for a wide variety of learning activities and coaching are available, and reinforcement of newly acquired knowledge and skills is provided.

The trainer should always keep in mind that the trainees are adults and thus have certain expectations from the training and have preferred styles and conditions under which they are most likely to learn. Adult learners generally want to improve and see the training as part of their key to better performance and subsequent career success. They need to feel that the training content is relevant to their work situations and setting. Many adult learners wish to be challenged and to be actively involved in the learning process. Trainers can meet adult learners' expectations by ensuring open communication, asking questions, providing a risk-free environment in which new skills can be practiced, and offering feedback and validation. The learning environment must be one in which active listening takes place and in which the trainee and the trainer can feel engaged.

Trainees and people in general are more apt to remember concepts, terms, or skills that they

- learned most recently,
- heard or saw more than once,
- are able to practice,
- can implement in their own setting,
- can use right away, and
- are encouraged or rewarded for using.

The Trainer

The person doing the training must also have a set of KSAs that support what he or she is seeking to accomplish. Because training is focused on the facilitation of learning, the trainer must have a good understanding of human behavior and adult learning theory. Many books and resources on these subjects have been written, and training-the-trainer programs designed to enhance the trainer's abilities are available. A trainer specifically must be highly skilled in interpersonal communication, active listening, questioning, and providing feedback.

Other critical capabilities of the trainer include an awareness to non-verbal communication or signals; strong knowledge base of the subject matter he or she is teaching; superb organization skills; ability to present materials in a fun, interactive, and creative manner; proficiency in various training methods; and a level of technological savvy. The credibility of the instructor is paramount to the trainee's willingness to learn, and a trainer's solid KSAs combined with his or her genuineness and helpfulness communicate to the trainee that a high level of efficacy can be expected from the training program. Ultimately the training must be useful in improving performance to achieve both individual and organizational goals.

Many times an organization hires outside consultants to conduct its training programs. Some advantages to this approach are that consultants bring in a fresh perspective, are responsive to tight deadlines, have expertise in specialized areas, and offer well-honed skills and well-developed programs that in-house trainers may not be able to provide. However, using outside consultants has some disadvantages as well. External trainers are less committed to the long-term goals of the organization, tend to be more expensive, and do not have an in-depth appreciation of the organization's culture.

Training Evaluation

As Bramley (1996) points out, the common view of evaluation is that it completes the training cycle. However, he suggests that it is an integral part of the cycle, not necessarily only a closer. Evaluation plays a key role in quality improvement in that it provides feedback on the following:

- the effectiveness of the methods being used;
- the achievement of the objectives set by both trainers and trainees; and
- the fulfillment of the performance discrepancies and gaps identified through the needs analysis process, both at the organizational and individual levels.

Goldstein (1993) defines evaluation as the systemic collection of descriptive and judgmental information to enable effective decisions related to selection, adoption, value, and modification of various instructional activities. Two broad categories of assessment—process and outcome—can be used to evaluate training. *Process analysis* examines how the training was designed and conducted, whereas *outcome evaluation* determines how well the training accomplished its objectives. Sources of data for process analysis are (1) the process before the training, including the setting of behavioral objectives, and (2) the instructional design features. Sources of data for outcome analysis typically comprise various outcomes such as reactions; learning; job behavior; and organizational results gleaned from questionnaires, interviews, focus groups, records, observation, and skill testing.

In addition to evaluating the process of training and its outcomes, the costs should be reviewed as well. A cost-benefit analysis should be undertaken to weigh the amount expended against the advantages that the effort brought to the organization. Many of these benefits, such as improved attitude or better interpersonal relations, are hard to measure but are nonetheless important outcomes. Similarly, a cost-savings analysis may be worthwhile as it will show the organization the money it saved in the form of reduced absenteeism, malpractice claims, or bad debt.

Knowledge Management

Knowledge management is the ability of an organization to capture, develop, organize, and apply the knowledge and learning that take place within its environment (Neese 2002). The efficiency of the systems, processes, rules, and information systems that an organization uses to manage knowledge directly affects the level of institutional knowledge and organizational learning. The more knowledge an organization captures and manages, the greater the organization's ability to access and use such knowledge, enabling the organization to devise strategies or improvements that take advantage of dynamic or ever-changing situations.

According to Neese (2002), an organization that is considering to develop or improve its knowledge management should keep the following questions in mind:

1. How does your organization's systems, processes, and information technology applications that capture, develop, organize, and use organizational knowledge and learning enable a stakeholder to access the knowledge when it is needed?
2. How does your organization develop a culture that encourages and fosters knowledge sharing across a wide range of specialty areas, shifts, and groups?
3. Because an organization is made up of individuals, what creates a culture of learning so that individual learning can be integrated into the learning of the organization as a whole?

In some cases, knowledge management is simple, with organizations routinely asking their employees to write down and flowchart the processes they use, the lessons they have learned, and the tricks of their trade. In certain ways, competency-based training and evaluations, such as those found in nursing sections in hospital wards, are a system of knowledge management in addition to functioning as accreditation documentation, individual evaluation of performance, and risk-management information. The complexity of knowledge management increases, however, when it is put in the context of capturing, organizing, managing, and using the knowledge across the entire organization. Knowledge management for the sake of capturing data is worthless; the purpose for it should be linked to the established mission, vision, culture, and strategy of the organization. The next section illustrates why this predetermined purpose of knowledge management is important.

Tension Between Learning, Innovation, and Knowledge Management

Learning, innovation, and knowledge management are each crucial to achievement of goals and improvement of performance. Learning allows the application of new and better KSAs. Innovation ushers in advances in systems, processes, services, and products. Knowing how systems work enables cross-training of employees, and this cross-fertilization of knowledge in turn allows innovation. An organization can be tightly coupled, loosely coupled, or anything in between these two extremes. The strength of the feedback loops determines organizational coupling: Stronger feedback loops imply tighter coupling, whereas weaker loops suggest loose coupling (Van de Ven and Poole 1995). Jelinek and Litterer (1995) suggest four criteria for determining the coupling status in organizations:

1. The closer the formal rules are followed, the tighter the coupling.
2. The greater the congruence among employees, the tighter the coupling.
3. The quicker feedback is given, the tighter the coupling.
4. The more attention, energy, and time that empowered individuals allocate to priorities in their areas, the tighter the coupling. (Participation, competence, and empowerment foster focused attention to areas of responsibility.)

Tightly coupled organizations have a greater ability to capture and manage organizational knowledge but encourage less learning and innovation. The important decision for leaders is to determine the level of coupling tight enough to capture and manage knowledge but also loose enough to allow learning and innovation. With the tension or trade-off between learning, innovation, and knowledge management in mind (see Figure 8.3), the organization must determine what and how much knowledge to manage, what level of innovation is desired, and how much organizational learning is required to achieve the goals and vision. The tightness or looseness of organizational coupling has a direct impact on organizational decisions and an indirect effect on other factors such as employee satisfaction.

Summary

Knowledge management as a strategy should be used to achieve a competitive advantage, to improve services and products, and to make operations more efficient and effective. Knowledge management, with consideration to learning and innovation, should create organizational wisdom—that is, a capable and trained employee (who is also motivated and empowered) is equipped with correct information that enables him or her to make a wise decision for the organization. When this occurs, decision makers at any level throughout the organization make wise, vision-seeking decisions that can be implemented. In short, *organizational wisdom* is produced through a thoughtful and active knowledge management strategy that has a defined component of learning and innovation that can be followed at the subordinate level.

As new methods of organizational development, training, and knowledge management are created, the range of options to develop strategies, deliver outcomes, and evaluate these systems will increase. This will pro-

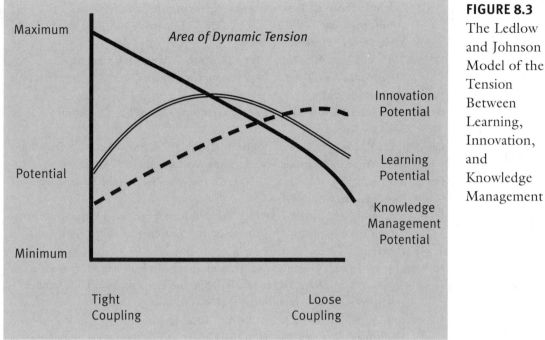

FIGURE 8.3

The Ledlow and Johnson Model of the Tension Between Learning, Innovation, and Knowledge Management

vide trainers and training departments with even more tools. However, until our full appreciation of human learning and learning-friendly environments is inculcated into our organizational cultures, these tools and techniques will have only marginal benefit. Ultimately learning organizations are those that "liberate the human spirit' (Bickham 1996) to achieve and accomplish creatively. The organization's goals are aligned with the individual's goals, and both entities work in unison to improve performance. Growth and learning become a continuous process that is rewarded and recognized for its value. Organizational development, training, and knowledge management then become vehicles designed to enhance the individual, the organization, and the communities served.[2]

References

Bennis, W. 1969. *Organization Development.* Reading MA: Addison-Wesley.

Bickham, W. 1996. *Liberating the Human Spirit in the Workplace.* Chicago: Irwin.

Blanchard, P. N., and J. W. Thacker. 1999. *Effective Training Systems, Strategies, and Practices.* Upper Saddle River, NJ: Prentice Hall.

Bramley, P. 1996. *Evaluating Training Effectiveness.* New York: McGraw-Hill.

Fried, B. 1999. "Human Resources Management." In *Handbook of Health Administration and Policy*, edited by A. Kilpatrick and J. Johnson. New York: Marcel Dekker.

Friesen, M., and J. A. Johnson. 1996. *The Success Paradigm: Creating Organizational Effectiveness Through Quality and Strategy*. Westport, CT: Quorum Books.

Goldstein, I. L. 1993. *Training in Organizations, 4th Edition*. Monterey, CA: Brooks-Cole.

Gordon, E., E. Morgan, and J. Ponticell. 1995. "The Individualized Training Alternative." *Training and Development Journal* 18 (9): 52–60.

Isaacs, S. L, and J. R. Knickman. 2001. *To Improve Health and Healthcare 2001*. San Francisco: Jossey-Bass.

Jelinek, M., and J. A. Litterer. 1995. "Toward Entrepreneurial Organizations: Meeting Ambiguity with Engagement." *Entrepreneurship: Theory and Practice* 19 (3): 137–69.

Johnson, J. A. 1996. "Organization Development in Healthcare Organizations." *Organization Development Journal*. See the Organization Development Institute at http://members.aol.com/ODInst.

Johnson, J. A., and V. Omachanu. 1999. "Total Quality Management as Healthcare Strategy." In *Handbook of Health Administration and Policy*, edited by A. Kilpatrick and J. Johnson. New York: Marcel Dekker.

Kent, T., J. A. Johnson, and D. A. Graber. 1996. "Leadership in the Formation of New Healthcare Environments." *Healthcare Supervisor* 15 (2): 28–29.

Kilpatrick, A. O., and J. A. Johnson. 1999. *Handbook of Health Administration and Policy*. New York: Marcel Dekker

Ledlow, G., R., D. M. Bradshaw, and C. Shockley. 2000. "Primary Care Access Improvement: An Empowerment-Interaction Model." *Military Medicine* 165 (2): 390–95.

Ledlow, G., M. Cwiek, and J. A. Johnson. 2002. "Dynamic Culture Leadership: Effective Leader as Both Scientist and Artist." In *Beyond Boundaries: Challenges of Leadership, Innovation, Integration and Technology*, edited by N. Delener and C. Chao, 694–740. Global Business and Technology Association International Conference.

Locke, E. A. 1968. "Toward a Theory of Task Motivation and Incentives." *Organizational Behavior and Human Performance* 3 (May): 157–89.

———. 1986. *Generalizing from Laboratory to Field Settings*. Lexington, MA: Lexington Books.

Locke, E. A., M. E. Gist, and M. S. Taylor. 1987. "Organizational Behavior: Group Structure, Process, and Effectiveness." *Journal of Management* 13 (2): 237–57.

Locke, E. A., and G. P. Latham. 1984. *Goal Setting, A Motivational Technique That Works!* Englewood Cliffs, NJ: Prentice-Hall.

Locke, E. A., K. N. Shaw, L. M. Saari, and G. P. Latham. 1981. "Goal Setting and Task Performance: 1969–1980." *Psychological Bulletin* 90 (1): 125–52.

McIlwain, T., and J. A. Johnson. 1999. "Strategy: Planning, Management and Critical Success Factors." In *Handbook of Health Administration and Policy*, edited by A. Kilpatrick and J. A. Johnson. New York: Marcel Dekker.

Neese, O. E. 2002. "A Strategic Systems Perspective of Organizational Learning: Development of a Process Model Linking Theory and Practice." In *Managing the Human Side of Information Technology: Challenges and Solutions*, edited by E. Szewczak & C. Snodgrass, Chapter 8. Hershey, PA: Idea Group Publishing.

Schein, E. H. 1999. *The Corporate Culture Survival Guide: Sense and Nonsense About Culture Change*. San Francisco: Jossey-Bass.

Senge, P. 1990. *The Fifth Discipline: The Art and Practice of the Learning Organization*. New York: Doubleday.

Tobin, D. R. 1998. *The Knowledge-Enabled Organization*. New York: American Management Association.

Van de Ven, A. H., and M. S. Poole. 1995. "Explaining Development and Change in Organizations." *Academy of Management Review* 20 (3): 510–41.

Notes

1. The address for further information and the international directory of services and members for the Organization Development Institute is O.D. Institute, 11234 Walnut Ridge Road, Chesterland, OH 44026-1299.

2. A good resource for organizational learning and knowledge management is Szewczak, E., and C. Snodgrass (eds.). 2002. *Managing the Human Side of Information Technology: Challenges and Solutions*. Hershey, PA: Idea Group Publishing.

Discussion Questions

1. Design a mock training program for a clinical unit of a hospital. Include training objectives and methods.

2. Describe an example of successful organizational development. What elements accounted for its success? How was the success measured? How was it sustained?

Experiential Exercise

Case   The leadership team of your organization has determined that achieving three goals, which are vastly different from past objectives, are critical for organizational success and survival:

1. Increase employee and provider diversity to better represent the community population it serves.
2. Provide excellent customer and patient service and physician support.
3. Improve the use of technology in both clinical and administrative areas of the operation.

The vision of the organization is linked to these goals: To become a healthcare organization of choice in the region by providing technologically superior healthcare, excellent patient service to customers, superior support to our physicians, and staff and caregivers who represent and celebrate the diversity of the community.

Case Questions

1. What organizational development strategies should be used by the leadership team? Changing the organizational culture clearly can contribute toward these goals. Organizational development, training, and knowledge management strategies can assist in accomplishing the changes necessary. Knowledge management is also useful in enabling the organization to be an excellent patient-service institution in that it captures patient information, which alerts staff and caregivers to the patient's service expectations, needs, and preferences such as for a private or semi-private room or for beans or broccoli.
2. How can frontline receptionists contribute toward these organizational goals? How will their culture, responsibilities, training needs, and skills change to meet expectations of the new vision? What new KSAs will they need to work with and serve diverse customers, to better support physicians, and to be proficient in more advanced technological systems?
3. How will you employ the concepts presented in this chapter to devise a planned strategy that will allow the organization to meet its new vision?

PERFORMANCE MANAGEMENT

Bruce J. Fried, Ph.D.

Learning Objectives

After completing this chapter, the reader should be able to

- define performance management, and describe the key components of a performance management system;
- discuss the reasons that organizations engage in performance management;
- identify the characteristics of good rating criteria for performance appraisal;
- enumerate various sources of information about job performance, and discuss the strengths and shortcomings of each;
- address the three types of information needed to assess employee performance;
- distinguish between rating errors and political factors as sources of distortion in performance appraisal; and
- conduct a performance-appraisal interview with an employee, taking into consideration the techniques that make such an interview successful.

Introduction

A central theme of this book is that the performance of individual employees is central to the long-term success of an organization. Human resources management (HRM) functions' ultimate goal is to enable high performance from individuals and teams. Selection, compensation, supervisory, and training procedures all have the ultimate goal of fostering high performance. *Performance management* comprises all of the organizational activities involved in managing employees, including measuring performance. Performance management can be viewed as a tool for evaluating and improving individual performance but also as a way to assess the success of other HRM functions. A well-functioning performance management system can provide insight into how effectively we select employees, whether our training is effective, and whether an incentive compensation system is successful in meeting its performance goals.

This chapter addresses performance management—a set of tools and practices that comprises setting performance goals with employees, monitoring employee progress toward achieving those goals, coaching by supervisors, and measuring individual performance. The term performance appraisal is often used to describe this process, but that term tends to limit the process to measurement. Performance management is more encompassing and includes improvement strategies as well as measurement.

Performance management makes sense. The adage "you can't manage what you can't measure" is very applicable to performance management. However, performance management has a well-deserved reputation for being very poorly implemented. It is perhaps the most misunderstood and misused HRM function. Measuring and improving employee performance is also among the most highly examined aspects of management, both in scholarly works and in the popular press. Perhaps because it has met with so much failure, it is also one of the areas of management most prone to passing fads, which have been widely adopted in the popular management literature and by countless consulting firms that seek to identify and promote the quick fix to improve employee productivity.

In this chapter, we describe the essential components of performance management and present the countless pitfalls in virtually every aspect of this process. To the extent possible, we avoid the jargon and fashions that come and go and maintain a focus on those structures and processes that are most likely to lead to improved employee performance. Specifically, we explore the following:

- reasons that organizations develop and implement performance management systems;
- the terms performance criteria, criterion deficiency, criterion contamination, reliability, and validity;
- sources of information about employee performance;
- the applicability of 360-degree performance appraisal;
- performance appraisal information based on individual traits, behaviors, and outcomes;
- advantages and disadvantages of common formats for collecting and summarizing performance appraisal information;
- common sources of errors and other problems in performance appraisal; and
- guidelines for conducting effective performance management interviews.

Every manager seeks to have employees who are highly motivated and productive. This is a challenging goal for a number of reasons. First, employee motivation is in itself a complex phenomenon and is influenced by many things outside of the manager's control. Second, whether or not managerial interventions are effective in improving performance is unclear. For instance, compensation clearly has some motivational potential for most employees, but money is not an effective motivator in all circumstances. In healthcare organizations with very small margins, the availability of performance-based rewards tends to be very limited. Third, employee performance is often difficult to observe and measure in a reliable manner, as the process involves multiple factors and organizations have developed systems to improve performance.

A performance management system monitors, measures, reports, improves, and rewards employee performance. As noted earlier, a performance management system does more than measure performance; it also includes procedures to feed performance information back to employees and to train and develop employees to perform at higher levels. As with all HRM functions, performance management activities are carried out within a legal context in that they consider how employment, equal employment opportunity, and labor-relations laws affect how performance management procedures are designed and implemented.

The Role of Performance Management

Performance management is a system that integrates the performance appraisal function with other human resources systems to help align employees' work behaviors with the organization's goals (Fisher, Schoenfeldt, and Shaw 2003). One of the most common misperceptions about performance management is that it focuses almost exclusively on the annual appraisal. Annual appraisals are necessary, but performance management is part of supervision that is carried out on a daily basis. An effective supervisor provides feedback continuously and addresses and manages performance problems when they occur. Performance management is an ongoing function that includes the following steps by managers:

1. Set performance goals and make development plans with the employee.
2. Monitor the employee's progress toward the goals.
3. Provide continual coaching and training/education as necessary.
4. Monitor the employee's performance progress.
5. Conduct annual performance appraisal against goals and development-plan activities, and establish a plan for next year (or other review cycle).

The annual appraisal may result in personnel decisions such as a promotion, change in compensation, disciplinary action, transfer, or recommendation for training. A performance management system typically requires defining performance, establishing a performance appraisal process, designing methods to measure performance, and developing a process for providing feedback and coaching (Fisher, Schoenfeldt, and Shaw 2003).

As illustrated in Table 9.1, performance management is highly interrelated with other HRM functions in that its activities affect and are affected by all other HRM activities. As such, for a performance management system to be effective, it must be integrated with other HRM functions.

Performance Appraisal

Organizations engage in performance management for a number of reasons, including the following:

1. To give employees the opportunity to discuss performance and performance standards regularly with their supervisors and managers
2. To provide managers the opportunity to identify strengths and weaknesses of employees
3. To provide a venue for managers to identify and recommend strategies for employees to improve performance
4. To provide a basis for personnel decisions such as compensation, promotion, and termination
5. To comply with regulatory requirements

A key element of performance management is performance appraisal. *Performance appraisal* is a formal system of periodic review and evaluation of an individual or team's performance. Remember that the collection of performance information is only one, albeit important, aspect of performance management.

In the healthcare environment, the Joint Commission on Accreditation of Healthcare Organizations (JCAHO 2003) requires accredited healthcare organizations to assess, track, and improve the competence of all employees (Decker, Strader, and Wise 1997). The 2004 JCAHO standards state that accredited healthcare organizations must provide evidence that "competence to perform job responsibilities is assessed, demonstrated and maintained" (HR. 3.10) and that "the organization periodically conducts performance evaluations" (HR. 3.20) (JCAHO 2003).

The requirements for healthcare organizations of the prestigious Baldrige National Quality Program (2004) include specific criteria for the

TABLE 9.1

Relationship
of
Performance
Management
to Other
Human
Resources
Management
Functions

HRM Function	Effects of Performance Management	Effects on Performance Management
Job analysis	Performance information may lead to redesign of jobs	Accurate information about jobs is key to develop criteria for performance appraisal
Recruitment and selection	Performance information lets managers know about the effectiveness of alternative sources of recruitment and the effectiveness of their selection criteria and procedures	Ability to recruit and select employees may affect the types of criteria and standards developed for performance appraisal
Training and development	Performance management systems provide information on employees' training and development needs; information on the performance appraisal systems assesses the effectiveness of training	Performance appraisal tools may be designed to assess the impact of training programs
Compensation	Compensation systems may be designed such that performance appraisal information has an impact on employee compensation	A fair and equitable compensation system may lead to higher levels of employee performance

TABLE 9.1 Relationship of Performance Management to Other Human Resources Management Functions

need for a performance management system with questions such as, "How does your staff performance management system, including feedback to staff, support high-performance work? How does your staff performance management system support a patient/customer and health care service focus?"

Use of performance appraisal can generally be broken down into two: administrative and developmental. Administrative purposes commonly relate to using performance information to make decisions about promotion and termination as well as compensation. To defend against charges of discrimination, organizations attempt to maintain accurate and current performance appraisal information on employees. Developmental purposes typically relate to using performance information to improve employee performance; appraisal information identifies employee strengths and weaknesses, which then become the basis for developing improvement strategies. Organizations can, of course, use appraisals for both administrative and developmental purposes. However, there is considerable debate about whether or not a manager or supervisor can actually conduct an honest developmental appraisal, considering that the results of the evaluation have an impact on the employee's income, promotion potential, and other bread-and-butter issues. This concern relates directly to the debate on whether or not linking pay with performance is the right thing to do, or whether it has an adverse impact on coaching and employee development.

The traditional assumption is that all levels of employees in the organization need a performance appraisal. However, some suggest that appraisal is not necessary for employees at certain levels (such as chief executive officers or senior leaders) and that the process may even be demeaning for these employees. Evidence in the literature indicates that the higher the position of an employee, the less likely that person will receive a performance appraisal. Appraisals conducted with employees at senior levels are usually poorly and haphazardly done. However, strong evidence also exists that indicates that executive-level employees have a strong desire to obtain information about their performance (Longenecker and Gioia 1992). The bottom line is that performance appraisal and performance management are for everyone in the organization. As discussed later, the types of performance information obtained may vary according to an employee's level and role in the organization.

Establishing Appraisal Criteria

As is the case with many other HRM activities, an effective performance management system must begin with clear job expectations and performance standards. Of particular importance is the need for managers and employees to agree on the content of the job description and to have a shared understanding of job expectations.

Once the job description and performance standards have been agreed on, employees and managers together must lay out the specific criteria by which performance will be evaluated. *Performance criteria* are measurable standards used for assessing employee performance. These criteria need to be job related and relevant to the needs of the organization. The development of criteria is a challenging task and requires the collaboration between the employee and the manager. Such criteria must be agreed on well in advance of a formal performance appraisal interview.

How should performance criteria be defined? What are useful criteria? First, criteria should have strategic relevance to the organization as a whole. For example, if patient satisfaction is an important organizational concern, then it makes sense to include patient-relations criteria for employees who interact with these customers. Criteria for individual performance appraisal are in many ways an extension of criteria used to evaluate organizational performance.

Second, criteria should be comprehensive and take into consideration the full range of an employee's functions as defined in the job description. *Criterion deficiency* occurs when performance standards focus on a single criterion to the exclusion of other important but less quantifiable performance dimensions (Barrett 1995; Sherman, Bohlander, and Snell 1998). For example, counting the number of visits made by a home care nurse may be relatively simple, but it is certainly more difficult (but no less important) to assess the quality of care provided during those visits.

Third, criteria should be free from contamination. *Criterion contamination* occurs when factors out of the employee's control influence his or her performance. In healthcare, this is a particular problem because of the complexity of patient care and the interdependence of the factors that affect patient care and clinical outcomes. Clinicians, for example, may have little control over patient volume or the speed with which laboratory test results are reported. Therefore, appraisal criteria should include only those items over which the employee has control.

Fourth, criteria should be reliable and valid. Reliability refers to the consistency with which a manager rates an employee in successive ratings (assuming consistent performance) or the consistency with which two or more managers rate performance when they have comparable information. Criteria can be made more reliable by selecting objective criteria and by training managers in applying the criteria. Validity is the extent to which appraisal criteria actually measure the performance dimension of interest. For example, if we are interested in measuring a nurse's ability to carry out the nursing role during emergency medical procedures, is it sufficient to assess knowledge of the role rather than performance under real emergency conditions? Questions of validity are also difficult when measuring attitudes deemed important for a particular job.

Collecting Job Performance Data

Traditional performance appraisal methods involve collecting information from the employee's supervisor. Typically, the supervisor observes the employee's performance using whatever format the organization has designed for performance appraisal (described later in this chapter) and records the appraisal information. Given the complexity of many jobs, however, it is often impossible for one individual to accurately describe each employee's performance. In recent years, a variety of alternative approaches to the collection of job performance data have come forth.

A *self-appraisal* is an evaluation done by the employee on himself or herself; it is generally done in conjunction with the manager's appraisal. This approach is very effective when a manager is seeking to obtain the involvement of the employee in the appraisal process. Because of the obvious potential for bias on the part of the employee, self-appraisals are almost always done for developmental rather than administrative purposes.

There are occasions when managers are concerned with how their performance is perceived by those whom they oversee. In this instance, the managers may ask for a *subordinate appraisal*, in which direct reports conduct an evaluation of their boss. This type is most useful for developmental purposes. Subordinate appraisal presents many benefits, among which are identifying the "blind spots" of managers and improving managerial performance. From the subordinate's perspective, this type of appraisal has obvious risks, as not all managers may take kindly to critiques and opinions and may retaliate toward the evaluator. Thus, such appraisals should be done anonymously; where this is not possible, the appraisal is unlikely to yield reliable results.

Team-based appraisal is beneficial in that it explicitly encourages teamwork—an important element in healthcare, where work is highly interrelated and interdependent. Team-based appraisal requires the identification of team goals and criteria for assessment. The assumption is that each team member will contribute to achieving team goals. This could become problematic as team member roles change and as members leave and new members join. Organizations may link team performance with pay, although it is not necessarily a component of team-based appraisal. This may exacerbate anxieties and frustrations with the "free-rider" syndrome, where one (or more) team members benefit from team rewards without putting forth corresponding effort. In using team-based appraisal, with or without compensation, it is critical that team members agree on behavioral- and outcome-based appraisal criteria.

Team members may also be involved in assessing the performance of other team members. This approach has the potential for building team cohesion and enhancing communication. Several questions need to be addressed, including the manner in which team members are involved in appraisals: Are all team members involved in appraising every other team member? Who should provide the feedback to members? While this approach may help build teams, there is also the risk of alienation and conflict if feedback is provided in a divisive manner. Therefore, whoever is selected to provide the feedback should be trained in interviewing and feedback techniques.

Perhaps the most useful form of appraisal is one that takes advantage of multiple sources of information about employee performance. Termed *360-degree appraisal* (or multirater assessment), this approach recognizes the fact that for many jobs, relying on one source of performance data is inadequate. To obtain a comprehensive assessment of performance, the perspectives of individuals from multiple levels of the organization must be solicited, including the manager or supervisor, peers, subordinates, clients, and even individuals external to the organization. This type of appraisal is typically done for developmental purposes, but it must be designed and administered with great care. A 360-degree appraisal can certainly be combined with other methods, and the benefits to the individual and organization are numerous (see Figure 9.1).

Regardless of where performance information comes from (supervisor, coworkers, and so forth), decisions need to be made about the types of information to be obtained in performance appraisals. In general, three types of information are possible:

1. Individual traits
2. Behaviors
3. Results or outcomes

Each of these three types of information can be obtained using the various methods explored in the following section. Each approach has its strengths and shortcomings and is useful for particular types of jobs and circumstances.

Graphic rating scales are any rating scale that uses points along a continuum and that may measure traits or behaviors (Cascui 1991). Graphic rating scales are the most common format used to assess performance, largely because they are easy to construct and can be used for many different types of employees. As shown in the example in Figure 9.2, such a scale aims to measure a series of dimensions through anchor points (i.e., 1 through 6) that indicate different levels of effectiveness. In this instance, both traits and behaviors of the employee are presented to be assessed. Note, however, that many of the items included in the figure, such as flexibility, are prone to subjective judgment.

Graphic Rating Scales

One of the drawbacks of graphic rating scales is that they are quite general, often not representing specific behaviors that illustrate positive or negative aspects of performance. The scale frequently does not yield information on how any item can be changed because the questions and statements for the behaviors or traits being rated are general. Because of this subjectivity, raters may be uncomfortable using this method of appraisal, particularly when ratings are linked with compensation. As discussed below, graphic rating scales can be improved by the use of behaviorally anchored rating scales. Specific behaviors are associated with each scale.

Perhaps the most important drawback of graphic rating scales is that they typically do not weight behaviors and traits according to their importance to a particular job. In Figure 9.2, for example, pace of work (ques-

FIGURE 9.1
Advantages of
Using 360-
Degree
Feedback

1. Defines corporate competencies.

2. Increases the focus on customer service.

3. Supports team initiatives.

4. Creates a high-involvement workforce.

5. Decreases hierarchies; promotes streamlining.

6. Detects barriers to success.

7. Assesses developmental needs.

8. Avoids discrimination and bias.

9. Identifies performance thresholds.

10. Is easy to implement.

Source: Adapted from Hoffman, R. 1995. "Ten Reasons You Should Be Using 360-Degree Feedback." *HR Magazine* (April): 82–85.

tion 1) may be extremely relevant to the job of some employees but relatively unimportant to others. Thus, ratings on this question may be irrelevant to the actual work performed. Another undesirable practice in using graphic rating scales is when an organization simply imports a scale used by another organization without giving consideration to the applicability of the scale to the organization or to its particular jobs.

Ranking   This method is used by a manager to rank employees from worst to best on an overall criterion of employee performance. Such a method is typically employed for administrative purposes, such as making personnel decisions on promotions and layoffs. The major advantages of the ranking method are that it forces supervisors to distinguish among employees and it does not have many of the problems associated with other appraisal methods. Among the disadvantages of ranking are as follows:

*   Focuses only on a single dimension of work effectiveness and may not take into account the complexity of work situations
*   Becomes cumbersome with large numbers of employees, forcing appraisers to artificially distinguish among employees
*   Simply lists employees in order of their performance but does not indicate the relative differences in employees' effectiveness
*   Provides no guidance on specific deficiencies in employee performance and therefore is not useful in helping employees improve

FIGURE 9.2

Example of
a Graphic
Rating Scale

Please answer the following questions about this employee.

Question	Scale
1. Rate this person's pace of work.	1 2 3 4 5 6 slow fast
2. Assess this person's level of effort.	1 2 3 4 5 6 below full capacity capacity
3. What is the quality of this person's work?	1 2 3 4 5 6 poor good
4. How flexible is this person?	1 2 3 4 5 6 rigid flexible
5. How open is this person to new ideas?	1 2 3 4 5 6 closed open
6. How much supervision does this person need?	1 2 3 4 5 6 a lot a little
7. How readily does this person offer to help out by doing work outside his or her normal scope of work?	1 2 3 4 5 6 seldom often
8. How well does this person get along with peers?	1 2 3 4 5 6 not very well well

One type of ranking that has come under a great deal of criticism is the process of *forced ranking*, or forced distribution. With this type of ranking, employees are not evaluated based on their own set of objectives but in comparison to other employees. Managers are instructed to force evaluations of employee performance into a particular distribution, which is similar to grading students "on a curve." For example, managers may be directed to distribute 15 percent of employees as high performers, 20 percent as moderately high, 30 percent as average, 20 percent as low average, and 15 percent as poor. Forced ranking has been rationalized in a number of ways: it has been used to (1) ensure that lenient managers do not systematically inflate appraisals, (2) push managers to distribute their rankings, and (3) limit bonuses and other financial payouts. Although these three uses have achieved their objectives, they corrupt the entire purpose of performance appraisal—to obtain honest information that can be used to development and implement improvement.

The most controversial use of forced distribution is as a way to force out poor performers, sometimes referred to as "rank or yank." For example, employees may be told that if they are in the lowest 15 percent of performers in two consecutive years, they will be terminated. At General Electric, supervisors identify the top 20 percent and the bottom 10 percent of managerial and professional employees every year; the bottom 10 percent are unlikely to stay (Abelson 2001). Lawsuits have been filed at companies such as Ford Motor Company and Goodyear to challenge the legality of this approach, claiming that the process discriminates against older workers. Interestingly, Ford abandoned forced distribution in 2001 and settled two class-action cases for about $10.5 million (Bates 2003).

Ranking employees for the purpose of deciding whom to let go is not performance management; rather, it is a method of distinguishing which employees to terminate at times of financial need. When this approach is used, it likely tarnishes and lessens the value of the overall performance management system.

Behavioral Anchored Rating Scales

Behavioral anchored rating scales (BARS) are a significant improvement over traditional graphic rating scales. A BARS provides specific behavioral descriptions of the different levels of employee performance—that is, poor, good, excellent, and so forth. Figure 9.3 is an example of a BARS that measures the performance of a nurse on the dimension of "patient relations." Using BARS, a manager is able to explain the reason behind the ratings, rather than vaguely state "unacceptable" or "average" on the performance criteria. With BARS, a manager can explicitly state his or her expectations for improved performance.

Among the advantages of BARS are as follows:

- Reduces rating errors because job dimensions are clearly defined for the rater and are relevant to the job being performed
- Clearly defines the response categories available to the rater
- Is more reliable, valid, meaningful, and complete
- Has a higher degree of acceptance and commitment from employees and supervisors
- Minimizes employee defensiveness and conflict with manager because employees are appraised on the basis of observable behavior
- Improves a manager's ability to identify areas for training and development

Developing a BARS for each job dimension for a particular job is not a trivial task. Among the disadvantages of BARS is the amount of time, effort, and expense involved in its development. Use of this approach is

FIGURE 9.3

A Behavioral
Anchored
Rating Scale
for the
Patient-
Relations
Dimension

Rating	Behavioral Description
Excellent	1. Employee always treats patients with dignity and cheerfulness, respecting their individual needs while performing professional duties. Employee receives frequent favorable comments from patients under his or her care.
Good	2. Employee treats patients with dignity and respect without becoming involved in their individual problems. Employee receives occasional favorable comments from patients.
Average	3. Employee is impersonal with patients, tending to their medical needs but avoiding personal interaction. Employee is the subject of few comments by patients.
Poor	4. Employee becomes impatient with patients and is concerned more about performing his or her tasks than being of assistance to patient's nonmedical needs. Employee generates some complaints from patients.
Unacceptable	5. Employee is antagonistic toward patients, treating them as obstacles or annoyances rather than individuals. Employee generates frequent complaints from patients and causes them considerable distress.

Source: Bushardt, S. C., and A. R. Fowler. 1988. "Performance Evaluation Alternatives." *Journal of Nursing Administration* 18 (10): 40–44.

most justifiable when there is a large number of jobholders for the same position. Finally, the use of BARS is most appropriate for jobs whose major components consist of physically observable behaviors.

A variation of BARS is the *behavioral observation scale* (BOS), a system that asks the rater to indicate the frequency with which the employee exhibits highly desirable behaviors. Desirable behaviors are identified through job analysis and discussions with managers and supervisors. Figure 9.4 is an example of a BOS for a manager for the performance dimension of overcoming resistance to change. As seen in the figure, six desirable behaviors are associated with this performance dimension, and the scale allows the rater to select the frequency appropriate for each item. As with the BARS approach, users of the BOS have a clear understanding of the types of behaviors expected.

**Behavioral
Observation
Scales**

FIGURE 9.4

A Behavioral
Observation
Scale for the
Overcoming
Resistance to
Change
Dimension

Item	Scale				
	Almost Never				Almost Always
1. Describes the details of change to subordinates.	1	2	3	4	5
2. Explains why the change is necessary.	1	2	3	4	5
3. Discusses how the change will affect the employee.	1	2	3	4	5
4. Listens to the employee's concerns.	1	2	3	4	5
5. Asks the employee for help in making the change work.	1	2	3	4	5
6. If necessary, specifies the date for a follow-up meeting to respond to the employee's concerns.	1	2	3	4	5

Source: Latham, G. P., and K. N. Wexley. 1994. Increasing *Productivity Through Performance Appraisal, 2nd Edition.* Reading, MA: Addison-Wesley.

Critical Incidents

Critical incident is a record of unusually favorable or unfavorable occurrences in an employee's work. This record is created and maintained by the employee's manager. A major strength of this method is that it provides a factual record of an employee's performance and can be very useful in subsequent discussions with the employee. The approach does require that the manager closely and continuously monitor employee performance, which is not always feasible, although linking a critical incident method with 360-degree feedback raises the possibility that incidents may be observed and recorded by a number of different individuals in the organization. Documentation of critical incidents need not be very lengthy, but it should be tied to an important performance dimension. An example of a critical incident for a mental health case manager is given below. This incident illustrates the employee's creativity and negotiation skills, an important performance dimension:

> In speaking with her client—an individual with severe mental disorder—the case manager discovered that the client was about to be evicted from her apartment for nonpayment of rent. She was able to work with the client and the landlord to work out a payment plan and to negotiate successfully with the landlord to have

much-needed repairs in the apartment done. She followed up with the client weekly regarding payment to the landlord and the home repairs, and positive outcomes have been achieved in both areas.

Management by Objectives

Management by objective (MBO) refers to a specific technique that has enjoyed substantial popularity. The basic premise of MBO is threefold: (1) the organization defines its strategic goals for the year, (2) these goals are then communicated throughout the organization, and (3) each employee in turn defines his or her goals for year based on the organizational goals. Achievement of these goals becomes the standard by which each employee's performance is assessed (Carroll and Tosi 1973).

MBO has three key characteristics (Odiorne 1986):

1. It establishes specific and objectively measurable goals for employees.
2. It establishes goals in collaboration with employees.
3. It allows managers to provide objective feedback and coaching to improve employee performance.

As with most managerial practices, MBO is most effective when it is supported by and has the commitment of senior management. MBO requires managers to obtain substantial training in goal setting, giving feedback, and coaching. While goal setting is central to MBO, the process by which goals are set is of great importance as well.

Depending on the position of the jobholder, organizations may use a variety of results-oriented methods such as the MBO. Such approaches are most useful when the work yields objectively measurable outcomes. MBO is most commonly used for senior executive positions (where objectively measurable bottom line concerns may be paramount), salespeople, and sports teams and individual athletes. The approach may be combined with other performance appraisal methods, particularly for jobs in which both the manner in which work is done and the outcomes are important and measurable.

The Cynicism About Performance Appraisal

Many managers and employees are quite cynical about performance management. This cynicism grows out of a belief that nobody likes performance appraisals: Managers are uncomfortable sitting down and discussing issues with employees, and employees may resent the paternalism and condescension that often accompany performance appraisals. This cynicism is clearly based in the reality that performance appraisals are traditionally punitive in nature and, particularly when tightly tied to employee compensation, have high emotional content.

Regardless of the type of data used in performance appraisal, there continue to persist what social psychologists call "rating errors." *Rating errors* refer simply to distortions in performance appraisal ratings—whether positive or negative—that reduce the accuracy of appraisals. The most common rating errors are as follows:

- *Distributional errors* come from the tendency of raters to use only a small part of the rating scale. These errors come in three forms:
  1. *Leniency:* some raters tend to be overly generous with giving positive ratings, and in being such they avoid conflict and confrontation with the employees being assessed.
  2. *Strictness:* some raters tend to be overly critical of performance, and in being such their ratings are deemed unfair when compared with the ratings given by managers without such a tendency.
  3. *Central tendency:* some raters tend to rate every employee as average, and in being such they avoid conflict.
- *Halo effect errors* result from the propensity of some raters to rate employees high (or low) on all evaluation criteria, without distinguishing between different aspects of the employee's work. This leads to evaluations that may be overly critical or overly generous.
- *Personal bias errors* arise because of some raters' tendency to rate employees higher or lower than is deserved because of the rater's personal like or dislike of the employee (Wexley and Nemeroff 1974).
- *Similar-to-me bias errors* stem from the likelihood of some raters to judge those who are similar to them more highly than those who are not. Research shows that the strongest impact of similarity occurs when manager and employee share demographic characteristics such as race and age group (Noe et al. 1996).
- *Contrast effect errors* are created when raters compare employees with each other rather than use objective standards for job performance.

The most important strategy for overcoming these rating errors is training. This typically helps to increase managers' familiarity with the rating scales and the specific level of performance associated with different points on these scales. The objective is to increase each manager's consistency in using rating scales and to improve the interrater reliability among managers. Training also typically focuses on minimizing managers' error rate. At a minimum, managers need to be aware of potential rating errors in performance appraisal. Strategies may be offered to help managers both identify their errors and develop strategies to avoid making errors in appraisal. For example, managers may avoid distributional errors by improving their awareness of the appraisal tool and their understanding of the objective standards used to evaluate performance. Of course, the success of training efforts is contingent on the existence of valid and reliable assessment instruments and clear performance standards.

Even with extensive training and well-tested appraisal tools, the "politics of performance appraisal" (Longenecker, Sims, and Gioia 1987) can rear its ugly head. Political considerations affect the appraisals given to particular employees. For example, managers are well aware of the fact that after an appraisal is completed, they must in most cases continue to work with their employees. Thus, many managers are lenient, believing that a negative appraisal will tarnish their relationship with their subordinates and perhaps hurt team dynamics and productivity. Many managers may also feel that a negative appraisal has a negative impact on an employee's career, or more immediately, on the employee's finances. One manager verbalizes the politics behind appraisals:

> "The mere fact that you have to write out your assessment and create a permanent record will cause people not to be as honest or as accurate as they should be. . . . We soften the language because our ratings go in the guy's file downstairs [the Personnel Department] and it will follow him around his whole career" (Longenecker, Sims, and Gioia 1987).

As a result of these and other pressures, managers may artificially inflate or deflate an employee's appraisal. Table 9.2 provides a summary of the political reasons that managers distort the assessment of an employee's true performance. Note that these problems with performance appraisal accuracy are more difficult to deal with than the errors discussed earlier, because these problems are deeply rooted in the organization and in the relationship between the manager and the employee.

Conducting Effective Performance Management Interviews

As noted earlier, the ultimate objective of a performance management system is to improve employee performance. Because performance management has historically focused on its evaluation or measurement aspects, relatively little attention has been given to its improvement aspects.

A key step in the improvement process is providing performance information to the employee. Many managers are reluctant to provide feedback because of the fear of confrontation and conflict. These are real concerns for both managers and employees, given most employees' experiences with performance management. In informal surveys we conduct with our

TABLE 9.2

Reasons Managers Inflate or Deflate a Performance Appraisal

Reasons to Inflate	Reasons to Deflate
Maximize merit increases for an employee, particularly when the merit ceiling is considered low	Shock an employee back on to a higher performance track
Avoid hanging dirty laundry out in public if the appraisal information is viewed by outsiders	Teach a rebellious employee a lesson
	Send a message to an employee that he or she should think about leaving the organization
Avoid creating a written record of poor performance that would become a permanent part of the individual's personnel file	Build a strongly documented record of poor performance that may speed up the termination process
Avoid confrontation with an employee with whom the manager had recently had difficulties	Promote an undesirable employee "up and out" of the organization
Give a break to a subordinate who had shown improvements	

Source: Adapted from C. O. Longenecker, H. P. Sims, and D. A. Gioia. 1987. "Behind the Mask: The Politics of Employee Appraisal." *The Academy of Management Executive* 1 (3): 183–93.

students, we typically learn that the great majority of them either rarely have a performance evaluation or have had a poorly done evaluation. Finding someone who has had a well-implemented appraisal is rare.

Following are techniques for conducting better performance evaluations:

1. *Do appraisals on an ongoing basis.* Checking on how an employee is performing should be a regular occurrence, not just done during the formal appraisal process. Giving continuous feedback is, after all, a key responsibility for managers. By providing ongoing feedback, surprises at the formal appraisal can be avoided.

   The frequency of formal performance appraisals depends to some degree on an employee's performance. For a high-performing employee, an annual appraisal (as well as ongoing informal feedback) may be sufficient. Such appraisals are usually done to reward good work and to reinforce existing levels of performance. For an average performer, more frequent appraisals may be necessary to ensure that improvement goals are on track and will be achieved. For marginal or low-performing employees, formal appraisals may need to be held monthly (or perhaps even more often) to provide an opportunity for closer coaching.

2. *Prepare for the performance appraisal.* The manager should be equipped with data, have a strategy for presenting performance information, expect employee reactions, and be ready to engage in problem solving and planning with the employee. An appropriate physical location should be found, and relevant supporting information should be available.

3. *Encourage employee participation.* The employee should believe that the performance management process is something that will be beneficial to him or her. The literature refers to two traditional modes of presenting performance information. The *tell-and-sell method* involves the manager presenting (telling) performance ratings and then justifying (selling) the ratings and encouraging the employee to use a recommended strategy for improvement. This type of strategy may be useful in situations where the manager must be very clear about expectations, or it may work with young employees who may not yet be ready to engage in self-evaluation (Downs, Smeyak, and Martin 1980). It may also be useful with very loyal employees who are strongly committed to the organization.

   The *tell-and-listen method* involves presenting (telling) performance information and then hearing (listening) the employee's side of the story and the employee's ideas for improvement. This type of approach is most useful for employees with a strong need to participate in their jobs, with employees who are close in status to the interviewer, and with highly educated employees (Downs, Smeyak, and Martin 1980).

   The most promising approach to participation is the *problem-solving method*, in which the goal of the interview is to help the employee develop a plan for improvement. This involves a partnership between manager and employee and requires an atmosphere of respect and support. Strong empirical support exists for this approach, indicating that employees are consistently satisfied with this method (Cederblom 1982) and that participation in feedback and problem solving is a key predictor of job satisfaction (Giles and Mossholder 1990; Noe et al. 1996).

4. *Focus on future performance and problem solving.* While it is important to review past performance during an appraisal, the emphasis should be on setting goals for the future and on generating specific strategies for meeting those goals. In many cases, the employee will identify factors outside of his or her control that may contribute to lower-than-expected levels of performance. These are certainly appropriate to discuss during performance feedback sessions. Follow-up sessions should also be scheduled as appropriate.

5. *Focus on employee behavior or results, not the personality.* In almost all cases, the purpose of performance feedback is to help the employee improve his or her work, not to change as a person. The performance feedback interview is not the time to change an employee's values, personality, motivation, or fit with the organization. If these are true problems, they should have been considered during the selection process. The manager should focus on behaviors and outcomes, not the value of the person. Condescending criticisms and reciting a litany of employee problems are rarely useful and are more likely to generate defensiveness and resentment from the employee.

6. *Reinforce positive performance.* Performance appraisal interviews have gained the reputation for being punitive and negative. One of the most effective ways that a manager can ally oneself with an employee is to ensure that the interview focuses on all aspects of performance, not just the negative. Reinforcing positive performance is essential.

7. *Ensure that performance management is supported by senior managers.* The best way to destroy any effort at implementing a performance management system is for word to get out that senior management is either unsupportive or ambivalent about the system. Senior management must assert and communicate that performance management is important to meeting organizational goals and that it needs to be done at all levels of the organization. If this message is absent or weak, the performance management system will either fade away or become a meaningless bureaucratic exercise.

Summary

In the past ten years, an important transition has taken place—performance appraisal turned into performance management. Historically, performance appraisal focused primarily on judging employee behavior. The process was viewed as negative and punitive in nature and was generally avoided by both managers and employees. Performance management, however, implies an improvement-focused process in which efforts are made not only to assess performance but also to develop specific collaborative strategies to improve performance. Recognizing that employee performance results from an employee's skills, motivation, and facilitative factors in the work environment, improvement strategies may include training, work process redesign, and other changes that are both internal and external to the employee.

References

Abelson, R. 2001. "Companies Turn to Grades, and Employees Go to Court." *The New York Times* (March 19): A1, A12.

Baldrige National Quality Program. 2004. *Health Care Criteria for Performance Excellence*. Gaithersburg, MD: Baldrige National Quality Program.

Barrett, R. S. 1995. "Employee Selection with the Performance Priority Survey." *Personnel Psychology* 48 (3): 653–62.

Bates, S. 2003. "Forced Rankling." *HR Magazine* 48 (6): 62–68.

Bushardt, S. C., and A. R. Fowler. 1988. "Performance Evaluation Alternatives." *Journal of Nursing Administration* 18 (10): 40–44.

Carroll, S., and H. Tosi. 1973. *Management by Objectives*. New York: Macmillan.

Cascui, W. F. 1991. *Applied Psychology in Personnel Management*. Reston, VA: Reston Press.

Cederblom, D. 1982. "The Performance Appraisal Interview: Review, Implications, and Suggestions." *Academy of Management Review* 7 (2): 219–27.

Decker, P. J., M. K. Strader, and R. J. Wise. 1997. "Beyond JCAHO: Using Competency Models to Change Healthcare Organizations. Part 2: Developing Competence Assessment Systems." *Hospital Topics* 75 (2): 10–17.

Downs, C. W., G. P. Smeyak, and E. Martin. 1980. *Professional Interviewing*. New York: Harper & Row.

Fisher, C. D., L. F. Schoenfeldt, and J. B. Shaw. 2003. *Human Resource Management, 5th Edition*. Boston: Houghton Mifflin.

Giles, W. F., and K. W. Mossholder. 1990. "Employee Reactions to Contextual and Session Components of Performance Appraisal." *Journal of Applied Psychology* 75 (4): 371–77.

Hoffman, R. 1995. "Ten Reasons You Should Be Using 360-Degree Feedback." *HR Magazine* 40 (4): 82–85.

Joint Commission on Accreditation of Healthcare Organizations. 2003. *CAMH 2004 Comprehensive Accreditation Manual for Hospitals: The Official Handbook*. Oakbrook Terrace, IL: JCAHO.

Latham, G. P., and K. N. Wexley. 1994. *Increasing Productivity Through Performance Appraisal, 2nd Edition*. Reading, MA: Addison-Wesley.

Longenecker, C. O., and D. Gioia. 1992. "The Executive Appraisal Paradox." *The Academy of Management Executive* 5 (2): 25–35.

Longenecker, C. O., H. P. Sims, and D. A. Gioia. 1987. "Behind the Mask: The Politics of Employee Appraisal." *The Academy of Management Executive* 1 (3): 183–93.

Noe, R. A., J. R. Hollenbeck, B. Gerhart, and P. M. Wright. 1996. *Human Resource Management: Gaining a Competitive Advantage, 2nd Edition*. Boston: Irwin McGraw-Hill.

Odiorne, G. 1986. *MBO: II: A System of Managerial Leadership for the 80's*. Belmont, CA: Fearon Pitman Publishers.

Sherman, A., G. Bohlander, and S. Snell. 1998. *Managing Human Resources, 11th Edition.* Cincinnati, OH: South-Western College Publishing.

Wexley, K., and W. Nemeroff. 1974. "Effects of Racial Prejudice, Race of Applicants, and Biographical Similarity on Interview Evaluations of Job Applicants." *Journal of Social and Behavioral Sciences* 20 (1): 66–78.

Discussion Questions

1. What is the distinction between performance appraisal and performance management?
2. Why does the Joint Commission now require hospitals and other healthcare organizations to have performance management systems?
3. What is the relationship between performance management and continuous quality improvement?
4. What are the advantages and disadvantages to including discussions of compensation during a performance management interview?
5. What is the difference between performance appraisal rating errors and political factors that influence the accuracy of performance appraisal information?
6. How does a manager decide how often to conduct formal performance management interviews?
7. Why is employee participation in the performance management process important? Under what circumstances is employee participation not necessarily important?

Experiential Exercise

Case   Summit River Nursing Home (SRNH) is a 60-bed nursing home serving a suburban community in the midwest. The facility provides a broad range of services to residents, including recreational activities, clinical laboratory, dental services, dietary and housekeeping services, mental health and nursing services, occupational and physical therapies, pharmacy services, social services, and diagnostic x-ray services.

The facility has a good reputation in the community and is well staffed. Licensed practical nurses (LPNs) administer medications and perform certain treatment procedures. Each nursing home resident receives at least two hours of direct nursing care every day. Certified Nursing Assistants (CNAs) perform most of the direct patient care.

A dietary service supervisor manages the daily operations of the food service department along with a registered dietitian. Activity coordinators provide nonmedical care designed to improve cognitive and physical capabilities. There are two social workers on staff who work with residents, families, and other organizations. An important part of their role is to ease residents and their families' adjustment to the long-term care environment. They also help to identify residents' specific medical and emotional needs and provide support and referral services.

Environmental service workers maintain the facility with a goal of providing a clean and safe environment for residents. Housekeeping staff also have considerable contact with residents on a day-to-day basis. SRNH has contractual relationships with a dental practice, physical therapists, a pharmacist, a psychologist, and a multispecialty physician practice.

The management team of the facility consists of an administrator, finance director, human resources (HR) director, director of nursing, and administrative support personnel.

There has recently been concern about quality issues in the nursing home. There have been several instances of communication breakdowns among staff and several instances of medication errors. A recent resident satisfaction survey also revealed problems, of which management had been unaware. Some of the problems concern contract staff who have not been included in the organization's performance management process.

After discussions with management and employees, it was established that the team atmosphere among staff was lacking. Each member of the management team was asked to develop a strategy that might help to improve the level of teamwork occurring in the facility. The HR director agreed to take action in three areas:

1. Ensure that all job descriptions addressed teamwork and that these changes are discussed with employees.
2. Develop and implement a team-building training program for all employees, including those on contract.
3. Revise the performance management approach taken by the organization so that it focuses on staff members' teamwork as well as on individual skills and accomplishments.

The first two strategies were relatively easy to complete. Job descriptions were revised, and supervisors met with employees to discuss these changes. With the assistance of an outside consultant, a training program was implemented to teach employees communication and conflict management skills. Several but not all of the contract employees attended the training program.

The third strategy created some difficulties. The current performance management system is traditional, using a 12-item graphic rating scale (some with behavioral descriptions) that measures such aspects of work as attitude, quality of performance, productivity, attention to detail, job knowledge, reliability, and availability. There is also room on the form for comments by both supervisor and employee. It was felt that this approach did not address team components of employees' jobs. An additional problem is that several staff members are on contract and are not fully integrated into the organization. These staff members are currently not included in the organization's performance management process.

The HR director would like to modify the performance management process so that it includes methods to assess and improve team performance and to include contract employees in the process.

Case Exercise

As a consultant to the HR director, your job is to develop a method by which teamwork may be assessed in the performance management process.

1. How would you proceed with the task of modifying the performance management process?
2. What specific strategies do you think should be considered?
3. What obstacles do you see in implementing your approach? How would you overcome these problems?

COMPENSATION PRACTICES, PLANNING, AND CHALLENGES

Howard L. Smith, Ph.D.; Bruce J. Fried, Ph.D.; Derek van Amerongen, M.D.;

and John Crisafulli, M.B.A.

Learning Objectives

After completing this chapter, the reader should be able to

- describe the purposes of compensation and compensation policy in healthcare organizations;
- distinguish between extrinsic and intrinsic rewards and the value of each to employees;
- understand the concepts of balancing internal equity and external competitiveness in compensation;
- enumerate the objectives of job evaluation, and discuss the comparative merits of alternative approaches to job evaluation in healthcare settings;
- discuss alternative types of incentive plans;
- articulate the challenges and problems faced in designing and implementing pay-for-performance plans;
- explain the rationale for indirect compensation and the various types of benefits and services provided to employees;
- understand how different practice settings affect physician income and physician compensation strategies;
- define the conflicts that can arise within different compensation models; and
- have an idea of the future direction of physician compensation.

Introduction

People work for a variety of reasons, although they may not be able to articulate them. These motivators have been studied for many years. Findings from research and practice suggest that several factors lead to job satisfaction and performance, including interest in work, competent supervision, and personal reward. Although "money is not everything," it is a significant motivator and a frequent measure of the value an employer places on jobs and jobholders.

Employees assess their own value in terms of the amount of money they receive for their work and in terms of how their pay compares with that of others. The compensation that people receive also sends a powerful message to employees about what their organizations value. Employees are very focused on whether their compensation is comparable to the rates offered in the general market and the rates given to coworkers who perform the same job.

A compensation system must be externally competitive and internally equitable to allow organizations to balance what they value with how they reward employees (Kaplan and Norton 1996).

Any compensation system must accomplish several objectives. First, it must fairly reward individuals for labor performed and expertise applied. Second, it must align incentives for workers with those of the organization. Third, it should reduce or eliminate undesirable behavior—that is, practices that prevent the successful accomplishment of required tasks and achievement of objectives. Fourth, it should be prepared for the evolution of a job or industry, particularly for those involved in a highly technical, complicated field such as healthcare delivery. Fifth, and of critical importance in healthcare, it should be comparable to or even exceed the compensation systems of similar organizations in the market to give the organization a competitive edge. Again, although compensation is not the only factor associated with attracting and retaining employees, it is unquestionably important.

As in many other economic sectors, in healthcare, employee compensation is a very significant human resources management (HRM) issue. The healthcare sector, however, presents complexities and nuances that often are not encountered in other service or manufacturing sectors. First, a substantial number of healthcare employees are professionals with advanced education and training who must obtain and maintain licensure. These employees' professional associations exert a strong influence over employees' compensation and benefits. Second, shortages of skilled professionals drive up salaries and wages, allowing healthcare professionals to enjoy both high mobility and lucrative compensation. Third, healthcare providers cannot always determine the price of services because of third-party payer reimbursement policies. Consequently, third-party payment confounds the need to meet rising wage and salary levels in the marketplace.

In sum, compensation always seems to be at the forefront of HRM in healthcare, requiring continuing vigilant attention from healthcare organizations and their managers. Healthcare managers can better respond to this challenge by understanding the basics behind compensation planning and policymaking as well as the unique compensation needs of physicians and other healthcare providers.

This chapter reviews the strategic role of compensation, considers operational issues involved in determining individual compensation, discusses the need for healthcare organizations to establish a process for determining the monetary value of jobs, describes common forms of job evaluation, examines different types of incentive compensation, defines the challenges encountered in developing and implementing compensation plans, and analyzes compensation practices unique to physicians and other healthcare personnel.

The Strategic Role of Compensation Policy

The healthcare environment is often extremely stressful. Those who work in the field are attracted by high pay levels commonly associated with high-stress occupations. However, a perception persists about people who work in the field: They do so primarily because of their intrinsic desire to help others. Evidence continues to confirm that nurses and physicians are attracted to their professions because of their altruistic nature (Kingma 2003), and many jobs in healthcare are intrinsically rewarding. Nevertheless, although most healthcare professionals are driven by the satisfaction they get from their work, they are also influenced to come to and stay with their organization by the financial rewards they receive for their efforts. A good compensation system is particularly important in an industry like healthcare in which professional shortages occur in a cycle, leaving organizations to vie against other providers for the limited supply of employees.

An employee's choice to stay or to leave is complex. Considerable inferential data on how and why this decision is made are documented in the literature (Bartol 1979; Capo 2001; O'Connor et al. 2002), but a reliable predictive model of employee behavior is elusive. Staff members cite factors such as compensation, match of personal needs, wants and expectations from the internal job environment versus external opportunities, job elements (e.g., responsibilities, goals, activities, tasks), organizational culture, and organizational structure as motivators (see Chapter 7 for a range of factors associated with retention). Figure 10.1 highlights the main findings of such a study.

In light of studies that confirm the importance but not the criticality of money in healthcare employees' decision to remain with their employers, organizations should develop a compensation policy that aims to enhance the other employee motivators. In addition, this policy should align employees'

FIGURE 10.1

Research
Finding:
Professional
Support, not
Compensation,
Is More
Valuable to
Nurse
Retention

William M. Mercer, one of the world's largest human resources consulting firms, conducted a study with healthcare executives from 185 organizations (93 percent of which were hospitals) to determine factors that contribute to nursing shortages. Their opinions are as follows:

- 30 percent of respondents said RN turnover is a "significant problem."

- 63 percent said RN turnover is "somewhat of a problem."

- 7 percent said RN turnover is not a problem.

- The biggest reason given for turnover problems is "increased market demand."

The results echo the argument that retention of good nurses depends on factors other than compensation: hospitals that retain more nurses "... have fewer patients in their workload, better support services, greater control over their practices, greater participation in policy decisions, and more powerful chief nurse executives. In addition, they [nurses] were less apt to burn out and twice as likely to rate their hospitals as providing excellent care." Although compensation is very important to every person, in healthcare delivery settings professional support is an even more important consideration in people's decision to stay.

Source: Egger, E. 2000. "Nurse Shortage Worse than You Think, but Sensitivity May Help Retain Nurses." *Healthcare Strategic Management* 18 (5): 16–18.

efforts with the objectives, philosophies, and culture of the organization, highlighting the employees' contributions when organizational goals are achieved. A strategic compensation policy that balances individual needs with organizational interests typically includes the following goals:

1. Reward employee performance.
2. Achieve internal equity within the organization.
3. Remain externally competitive in relevant labor markets.
4. Align employee performance with organizational goals.
5. Attract and retain employees.
6. Maintain the compensation budget within organizational financial constraints.
7. Abide by legal constraints.

The strategic contribution of compensation is apparent in these goals. Compensation directly affects an organization's ability to achieve its fundamental missions and strategic objectives, to maintain fiscal integrity while delivering high-quality services, and to ensure customer satisfaction.

Compensation Decisions and Dilemmas

These compensation goals may come into conflict in certain situations. For example, higher compensation offered to attract certain types of employees can disrupt internal equity. Recruiting physical therapists is a case in point. Physical therapists are in short supply in many parts of the United States; therefore, offering compensation packages that are inconsistent with existing pay rates in the organization may be necessary. The discrepancy between an employee's worth (relative to other employees in the organization) and the amount that employee is paid is often determined by the market. This conflict between the goal of internal equity and external competitiveness is one of the major challenges in establishing an enlightened compensation policy, a conflict that is particularly acute in healthcare because of periodic shortages of professionals. In certain communities where competition for employees is very acute, organizations watch compensation levels carefully (often on a weekly basis) for key professional groups.

Organizations must make a number of other decisions when developing a compensation policy, which in turn may affect the goals and architecture of their current compensation programs. First, a determination must be made on whether to pay above, below, or at prevailing rates; this decision may be made explicitly or implicitly. Typically, organizations earn a reputation for the amount they pay employees. Second, the types of employee performance, practice, or contribution that are rewarded must be identified. This decision may seem trivial, but the factors chosen to be rewarded usually signal what the organization values. For example, annual raises that are not explicitly tied to performance tend to reward longevity and seniority in an organization. Rewarding longevity seems to contradict the general movement toward a pay-for-performance culture; however, the goal of retaining employees may be as important as providing incentives for high performance. Retention bonuses in fact aim to encourage longevity in the organization.

The trend toward paying for performance appears to be a permanent fixture in healthcare. The idea behind a pay-for-performance system is not only to compensate employees for their contributions but also to encourage good performance for the sake of maintaining and attracting high-level service reimbursements for the organization. This system is being enacted in the hospital sector and is seriously discussed in seminars and formal education programs. One of the criticisms of organizational "reimbursement" for performance is that payers are possibly rewarding high level of performance that is the result of environmental circumstances rather than the specific strategies undertaken by the organization to engender high performance. Managers in poorly performing hospitals (and educators in poorly performing schools) argue that punishing poorly performing organizations only reinforces historical inequities that may have caused differences in performance in the first place. For example, organizational performance is affected by factors outside of the institution's control such as being located in a community with high numbers of uninsured people. The dilemmas that plague organization-level pay for performance parallel those for incentive schemes for employees.

Among the first decisions necessary in designing a pay-for-performance system is establishing the performance criteria to be used in determining compensation. Furthermore, organizations must explore the unanticipated consequences of rewarding certain aspects of performance. Managers must be especially vigilant about the causal relationship between compensation and outcomes: When excessive emphasis is placed on fiscal concerns, especially cost containment, an imbalance can result in other critical outcomes such as quality, access, and consumer satisfaction. This necessitates careful attention when defining performance criteria as well as caution in establishing prudent measures and data collection. Additionally, managers must extrapolate from intended policy to see results and must anticipate dysfunctions associated with policy.

Other concerns are inherent when designing, improving, and implementing compensation programs. First, the worth of individual jobs must be determined. Second, the value that an employee's education and experience contribute to the position must be assessed. Third, guidelines on keeping salaries, benefits, and incentives confidential to the recipient and managers must be formulated and communicated to all concerned.

The point here is sobering: Creation of and improvement in employee compensation policies and practices is a never-ending challenge. Changes in the marketplace, trends within the healthcare professions, redirection of organizational goals and objectives, and other factors suggest that compensation policies and plans are seldom, if ever, stable, reinforcing the fact that compensation is a critical strategic issue in organizations.

Intrinsic Versus Extrinsic Rewards

Rewards can be intrinsic (internal) or extrinsic (external). *Intrinsic compensation* is intangible and may include recognition such as praise from a supervisor for completing an assignment; for meeting established performance objectives; or for having feelings of accomplishment, recognition, or belonging in an organization. *Extrinsic compensation* is tangible and may include both monetary and nonmonetary rewards such as salary, benefits, payment for time not worked (e.g., vacation pay), and stock options.

Determining which type of reward drives each employee is difficult because in most instances employees are motivated by a combination of intrinsic and extrinsic rewards. In one early approach to defining reward systems and understanding motivation, Herzberg, Mausner, and Snyderman (1959) suggested that employees first must have their basic "hygiene" needs met. Fulfillment of these needs does not produce employee motivation or job satisfaction but is a precondition that ushers in motivation. Thus, extrinsic rewards (most notably remuneration and satisfactory working conditions) are necessary but are insufficient elements for encouraging employees to contribute and subsequently feel a sense of accomplishment. The presence of extrinsic factors may prevent dissatisfaction but does not necessarily lead to satisfaction. This perspective is similar to Maslow's (1970) view that individuals must have their basic needs met (biological and safety) before they are able to achieve high esteem and fulfillment goals that are usually associated with high levels of performance. Managers, therefore, need to be cognizant of these two types of rewards and understand their functions and limitations.

The distinction between intrinsic and extrinsic rewards has substantial implications for managing healthcare professionals and support staff. It is not enough for managers to simply devise a well-orchestrated plan for compensation because pay in and of itself is only part of a complex equation that affects employee satisfaction. Managers must also attend to rewards that may not require fiscal resources. Encouraging employees, establishing a collegial practice environment, consistent setting of performance objectives, and conducting periodic performance assessments are all strategies that cost time rather than money. Assuming a prudent span of management, these are strategies that fiscally challenged healthcare providers can pursue in establishing a fertile reward environment. See Figure 10.2 for an example of balancing intrinsic and extrinsic rewards for academic physicians.

Low- or no-cost rewards are particularly of interest to nonprofit and financially strapped healthcare organizations with adverse budgets. In these circumstances managers should be especially mindful of the potential for using intrinsic rewards to supplement limited extrinsic rewards. This is a delicate balancing point that eventually may result in employees perceiving that their salaries are not comparable to the pay given in other provider organizations. How much of an imbalance that staff members will tolerate is never certain. It behooves fiscally challenged organizations to pursue intrinsic rewards to the greatest extent possible to minimize turnover and its associated costs.

FIGURE 10.2

Balancing
Intrinsic and
Extrinsic
Rewards in
Academic
Medical
Settings

Academic physicians have traditionally been drawn to universities because of opportunities to combine education and research with clinical care. Fiscally strapped academic medical centers and schools of medicine have progressively asked faculty to provide more clinical service as a means to raise revenue. So-called revenue-based compensation (RBC) pays academic physicians according to the clinical revenue they generate, thereby raising faculty members' income as well as that of the medical center and rewarding physicians who generate high revenue.

Richard Gunderman (2004) of the School of Medicine at Indiana University argues that RBC is insidious as far as the intrinsic rewards of academic medicine are concerned. He underscores that RBC can distract faculty members and encourage them to focus on remuneration, eroding their commitment and loyalty to the academic mission. Specifically there is potential erosion under RBC in the following intrinsic rewards:

1. Institutional prestige

2. Intellectual discourse

3. Opportunities for collaboration

4. Quality of intellectual discourse

5. Infrastructure

The end result is greater potential for faculty to migrate out of academic medicine.

The solution? Gunderman suggests that RBC plans should define revenue in measurable and objective terms, that expectations should be transparent, and that compensation plans should promote the mission of the medical school and the academic departments. These strategies will ensure that compensation is balanced with intrinsic aspects of the academic role.

Internal Equity and External Competitiveness

Every organization must maintain a delicate balance between internal equity and external competitiveness in its reward system. *Equity theory* (Homans 1961; Adams 1963) is a useful and well-tested framework for understanding the impact of perceived equity and inequity on individual motivation and performance. Equity is the perceived fairness of the relationship between what a person contributes to an organization (inputs) and what that person receives in return (outcomes). Inputs refer to such things as an individual's education, seniority, skills, effort, loyalty, and experience. Outcomes include pay, benefits, job satisfaction, opportunities for growth, and recognition.

According to equity theory, employees calculate the ratio, or balance, between their outcomes and inputs. They then compare their own ratio to the ratio of other people (referent others) in their organization or another organization. Particularly where professionals are concerned, comparisons may be made to people holding similar jobs in other organizations. For example, an operating room nurse in a hospital will likely compare his or her ratio with the ratio of other operating room nurses in the same hospital, with other nurses performing different tasks, with other types of staff members (to determine the comparability of their outcomes in relation to their inputs), and with nurses who perform similar work in other organizations. The result of this comparison is a belief by the employee that he or she is either being treated equitably or inequitably.

We can think of two types of perceived inequity. *Overpayment inequity* is a person's belief that his or her ratio is greater than that of the referent. Depending on the person's predisposition, overpayment inequity may lead to feelings of guilt, which can result in efforts to restore equity such as putting in greater effort. *Underpayment inequity* is a perception that occurs when an employee finds that his or her ratio is smaller than the referent's. In such a situation, an employee is likely to attempt to restore equity either by lowering inputs or by increasing the outcomes received from work. With these perceptions, employee motivation, morale, and performance are likely to decline.

This "comparing" feature of equity theory is pervasive in all organizations. Consider, for example, the interest generated when the salaries of senior executives in *Fortune 500* firms are publicized in the media. Of course, the comparative judgments made by employees may be highly subjective and based on limited or inaccurate information. Regardless of how subjective we think these assessments are, managers must contend with these perceptions because they affect motivation and performance. Managers must be attentive not only to the fairness of the reward system but also to *perceptions* of the fairness or equity of rewards. Perception, rather than reality, is what affects motivation.

Healthcare managers face a substantial challenge in addressing pay equity. Salaries and wages in most of the healthcare professions are common knowledge, as they are widely communicated for the purpose of recruitment. Consequently, some staff will allude to these differentials as a strategy to seek higher compensation. In addition to demonstrating great patience, managers can emphasize and develop the intrinsic rewards offered by their organization. This may help to defuse that differential and encourage staff to focus on the bigger picture, an approach that is especially appropriate to the professions.

Equity issues are particularly troublesome because of shortages in certain healthcare professions. Newly graduated nurses, for example, may be hired at a salary level that approaches the compensation of well-seasoned and experienced nurses. While the experienced employee may have a cognitive understanding of the market-based reasons for this inequity, the impact of this inequity is likely to remain. Such an employee is faced with several choices: accept the situation, seek additional compensation, change jobs within the organization, take on additional responsibilities, or move to another organization to achieve the financial benefits of being newly hired. In some markets, job hopping is a tried-and-true method of increasing one's compensation.

As mentioned earlier, employees who perceive inequity may attempt to equalize the situation through two ways: (1) increase their outcomes or (2) decrease their inputs. The first way can be accomplished by working harder and perhaps, as a result, obtain additional compensation or a promotion (note that working harder may also increase the "inputs" side of the ratio); by organizing other employees, possibly in the form of unionization; and by engaging in illegal activities such as theft or false reporting of hours worked. The second approach can be done through working fewer hours (e.g., coming in late, leaving early, or being absent) and putting forth less effort. Employees may also attempt to restore a sense of equity by changing their perceptions of the inputs or outcomes of others. For example, an employee may convince herself that the referent employee has more experience and is therefore entitled to a higher level of rewards. Similarly, an employee may conclude that while his salary may be lower than that of a referent, working conditions are much better at his organization than at other organizations. In other instances, employees may simply change their frame of reference—that is, the person with whom they compare themselves.

While organizations seek to ensure internal equity, they must also pursue external competitiveness to recruit staff. To be externally competitive, organizations must provide compensation that is perceived to be equitable to the salary given to employees who perform similar jobs in other organizations. If an organization is not externally competitive, it is likely to face problems of turnover and staff shortages, particularly in geographic areas where the supply of certain professionals may be scarce.

Healthcare employers have traditionally faced tight labor markets for physicians, nurses, and medical technicians, which lead to the difficulty in attracting and retaining these and other clinical providers. This competition results in an ascending spiral of wages, salaries, benefits, and other forms of compensation that the market cannot afford and that inflate organizational cost structures and eat away at margins. In such a situation, emphasizing intrinsic rewards or intangible incentives can contribute to attracting and retaining high-quality staff.

When confronting a tight labor market, organizations should formulate specific strategies to position themselves in the labor market. As far as pay is concerned, these positioning strategies typically follow a quartile strategy. Most employers seek to position themselves in the second quartile (the middle of the market) or higher, a position that is preferred by other employers according to survey data. By choosing this position, organizations can balance employer cost pressures with the need to attract and retain employees.

An employer that uses a first-quartile strategy, on the other hand, is choosing to pay below-market compensation. Employers take this position for several reasons. First, shortage of funds or an inability to pay more may converge with the need to continue to meet strategic organizational objectives. Second, if a large number of applicants with lower skills are available in the labor market, this strategy can be used to attract sufficient workers at a lower cost. A major disadvantage of using a first-quartile strategy is high turnover, and, if the labor supply tightens, the organization may have difficulty attracting and retaining workers. Quality-of-care ramifications in nursing homes that operate in the lower quartile are illustrated in Figure 10.3.

A third-quartile strategy, in which employees are paid above-market value, is more aggressive. This strategy may be used to ensure that a sufficient number of employees with the required capabilities are attracted and retained; it also allows an organization to be more selective. However, the expectation in most organizations is that those employees who are paid above-market rates must be more productive and must deliver higher-quality services and products.

Determining the Monetary Value of Jobs

Job evaluation is a formal process for determining the value of jobs in monetary terms. Development and maintenance of an intelligent wage-and-salary system begin with accurate job descriptions and job specifications for each position. This information is used to perform a job evaluation and to conduct pay surveys. These activities ensure that a pay system is both internally equitable and externally competitive. Data gathered in the job-evaluation process and pay surveys are used to design, or improve, pay structures, including pay grades and pay ranges.

In theory, job evaluation is used to obtain an objective assessment of a job's worth or contribution to the organization. This level of contribution is then translated into monetary terms. After this monetary value is determined, compensation levels may be adjusted to better reflect compensation levels in the marketplace. However, in tight labor markets, the use of job evaluation information for setting compensation levels may be of limited use. In particular jobs, information from wage and salary surveys may be more

FIGURE 10.3

Quality-of-Care Ramifications of a Low-Quartile Position

Mohr and colleagues (2004) studied nursing homes in the lowest tier—that is, facilities that house mainly (>85 percent) Medicaid residents. They note that nursing homes with high proportions of Medicaid patients have correspondingly fewer resources to hire staff and that poor, frail, and minority residents in these facilities tend to receive substandard care. In particular, their analyses suggest that staffing intensity is statistically lower in Medicaid-dominated nursing homes. Fewer registered nurses are found on staff in lower-tier nursing homes, but not fewer licensed practical nurses. This led the authors to conclude that less-expensive and less-qualified staff is used as substitutes for higher-trained staff by fiscally constrained Medicaid facilities. Physician extenders and administrators are also less prevalent in lower-tier nursing homes.

Quality-of-care indicators suffer in lower-tier nursing homes, according to the study. Medicaid-dominated facilities report higher incidences of pressure ulcers, higher use of physical restraints, and higher use of antipsychotic medications. Clearly, poor quality of care is associated with restricted use of registered nurses as well as limited administrative resources and physician extenders. Mohr and colleagues acknowledge that lower staffing intensity is accompanied by fewer resources to hire and train clinical and administrative staff. In sum, economic constraints lead to higher turnover, lower retention, and ultimately lower quality of care.

useful in setting compensation levels and may in fact be the sole determinant of salary levels. Periodic job evaluations may be conducted, but over extended periods (often several years), salary decisions may be made almost exclusively on market information. Our discussion, therefore, needs to be placed in the context of volatile and unpredictable labor markets.

During job evaluation, a job is examined and ultimately priced according to each job's relative importance to an organization; the knowledge, skills, and abilities each job requires; and the difficulty of each job. The premise of job evaluation is that jobs that require greater qualifications, that involve more responsibility, and that assign more complex duties should pay more than jobs with lower requirements or lesser tasks (Martocchio 2001). Job evaluation is also a way of ensuring that employees perceive equity in the compensation system. To motivate staff, it is essential that a fair pay value be assigned to each job.

When conducting a job evaluation, benchmark jobs are identified. These benchmarks require similar knowledge, skills, and abilities and are performed by individuals who have been assigned relatively similar duties. Benchmark jobs are used to establish a basis on which other comparable jobs are evaluated.

Methods of Evaluating Job Value

Ranking Method

Perhaps the simplest job value assessment technique, the *ranking method* lists jobs in order of their inherent value to an organization. The entire job, rather than individual components of the job, is considered. Those who rank jobs use their judgment when ranking, and consequently this method is extremely susceptible to subjectivity. Managers may have difficulty explaining why one specific position is ranked higher than another. Additionally, this method is very cumbersome to do in large organizations because of the sizeable number of jobs in such institutions.

Job Classification

Job classification is a system of categorizing jobs based on predetermined requirements. This approach is most common in the public sector, where jobs are classified according to the federal government's General Schedule (GS) of 18 grades. In the GS system, each job is classified into one of these 18 grades based on knowledge requirements, responsibilities, physical effort, and working conditions. Each grade is associated with a salary range, which varies by geographic location.

Similar to ranking, job classification is subject to considerable subjectivity and is vulnerable to manipulation. Jobs can be misclassified, or perceived as misclassified, because of assumptions made by the job analyst. Job classification is problematic when applied to multisystem organizations, because two jobs with the same title may entail very different responsibilities in different settings. For example, a registered nurse in a skilled nursing facility performs roles that are substantially different from those performed by a registered nurse in an outpatient surgery center.

Broadbanding

Job classification systems assign jobs to categories known as pay bands. The *broadbanding* approach to compensation is a response to the constraints imposed by rigid classification systems in which an employee's maximum compensation is limited by a very narrow salary band. Traditional classification systems have very narrow ranges of pay for a job classified in a particular category. If we wish to provide additional compensation to an employee who assumes new responsibilities or learn new skills, traditional classification systems provide little flexibility in how this person is compensated; promotion to a new position and reclassifying the position are the main options. Broadbanding involves enlarging these pay bands for jobs in such a way that there is more flexibility in compensation for a particular job.

A broadband is a single, large salary range that spans pay opportunities formerly covered by several separate small salary ranges. Several jobs and salary levels can be included within a single broadband. A major advantage of broadbanding is that it provides more flexibility when managing an employee's compensation within a particular pay range. Levels of compensation can be changed without the necessity of changing job titles or reclassifying jobs. Individuals can be moved between jobs without concern for dramatic changes in salary. For example, an employee may be reluctant to move into another position because of the possibility of a salary decrease. With broadbanding, both jobs may be in the same salary range, allowing for stability in salary. Employees can also be more easily rewarded within a broad pay grade for taking on new responsibilities or obtaining new skills. For the employee, career growth can be thought of in terms of increased responsibilities rather than promotion (Wagner and Jones 1994).

Broadbanding is becoming a more popular approach to valuing jobs. A 1996 survey of 380 large companies by Buck Consultants in New York found that 29 percent of these companies were using or implementing broadbanding, up from 16.7 percent in 1994. In addition, 27 percent of the respondents who had not used a broadband approach indicated they were considering making the change (Jacobs 1997). In fact, a growing number of organizations are looking for alternative pay structures to fit new organizational structures driven by competitive environments. Broadbanding is especially appropriate because it is consistent with trends toward flatter, less hierarchical organizations and the use of cross-functional job positions. Cross-functional positions enable organizations to respond quickly to competitive pressures. With broadbanding, employees can more easily shift responsibilities as market and organizational requirements change.

Broadbanding offers other advantages. It enables companies to base compensation decisions on characteristics of people who perform jobs rather than on characteristics of the job alone. Authority for compensation decisions is largely decentralized to operating managers. Therefore, managers find it easier to gain approval for changes in compensation because broadbanding enables them to reward employees without going through myriad justifications required in a traditional classification system. Additionally, the wider spread between pay grades gives managers more flexibility to recognize and reward different levels of individual contribution.

Because broadbanding results in fewer pay groupings, job evaluation is potentially simpler because organizations no longer need complex job evaluation schemes. Managers can encourage employees to move into other job areas that may broaden knowledge, skills, and abilities. Finally, broadbanding allows employees to evaluate their own skill acquisition and cross-training opportunities in terms of professional development and personal growth, rather than focus on pay grades.

However, broadbanding is not appropriate for every organization and organizational culture. The narrow range of the traditional pay system may serve as an automatic cost-control mechanism that keeps compensation expenses in check. With broadbanding, all employees may potentially float to the maximum pay level within their band, resulting in higher-than-market compensation for many or most employees. New employees who replace those with seniority may discover that they are paid at significantly lower levels, an artifact of time on the job of their more senior counterparts. However, such an explanation may provide little solace. Perceptions of inequity may become an irritant and may lower morale.

The most difficult aspect of implementing broadbanding is helping employees to think differently about how they are paid. Pay grades have long been used to determine status, titles, and eligibility for perquisites. Consequently, employees sometimes have difficulty relinquishing these preconceptions. Broadbanding also implies fewer upward-promotion opportunities. With a smaller number of bands, employees recognize that promotions to a higher grade level will occur less frequently than before. Employees must assume significantly greater job responsibilities to warrant placement in a higher band (Jacobs 1997).

Point Method

The *point method* is the most widely used job-valuation tool. A basic assumption behind this method is that organizations do not pay for jobs but for specific aspects of these jobs, known as *compensable factors*. Examples of compensable factors include knowledge and skill requirements, job experience, accountability, supervisory responsibilities, and working conditions. These compensable factors are determined through job analysis and are then assigned values or weights—points—based on the extent to which each factor is present. Compensation levels and pay ranges are then linked to these points, although actual compensation for a particular job may vary based on market and other factors.

The point method is popular because it is relatively simple, is based on job analysis, may be used for many jobs, and once established is relatively easy to update. However, this method does have several drawbacks, including the amount of time needed to develop the system and the tendency to reinforce traditional organizational structures and job rigidity. Further, as discussed earlier, compensation levels for particular jobs may be based more on salary survey data than on the results of job evaluation. Often, very significant differences exist between compensation levels derived from job evaluation and levels according to market pay rates.

The following are necessary in developing a point system (Hills, Bergmann, and Scarpello 1994):

- Compensable factors must be acceptable to all parties.
- Compensable factors must validly distinguish among jobs.
- Compensable factors must be relevant to the jobs under analysis.
- Jobs must vary on the compensable factors selected so that meaningful differences in jobs can be identified.
- Compensable factors must be measurable.
- Compensable factors must be independent of each other.
- Job evaluation and market pay rates must be reconciled.

Factor-Comparison Method

The *factor-comparison method* is a combination of the ranking and point methods. It differs from point system in that compensable factors for a job are evaluated against compensable factors in benchmark jobs in the organization. *Benchmark jobs* are important to employees and the organization, vary in their requirements, have relatively stable content, and are used in salary surveys for wage determination.

Benchmark jobs are typically evaluated against a set of compensable factors such as skill, mental effort, physical effort, responsibilities, and working conditions. A pay rate is assigned to each compensable factor for each benchmark job. For example, the job of emergency room (ER) nurse may be identified as a benchmark job. Analysis determines that of the $17 hourly wage paid to an ER nurse, $5 is paid for mental effort, $3 for responsibility, and so forth. Similarly, we may use a hospital medical technologist's job as a benchmark, and we may decide that of the $15 hourly wage paid to this individual, $4 is paid for mental effort, $2.50 for responsibility, and so forth. A factor-comparison scale is developed to evaluate other jobs in the organization. Thus, if we are attempting to evaluate the job of an occupational therapist, the mental effort, skill, and other factors of that job are compared to that of the ER nurse and the medical technologist.

A key advantage of the factor-comparison approach is it can be tailored to one organization, and it indicates which jobs are worth more and how much more, making factor values more easily converted into monetary wages. Disadvantages of this method are complexity, time required to establish comparable factors, and difficulty explaining the methodology to employees.

The Impact of the Market

The approaches to valuing jobs discussed in this section focus almost exclusively on ensuring equity within the workplace. However, clearly, particularly in healthcare, the compensation that an organization offers is often heavily dependent on labor supply and market wages. We learn about market wages largely from salary surveys, and salary surveys are carried out by organizations, government, associations, and external consulting firms. Annual surveys are conducted by the Bureau of Labor Statistics on area and industry wages, as well as surveys of professional, administrative, technical, and clerical positions. Private consulting firms that conduct salary surveys include The Hay Group, Heidrick & Struggles International, Inc., and Hewitt Associates. The Society for Human Resource Management and the Financial Executives Institute also conduct wage surveys. In the healthcare sector, the American Hospital Association conducts a series of annual healthcare-specific wage and salary surveys. Finally, the Internet may also be used to obtain market salary information (see, for example, http://salary.com).

Variable Compensation

Team-Based Compensation

Healthcare providers increasingly structure service delivery around work teams, stimulating HR managers to consider compensation systems that reward team performance. Unfortunately, the actual development of *team-based compensation* systems is often constrained by the need to reward individual performance.

A care delivery team made up of an obstetrician, a case manager, a social worker, and a nurse's aide may be rewarded for a productive performance such as delivering more infants than other teams and experiencing minimal adverse cases and high patient satisfaction. However, what level of reward should be assigned to the team? What percentage of the respective base salaries of each team member will the reward constitute? Will inequities in rewards cause some team members to work less in achieving team objectives? These are representative questions that must be addressed before implementing a team-based compensation system.

Healthcare organizations that are interested in rewarding team performance need to strike a balance between individual and team rewards. Paying the same amount to everyone on the team regardless of his or her competencies or contributions may create pay-equity problems. Team incentives are most commonly incorporated as variable pay—that is, a team-based incentive is added to base pay. While base pay is determined by job evaluation and market information, variable pay is added according to team performance.

Skills-Based Pay

In *skills-based compensation* systems, employees are paid according to work-related skills and competencies. The reward structure of this approach is based on the range, depth, and types of skills that individual employees possess. Compensation is increased after an employee demonstrates the ability to perform specific, desired skills. This compensation approach is based on the idea that employees with a broad range of skills provide the organization with more flexibility in its deployment of staff.

Typically, an employee is hired and is provided training for that job. The employee may then join a work team and be given the opportunity to learn new skills through additional training and on-the-job experience. As the employee learns new jobs, his or her compensation is increased. This approach reinforces the concept of the autonomous work group, where members work interdependently.

Skills-based pay can follow a stair-step approach, in which a logical well-defined progression is followed in skills development. Pay is increased as skills are mastered. A job-point accrual model is used when there is a variety of jobs for which an employee may be trained. Jobs are given a point rating that is based on the difficulty of mastering job skills, and compensation is increased in accordance with points earned. A cross-department model is one in which employees may be trained to work in jobs in other parts of the organization, and compensation increases as the employee masters these jobs (Bunning 1992).

Pay for Performance

Pay-for-performance systems are built on the principles that good work deserves to be rewarded and that pay based on good work produces improved performance. In a pay-for-performance system, managers evaluate the work of their employees based on preestablished goals, standards, or company values. Based on this judgment, employees are given variable or contingent financial rewards. Individual compensation is directly linked to personal performance and attainment of objectives consistent with the organization's mission. This approach is intended to motivate employees to perform at the highest level regardless of their particular role or specialty (Grib and O'Donnell 1995).

Pay for performance may be structured in a variety of ways. Piece-rate incentives reward employees for each unit of output produced, whether this unit is a product or service. Commissions are most common in sales and are structured so that employees receive a percentage of their gross receipts. Bonuses are one-time financial rewards to recognize individual and/or organizational performance.

Other incentive systems are based on encouraging team or organizational performance. Profit-sharing plans enable employees to share in the organization's profits, and gain-sharing plans allocate to employees a portion of the gains made by the organization as a result of increased efficiency or productivity. This sharing approach has manifested itself in a number of forms such as the Scanlon Plan, the Rucker Plan, and Improshare.

In incentive-based compensation systems, pay is tied to the accomplishment of goals that are established with employees prior to the performance period for which employees will be evaluated. The focus is on specific actions that employees have performed in pursuit of these set goals (see Figure 10.4, for example).

Some argue that pay-for-performance systems decrease the focus on customer needs, increase the loss of accurate information about defects and improvement opportunities, discourage achievement of stretch goals, and reduce risk taking and innovation. These disadvantages have been cited because pay-for-performance systems make the supervisor the most important customer; employees, it is claimed, play to their supervisors rather than to external customers or patients. The system also deprives providers of essential information because managers learn less about defects and changes that need to be made. Under a pay-for-performance plan, employees may be reluctant to report problems because doing so may have a negative impact on their compensation. Pay-for-performance approaches may also encourage employees to set lower goal aspirations. When goals are set in advance, employees may argue for less ambitious goals than for stretch goals to ensure that they receive performance-related rewards. Finally, pay-for-performance systems may hamper change because innovation disrupts tried-and-tested ways of delivering services, thus lowering efficiency and affecting goal accomplishment. This is especially detrimental in healthcare because constant breakthroughs in performance require substantial changes in the way employees do their work (Berwick 1995; Pfeffer 1998). Pay-for-performance plans may discourage risk taking and reduce creativity because the fear of not getting the reward makes people less inclined to take risks or explore alternative approaches to work. Thus, the efficacy of incentive plans is a topic of considerable debate.

Those who support incentive plans point to the fact that most of us are, in reality, motivated by money. In other words, most people would rather have more money than less money; therefore, money can be used to change employee behavior. Supporters of pay for performance assert that behaviors that are rewarded are repeated and behaviors that are punished are eliminated. People tend to set aside behaviors for which they are not rewarded. This suggests that, when rewarding behaviors, organizations

FIGURE 10.4

Financial
Incentives for
Physician
Productivity

In 2002, Conrad and colleagues explored the relationship of financial incentives with physician productivity in 102 medical groups and 2,237 physicians in the Medical Group Management Association (MGMA). The sample is admittedly a very small proportion of MGMA's membership of 5,725 practices (there are 19,478 medical groups in the United States); however, the advantage of this study group is the valuable information it supplied on resource-based relative value scale units produced in 1997. Data were derived from MGMA's annual surveys—the Compensation and Production Survey and the Cost Survey.

The conceptual basis underlying this study relates back to a seminal analysis that Gaynor and Pauly (1990) completed on medical group partnerships. These researchers discovered that physician productivity is extremely sensitive to individual compensation. Tying compensation completely to productivity (i.e., productivity determines 100 percent of a physician's total salary) increased productivity by 28 percent. In practical terms, physicians respond very favorably to incentive-based compensation.

Conrad and colleague's findings reaffirm those of Gaynor and Pauly. Physicians for the medical groups that base pay on individual performance are more productive than individual physicians. Moreover, the results suggest that bonuses heighten the productivity effect. The individual characteristics of the physicians also play a role in responses to incentives, according to further in-depth study. Physician experience is associated with modest increases in productivity. Gender appears to have some impact, although the statistical results in the Conrad study are affected by the fact that female physicians tended to work fewer hours per week than did their male counterparts.

Turning to incentive effects on each group as the unit of analysis. The findings suggest an inverse relationship with group size—that is, as the size of groups becomes larger, the impact of incentives dissipates. The sense of participating in a cohesive, close-knit professional team seems to be adversely affected by a larger number of providers. In effect, physicians may be less motivated psychologically because they are only one provider among many in a large group practice, possibly leading them to remain at the average production capacity rather than strive to exceed this average. These are important findings because they indicate that large, vertically integrated delivery systems can be inimical to high productivity.

Conrad and colleagues' study has very important practical implications for all healthcare providers. It infers that production of services is linked to the availability of incentives. As healthcare costs continue to escalate and healthcare organizations seek higher productivity from clinicians, the scope and depth of incentive compensation plans will likely continue to grow.

must ensure that all relevant aspects of behavior are measured. Incomplete measurement may result in incomplete performance, with employees only doing those tasks or engaging in those behaviors that are rewarded. Rewards also provide an opportunity for management to communicate values to employees. Numerous studies suggest that financial incentives do improve work quantity. Too few studies exist, however, to determine their effect on performance quality (Gupta and Shaw 1998).

Under continued pressures for efficiency, the adoption of pay for performance continues to increase in the healthcare sector. In many settings, physicians are under pressure to meet production targets, achieve quality and outcome goals, and abide by critical pathways (Berkowitz 2002; Rost 2002). Pay for performance is one strategy to focus physicians and other clinicians on performance.

The Future of Variable Compensation Arrangements

In an effort to achieve greater levels of effectiveness and efficiency, we will likely continue to witness a variety of new compensation arrangements in healthcare. Change can be good, but healthcare managers should proceed cautiously because compensation is a very charged topic. Tampering with compensation arrangements can have disastrous effects, so consequences cannot be overlooked or undermined. Nonetheless, the difficult constraints facing healthcare providers call for taking bold action. Perhaps the most important element in ensuring success in this regard is to involve employees at all levels in the design and implementation of compensation plans. In this way, the plan is more effective and meets broader acceptance.

Indirect Compensation

Indirect compensation refers to a wide range of benefits and services provided to employees. Benefits and services account for a very significant portion of total compensation—almost 40 percent of wages and salaries. This proportion has increased steadily, largely because of the rising cost of healthcare and higher employee demands and expectations for improved benefits. In this section, we review the rationale for providing benefits and services and describe the various types of benefits provided to employees, along with issues regarding compensation administration.

The origin of indirect compensation dates back to periods of wage and salary controls, which were instituted to control inflation. In lieu of additional compensation, employers developed alternative ways of rewarding employees. Healthcare benefits were among the firsts of such strategies.

In recent years, a number of factors have come to affect the types of benefits offered and the extent to which companies provide benefits.

Through the years, indirect compensation has become the norm in most medium- to large-size organizations. Benefits are now used to attract and retain employees and to increase staff job satisfaction and morale. On a more general level, compensation and benefits may be used to improve the reputation of the organization in the larger community. Presumably, the organization's favorable reputation may lead to the organization being viewed favorably in the labor market.

Tax laws also have an impact on indirect compensation. Companies naturally prefer to provide those benefits that can be counted as business expenses, and employees seek to obtain benefits that are exempt from taxation. Other factors, such as salary, work location, and opportunities for promotion, may play a larger role in employee satisfaction than benefits packages. Particularly in larger organizations, employees have come to expect benefits as part of their employment. In unionized organizations, employee benefits are routinely negotiated between the employer and employee groups. To remain competitive with unionized organizations, nonunionized facilities may need to match or exceed benefits offered by their unionized counterparts.

Benefits may also be offered according to the philosophy, culture, and values of the organization. For example, some organizations, seeking to reinforce an egalitarian culture, may develop a benefits policy that gives all employees the same package. Other firms may use a strategy that differentiates benefits on the basis of one's level in the organization.

Forms of Indirect Compensation

Figure 10.5 lists the variety of benefits and programs offered by organizations to employees. Some of these benefits are explored below.

Mandatory Benefits

These benefits are provided because they are required by either federal law or state law. Perhaps the most well-known of these are employer and employee contributions to Social Security, specified by the Federal Insurance Contribution Act (FICA). The Social Security system provides retirement benefits, survivor's benefits, and disability payments. Mandatory contributions are also made to the Medicare program.

Unemployment compensation insurance is also a required benefit under the Social Security Act and is administered by states in accordance with federal guidelines. Because of variations in income among states, unemployment compensation payments vary by state. All states have some form of worker's compensation insurance, a no-fault insurance program that

- *Health, dental, vision and prescription coverage*

- Cafeteria/flexible benefit options

- Life, accidental death, travel insurance

- Short-term and long-term disability insurance

- Sick, vacation, personal, holiday leave

- Pension and retirement savings plans

- Stock purchase plans/options

- Training and education programs

- Membership in associations, clubs

- Wellness, smoking cessation, weight-loss programs

- Recreation, fitness centers, special events

- Employee assistance program

- Legal and financial services

- Credit union, financial/retirement planning

- Transportation subsidies, parking

- Housing subsidies, relocation benefits

- Flexible work environments and schedules

- Casual dress

- Dependent care subsidies, referrals, services

- Childcare, elder care, long-term care

- Food service, concierge service

- Discounts on company services/products

FIGURE 10.5

Indirect Compensation Provided by Organizations

provides benefits to workers who are injured or killed on the job. The federal government does not get involved in worker's compensation and does not offer guidelines. The program is handled entirely by the states.

Compensation for Time Not Worked

Virtually all employers provide full-time employees with various forms of compensation for time not worked. Among the most common of these are payment for holidays, vacation, sick leave, bereavement, and personal days. Most organizations also provide paid days to allow employees to tend to civic obligations such as jury duty, voting, and military duty and to personal matters such as funerals and family emergencies.

The Family and Medical Leave Act (FMLA) requires employers to provide unpaid leave of up to 12 weeks per year for a variety of family-related and medical situations. The FMLA is the only law that mandates a particular type of payment for time not worked, and it provides specific guidelines for defining situations that can be considered under FMLA leaves. Among the requirements for eligibility under the FMLA is that an employee must have worked at least 1,250 hours in the previous 12 months with the current employer. Employers have several responsibilities under the FMLA as well, including guaranteeing the employee the right to return to his or her previous job or to an equivalent position (with exceptions for certain employees) and maintaining health benefits for the employee on FMLA leave.

Organizations may, of course, provide leave for other reasons such as birthdays and employment anniversaries.

Optional Benefits

Certainly the most common and costly optional benefit is health insurance. In 2004, three-fifths of private establishments offered health insurance to employees. Among all benefits, health insurance is the most hotly debated, particularly in relation to issues such as covered services (prescription drugs), cost sharing, limits on utilization, and cost-control measures. Health insurance may also cover dental care, mental health services, vision care, and chiropractic care as well as specialized insurance for intensive care, long-term care, critical illness, and cancer. Health insurance benefits come in multiple forms of copayment, deductibles, limits on utilization, and other cost-sharing and cost-cutting arrangements.

Organizations have expanded into multiple other areas of healthcare benefits, including preventive care and wellness programs (e.g., onsite vaccinations, CPR/first aid training, health screening programs, employee assistance programs) and nontraditional healthcare benefits (e.g., acupuncture, alternative/complementary medicine, coverage for experimental drugs).

Flexible spending accounts for healthcare expenses are particularly popular among employees, as they typically allow employees to pay for healthcare services with pretax earnings. As with many benefits programs, healthcare benefits are subject to much regulation. For example, COBRA (Comprehensive Omnibus Budget Reconciliation Act) requires employers to extend group medical benefits to terminated employees. Some states have passed legislation that mandates minimal coverage for certain conditions (e.g., childbirth). National legislation also sets minimum mental health care benefits.

Health Savings Accounts

One of the newest variations of healthcare accounts is the health savings Account (HSA), established by H.R.1 through the Medicare Prescription Drug Improvement and Modernization Act of 2003 to be used in conjunction with a high-deductible health plan. An HSA allows individuals to pay for current healthcare expenses and to save for future qualified medical and retiree health expenses on a tax-free basis.

Contributions to HSAs may be made by the employer, employee, or both and may be used for qualified medical and other expenses. Amounts contributed to an HSA belong to individuals and are completely portable. Every year the money not spent stays in the account and gains interest tax-free, similar to an individual retirement account. Unused amounts remain available for later years, in contrast to Flexible Spending Arrangements in which money not used by the end of the year is forfeited.

Flexible Benefits

Because employees often have different benefits preferences, many organizations have implemented flexible benefits plans, sometimes called cafeteria benefits plans. In a flexible benefits plan, the employee is given a fixed fund budget and allowed to allocate benefit dollars in a matter suited to his or her needs. Another common benefit is life and disability insurance. An advantage of employer-sponsored plans is that the employer is able to obtain coverage at the rates far lower than are available to individuals.

Many organizations offer private pension plans, which are sometimes funded entirely by employer contributions but are more commonly funded jointly by employer and employee. Invested funds yield dividends and grow, providing retirement income. An important advantage of employee pension plans is that employee contributions are a means of deferring income.

There are several types of retirement plans. A defined benefit plan is one in which a retired employee receives a specific amount based on salary history and years of service. Contributions, based on actuarial calculations, are made by the employee, the employer, or both. An advantage is that the employees know the amount of their retirement benefits prior to retirement. Because of this, unions tend to favor this type of plan. A defined contribution plan is one in which an employee defers some part of his or her salary, investing that portion in a pension plan in which the employee assumes the risk. Among the most common defined contribution plans are 401(k) and 403(b) plans. Retirement plans are highly regulated by the government; the first piece of legislation regarding this is the Employee Retirement Income Security Act of 1974 (ERISA). ERISA requires that employer-sponsored pension plans must be made available to employees after one year of service or at age 25. Detailed regulations regarding vesting, or the period of time when employer contributions can belong to the employee, are also included in this act.

Another set of benefits comprise those related to the work environment and the work-family interface. These types of benefits may be related to the manner in which work is structured or may be specific to family-focused services. Among the most common are flexible spending accounts for dependents, life insurance for dependents, family leave outside of FMLA requirements, healthcare benefits for dependent grandchildren, childcare services, telecommuting, domestic-partner benefits, and compressed workweeks.

Problems with Indirect Compensation

Indirect compensation is a significant, costly, and somewhat unpredictable expense for employers. Employers face many problems with indirect compensation. First, the cost of providing healthcare benefits is staggering. Increasingly, employers are shifting the cost of healthcare to employees, which is partly a result of the negative reaction to managed care and its associated cost-control mechanisms. Second, it is hard to measure the effectiveness and cost effectiveness of many benefits programs. Third, complying with regulations that govern benefits programs is a complex task. Fourth, balancing the need to control organizational expenses with the need to attract and retain employees is difficult.

Special Considerations for Compensating Physicians

Before World War II, most physicians were general practitioners who delivered care in independent practices on a fee-for-service basis (Starr 1982). Medicine was considered one of the more successful cottage industries. This changed radically after the war, with an explosion of medical subspecialties nurtured by battlefield needs, the rise of care within hospitals instead of at home, and the advent of employer-based medical insurance. Once consumers of care (patients) were no longer directly responsible for the cost of care they received, payers of the services (i.e., employers or government) and the deliverer of care (i.e., physicians) were no longer obliged to justify costs to consumers. The checks and balances that typically exist in any economic interaction were lost. The result was a system that paid physicians whatever they requested, without the system attempting to validate the appropriateness of those services. This series of events led to the managed care movement (Burchell, Smith, and Piland 2002).

With the development of managed care, attention shifted to using payment mechanisms as a means to modify clinical behavior. Analysts have expressed concern that medical evidence is infrequently used in treatment decisions (Winslow 2000). For example, two patients with the same condition may receive vastly different therapies, or two patients with very different diseases may be treated virtually the same. Allowing for the so-called "art of medicine" does not explain the inconsistent use of clinical practice guidelines that have been shown to improve outcomes. Furthermore, variation in practice is widespread and is not linked to medical differences in populations. Two adjacent communities, with similar populations and demographics, may have dramatically different rates of surgery or use of certain modalities. Scientific justification for such discrepancies usually does not exist, suggesting that differences in care come from physician choice and habit, not medical data.

A key objective of health policy in the early 1990s was to leverage reimbursement mechanisms to address variation in treatment processes and outcomes. However, the track record for reducing practice discrepancies or improving practice behaviors in the last ten years has been disappointing. Modifying physicians' use of various forms of reimbursement has been a notable failure. Capitation is a system that pays a physician a certain amount for each patient assigned to his or her panel or list of patients. The fee is meant to cover professional services required to care for each patient. The challenge for the practitioner is to provide these services within the limits of capitated payment. As an incentive, any funds left over after delivering care revert to the physician as revenue.

Capitation was initially seen as a way to provide incentives to physicians to perform the appropriate level of care without generating excess costs. In contrast, fee-for-service encourages the use of (and reimbursement for) excessive services and the tendency to neglect preventive measures. The argument was that compensating physicians a set amount per patient (a capitated payment) would encourage them to do as much as possible to keep patients healthy, thereby avoiding the need for expensive services.

The Achilles' heel of capitation was that it put physicians at risk for patients who have preexisting conditions or medical predispositions over which physicians have no control. Capitation also rendered physicians responsible for patients whom they had never seen before. While many physician groups initially were enthusiastic about accepting risk payment, mainly because of the increased payments it brought, they usually failed to understand the full implications of being responsible for a population, versus caring for individual patients. Bankruptcies of medical groups were not uncommon because of their inability to manage the very problems with physician behavior that capitation was supposed to solve. As a result, risk payment methods became increasingly unpopular as a payment option. Because of capitation's inability to change practice patterns (Grumbach et al. 1999; *Managed Care Outlook* 1999) and its adverse impact on both physician group viability and the willingness of groups to participate in such plans, other compensation approaches have surfaced.

An important element affecting the potential for compensation models to change behaviors is the continued growth in physician income. In the early 1990s, the general belief was that by putting the brakes on the rise in salaries, physicians could be brought in line with the directions that health plans and employers wanted them to go. This concept is frequently referred to as aligning incentives. However, numerous studies (Thompson 2000; Kilborn 1999) have demonstrated the surprising ability of physicians to continue to increase their incomes, albeit at lower rates of growth than in the 1980s. Nevertheless, with most specialists making well over $200,000 per year, using income as a tool for change has become difficult.

The ability to increase volume even as the cost per unit decreases has largely protected most physicians from experiencing radical shifts in income. Furthermore, unlike other professions, an increased supply of physicians has actually led to higher levels of health spending. Unlike in other industries in which more suppliers typically result in lower overall costs and revenues, in healthcare, competition has had minimal impact on total costs.

An additional issue to consider is the backlash against managed care. Managed care organizations (MCOs) and medical groups have been accused of skimping on patient care to increase revenues. Numerous lawsuits have been initiated against managed care companies (Mariner 2000), and more suits are likely in the future. An important issue for, Congress will be deciding on the level of liability appropriate for MCOs. Regardless of Congressional action, creative lawsuits will continue to be filed against MCOs. Consequently, physician compensation models and managed care plans must anticipate the potential for legal action. This undercuts the willingness of employers, who ultimately pay most of the costs for medical care, to aggressively promote such models.

Payment Mechanisms Associated with Practice Settings

Most variations in how doctors are paid come from settings in which doctors practice or are employed. Each setting offers benefits and drawbacks to compensation, depending on the goals of the particular practice. It is helpful to understand where they have been to help us better understand how practice settings will continue to evolve.

Office-Based Practices

Three broad categories of office practice are solo, group, and independent practice association (IPA). The solo practitioner practices alone, and the group practice may consist of several partners or a larger group of physicians who have established a legal entity to deliver care. The IPA usually consists of a collection of practices, including both solo and group practitioners who join forces in taking advantage of economies of scale for contracting, business services, or ancillary services (such as laboratory). The IPA may negotiate on behalf of the members and typically has signature authority to establish contracts and distribute reimbursements.

Office-based physician practice is the classic model in which two or more physicians work together in an office setting. The degree of affiliation between the physicians can range from tight to very loose. A closely knit group comprises physicians seeking to practice with a common philosophy and approach; this closeness may include both business and clinical functions. A loosely connected group has physicians sharing some common office services, such as clerical and billing, but practicing independently in all other regards, especially concerning fiscal matters.

For solo and group practice physicians, the dominant reimbursement mode is pure fee-for-service (FFS). Fee schedules used in determining payments have been significantly reduced by private payers and the government in recent years. An unintended, but not unexpected, consequence has been an increase in utilization of services so that even as the price of each unit of service has declined the number of units provided has increased. This increase in service has further resulted in higher incomes for many specialties even as fee schedules are driven lower. As fee schedules are lowered, or discounted, physicians have an incentive to increase volume to make up the difference in their income.

Discounted FFS is not likely to change in the foreseeable future. Solo physicians and smaller groups are not good candidates to accept risk structures. Rather than set such practices up to fail—leading to network disruption and the dissatisfaction of patients, physicians, and employers—

most payers will continue to reserve risk contracts for the few large, highly integrated groups that can handle them. Discounted FFS is simple and straightforward in contrast to risk models. It is also much easier for most health plans to administer.

IPAs may seek risk contracts from a payer, particularly if the IPA is large and well integrated. This implies a shared philosophy of care among physicians, with a high degree of self-discipline. Such groups actively monitor utilization internally, usually comparing it to national standards and scientifically validated treatment guidelines. Physicians who deviate significantly from these norms are either reeducated by their peers or are asked to leave the group. Frequently, a sophisticated information-gathering system is in place within the group to facilitate monitoring of outcomes and utilization. Information allows a group to control costs and to maximize efficiency. This creates a climate for accepting financial risk.

Few IPAs have the ability to accept significant risk projects and make them work. More typical is the IPA that is paid from a discounted FFS schedule and has some sort of incentive program to add dollars to the total reimbursement for the group. Such incentive plans may award a portion of any savings to physician members if the group achieves targeted utilization in areas such as use of pharmaceuticals or lab tests. Incentives may consist of simply a bonus, or they may be more complicated. Money may be put aside to be shared if targets are met, or a percentage increase in the fee schedule may occur if the group successfully manages its patients. The key point is that incentives are designed to encourage the group to perform at a higher level, but regardless of the success in reaching these goals, the physicians are still paid for each service provided.

Staff-Model Groups

Some medical groups or HMOs employ physicians on a straight salary basis or staff model—a model common in the late 1970s and early 1980s. Many early HMOs, such as Prudential and Humana, formulated the staff model as their primary method of caring for their members. Under a staff model concept, physicians employed by a care delivery organization are not distracted by concerns of generating revenue to cover practice expenses. They are able to focus on practicing medicine.

There are several drawbacks to the staff model, especially the difficulty in recruiting physicians who want to be employees. Most physicians enter medicine to practice independently, not to be under an employer's control. Despite having an employed group of doctors who theoretically have their personal goals aligned with an organization, many HMOs found physician utilization to be as high and as variable as use of physicians in private practices.

The work ethic of employed physicians was a significant factor in determining the fiscal success of the staff model. Many medical directors of staff-model HMOs were frustrated by the difficulty in motivating salaried physicians to extend themselves beyond prescribed hours and tasks. As a result, the staff model withered in the last decade. However, the model is still a force in California because of the strong presence of the Permanente group, the staff-model organization that serves Kaiser HMO. Elsewhere in the country, isolated staff-model groups remain as relics of the past, supported primarily by a loyal base of long-time patients. However, the era of the salary-based physician practice has probably come and gone, and with it are significant losses as noted in Figure 10.6.

Hospital-Based Physicians

A large cadre of physicians—pathologists, radiologists, and anesthesiologists, among others—practice almost exclusively within the confines of nonacademic hospitals. In the past, many were directly employed by hospitals and received a straight salary. Recently, however, these physicians have formed professional corporations that contract with hospitals for services, often on an exclusive basis. For instance, a hospital may contract to have services provided by a group of emergency medicine physicians. This group will staff the emergency room, be paid on a contractual basis, and may even take over the administration of the unit. The basis for the contract is typically some formula that represents the billings the unit generates, with an additional amount included for such items as administration, participation on hospital committees, and so forth. The same model can apply to other specialties as well. The key interaction from a reimbursement perspective occurs between the administrators of the hospital and the physicians' organization. The doctors function as independent contractors within the hospital; they are "in it" but not "of it."

The scenario changes somewhat for physicians in the academic, tertiary care medical center. Several unique aspects of these institutions must be considered. A large percentage of physicians in this setting are in training as residents or fellows. Their salaries are paid in large measure from Medicare reimbursements received by the medical center for the purpose of supporting graduate medical education. Thus, their salaries are not linked to their clinical performance, number of patients seen, rate of procedures performed, or other measures of productivity or quality. For staff or faculty physicians, salary is also the rule (because typically these physicians receive a straight salary that is not based on productivity), although the role of clinical activity is often figured into it.

The mission of the academic physician may be summarized as a combination of teaching, research, and patient care. With decreased

FIGURE 10.6

Outfall from
the Demise of
Staff-Model
Groups

For several decades, the Group Health Cooperative of Puget Sound, a staff-model HMO based in Seattle, Washington, has participated with several other HMOs in providing managed care data for public health research. The advantages of a defined population and provider group offered by Group Health have enabled health services researchers to suggest policy improvements in care delivery. Breast cancer screening, sexually transmitted disease, adverse pharmaceutical effects, smoking mortality, and periodic health checkups illustrate areas to which health research has contributed to improve service delivery.

The so-called HMO research network has been supported by staff-model groups, including The Meyers Primary Care Institute (Massachusetts), Group Health, Harvard-Pilgrim Health Plan, Health Partners (Minnesota), Henry Ford Health Systems (Michigan), Kaiser (Georgia, Hawaii, Northern California, Rocky Mountain Region, Southern California Region, Northwest Region), and Prudential. These groups have progressively improved their data systems to the point that large-scale collaborative investigations have been facilitated. Research has focused on both quality of care and fiscal issues.

According to Fishman and Wagner (1998) at Group Health Cooperative's Center for Health Studies, desirable research possibilities may soon deteriorate. They cite the growing transition to IPAs—network organizations where loosely affiliated physician groups do not have strong incentives to partake in research. Cost-savings concerns by IPAs further diminish the potential for research as there is less investment in data systems. Thus, the clinical outfall from the demise of staff-model groups is less high-quality data for disease management.

reimbursements to hospitals, the need for these physicians to perform more clinical work has grown. This may or may not be accompanied by an increase in salary and often depends on whether a "faculty practice plan" exists. This is essentially a group practice consisting of the faculty of the medical center. Such a group is created as a way to leverage the billings generated by faculty into some sort of shared distributions, or at least a higher salary for those physicians who produce high clinical volumes.

The amount of additional income flowing from the faculty practice plan is usually not great except for subspecialties; the principal source of income for an academic physician remains the salary from the institution. These salaries are invariably lower than those in the private-practice sector and reflect the typical differential for salaries between the academic and commercial environments. Some physicians within the academic setting may see no patients at all but focus entirely on research. Many of them derive the bulk of their salaries from grants they are able to secure from outside agencies; the remainder may come from the university. As a result, the longevity of a researcher in this environment may well depend on his or her skill at preparing grant applications and performing research that is deemed worthy of outside support.

A growing mode of practice for physicians is working in temporary staffing arrangement, or locum tenens. *Locum tenens* physicians refer to any temporarily employed physician, who is typically paid a fixed amount for services provided. This increase in temporary work arrangements has been linked to the increase in female physicians (Croasdale 2002), the persistence of physician shortages, an increase in the number of partially retired physicians, and lifestyle considerations favored by a growing number of newly trained physicians. Physicians move into these positions by arranging a position through personal contacts or advertising and by being assigned by a physician staffing service (Simon and Alonzo 2004). The use of locum tenens physicians is likely to increase because of the flexibility given the physician and the organization. This is also part of a significant national trend across industries—the use of contingent workers.

Physicians in Management and Administration

One interesting trend over the last decade has been the rise in the number of physicians who are employed full time as medical directors, consultants, and administrators. Aside from those working for managed care organizations, health insurers, and large provider groups, many physicians are now working for large employers who want to better understand and control the resources devoted to healthcare benefits. These physicians fill critical roles as internal experts on medical care and health policy. By functioning as internal experts attuned to the unique problems of their employer, these physicians help benefits coordinators and HR administrators address the complex issues that arise for employees. They also serve as liaisons between the benefits and HR personnel of the company and external vendors such as health plans, large provider groups, and ancillary providers.

Medical directors are also increasingly found in important roles in state and federal agencies for the same reasons. As healthcare costs continue to escalate, this trend will likely continue. Medical directors are typically salaried and given the same sorts of benefits and incentives offered to executives in most companies.

Difficulties and Conflicts in Compensating Physicians

The most contentious issues that employers face with salaried physicians, whether in an academic medical center, a large provider group, or a large system, are the same as for any other employees: benefits, perquisites, and salary levels. A very difficult challenge in determining physician pay is assessing the parameters based on productivity. Even for a medical group of two physicians, the potential exists for disagreements over what constitutes productivity levels. The following illustrate the complex issues behind the arguments:

- If a patient new to the practice is "counted" at a higher value than a returning patient, what defines a new patient? Someone who has never been seen before? Someone who has not been seen within a given time frame? Someone who has not been seen for a non-acute visit?
- For a procedure-based specialty such as gastroenterology, does the physician who performs the procedure get full credit for it, or should partial credit go to the physician who has seen the patient most frequently over the past year?
- For an obstetric practice, should the physician who performs more vaginal deliveries (which represent more time at the bedside) receive more credit than a physician who has a higher rate of Cesarean-section operations (which produce a higher fee for the practice)?

The details or fine points of a case may seem unimportant, but they are worth careful consideration because they are linked to a dollar value. This can make a significant difference in overall compensation for a physician. Add elements as seniority in the group, the number of call days taken, or outside activities such as service on hospital or medical society committees, and one can appreciate the dilemma many practices face in dividing up practice revenues.

Many medical groups have attempted to address these problems by designing formulae that incorporate multiple contributing factors to be considered when calculating compensation. By their nature, these formulae can become extremely complex in that they try to account for a number of unrelated items that are often difficult to accurately measure. For example, surgical groups may try to include the number of cases seen with various weightings based on the severity of illness of the patient as well as a factor for covering the emergency room, teaching residents at the medical school, and the number of holiday calls taken. Such projects take an inordinate amount of time to devise but typically end up affecting a small fraction of the total income of the physician. A further problem is the inability of any complicated payment scheme to either reinforce behavior desired by the practice or to extinguish undesirable behavior. Problems in defining incentive pay systems are further described in Figure 10.7.

While employed physicians in large medical groups may not be directly affected by such productivity questions, groups are highly dependent on medical staff members for their contributions in attaining efficiency while upholding high quality of care. For many groups that went on a hiring

Epstein, Lee, and Hamel (2004) cite the increasing prevalence of pay-for-performance schemes for physicians. They observe that physicians are more likely to experience schemes that encourage them to improve quality of care and patient satisfaction than utilization. Despite the relatively unsophisticated nature of these approaches (often based on questionable patient survey data), the authors conclude that the magnitude of financial incentives for physician performance is growing. They review three examples to illustrate the diversity of physician compensation approaches.

1. *Bridges to Excellence*. General Electric and other employers in Massachusetts partnered with Tufts Health Plan, the Lahey Clinic, and Partners HealthCare to create an incentive of $55 per patient per year for physician offices that maintain systems for improving care (e.g., registries and electronic medical records). An additional $100 is awarded to physicians who qualify for the American Diabetes Association's Provider Recognition Program. The diabetes module of Bridges to Excellence now exists in several other cities, including Cincinnati and Louisville, with Humana and GE as codevelopers. Close to $80,000 in incentive rewards were distributed in Cincinnati in 2004, with more than 3,000 participating diabetic patients. Of great significance is the fact that the program has been successfully implemented in a community setting, moving beyond the large academic environment.

2. *Integrated Healthcare Association's Physician Payment Program*. Six health plans in California, known as the Integrated Healthcare Association, issue a physician performance scorecard incorporating clinical measures, patient ratings, and information technology. Clinical measures account for 50 percent of the rating, but other measures constitute the remaining 50 percent. This incentive plan is estimated to result in the distribution of $100 million in 2004.

3. *Anthem Blue Cross and Blue Shield Plan*. This New Hampshire health plan rewards physicians who provide preventive services linked to HEDIS (Health Plan Employer Data and Information Set) measures. Physicians in the top performance group receive $20 per patient per year. The average award for all levels of performance per practice is $195.

According to Epstein, Lee, and Hamel, current systems for measuring performance are either lacking or need improvement to align incentives with outcomes.

FIGURE 10.7

Trends in Physician Pay Systems

binge in the mid-1990s, as well as hospitals that adopted practices to lock in patient referrals, the assumption often was that employed physicians would maintain the same high productivity rates they delivered when they were self-employed. However, many physicians sold their practices to reduce their workload, leading to a dramatic drop in patient volumes. As a result, healthcare organizations that employ physicians have been faced with large deficits from their staffs of providers, which have led to severe financial strains.

Future Directions for Physician Compensation

The current framework for compensating physicians has not substantially changed medical practice. The advent of capitation and the use of incentives were assumed to initiate a revolution in how physicians treat patients as well as how physicians would be paid for their services. After a decade of change in the healthcare industry, the vast majority of practicing physicians continue to be paid on some sort of fee-for-service basis. Rather than this number decreasing as a result of the expansion of managed care, it is actually growing as more health plans move away from risk-based contracts in a tacit acknowledgment of their failure to substantially modify physician behavior (*Managed Care Outlook* 1999). As such, new compensation methods are necessary to transform patterns of medical practice. Proposed changes to medical care delivery cannot be successful unless physicians support them. This support depends on making certain that physicians are fairly and adequately compensated.

In the coming years more opportunities for innovation will surface as the healthcare field searches for new paths to follow. These include the following:

- Physicians will become more creative in defining their fee and payment structures. The leaders in this area have been cosmetic surgeons who have always been paid out-of-pocket for the bulk of the work they do. They were among the first physicians to make payment for services with credit cards possible and to set up payment schedules in advance of surgery. While these payment options were commonplace in the rest of the economy, in medicine they were revolutionary.
- Reproductive endocrinologists are now asking for a fee up front— say $30,000—to cover three cycles of in vitro fertilization. If the patient does not conceive at the end of the third cycle, the fee is refunded except for a small amount to cover costs. Patients are thus provided with a quasi money-back guarantee. By seeking flexibility in payment, recognizing that their services are expensive, and making services more accessible to those without insurance coverage, these specialists have found new ways to secure their revenue stream.
- Americans spend more than $13 billion per year on complementary and alternative medicine modalities, such as acupuncture, massage therapy, homeopathy, and biofeedback. Almost 100 percent of this alternative medicine expenditure is usually not covered by insurance. The public seems to have an insatiable demand for these therapies, and physicians will seek to capture some of this huge volume of care

by offering more options to receive alternative medicine within the context of their (traditional) medical practices. Because this care occurs outside of a fee schedule negotiated with a payer, it may well come to represent a large portion of some doctors' incomes in the future.

- For physicians who are still paid primarily by third-party payers, reimbursement will be tied to performance. Tools for assessing outcomes of care tied to such parameters as patient satisfaction and use of various treatments will increase in number and utilization. Report cards on doctors' practice patterns and performance will become more widely available. Just as consumers now go to a variety of sources, especially the Internet, to research the purchase of a new car or house, they will be able to do the same for selecting their physicians and hospitals. Once chosen, the level of reimbursement will be more related to reported performance. Providers who perform at a high level will be paid at a higher level than those who do not perform as well.

- Employers are nearing the end of their 50-year run as the source for most Americans' health insurance. In the next few years, a sea change will occur, with more and more employers divesting themselves of this responsibility and returning it to the individual. Patients/consumers will then be accountable for making the kind of healthcare choices currently left up to benefits managers at work. Having this freedom to choose will require consumers to become more educated in managing their own health. This will be facilitated by the creation and availability of thousands of web sites devoted to medical topics. In turn, physicians will see their patients become more informed and discriminating consumers. They will need to provide their patients with the type of service and quality that will lure them back for a second visit and will represent value to them as the ultimate payer. Price will certainly be part of this value equation, and physicians will need to respond to price in ways they have never contemplated.

Summary

Note that all the options discussed in this chapter revolve around some variation of the fee-for-service (FFS) model, which will continue to be the primary method for paying for medical services. Ironically, after an intense decade of experimentation with novel methods of reimbursement, we return to the time-tested FFS structure. Yet important differences exist between the models represented in 2004 and those used in 1985. FFS payment levels will no longer be dictated by "usual and customary" rates that were established by a de facto agreement of practicing physicians. They will instead be based on a market formulation that relates to the value of services as perceived by patients/customers. Therefore, physicians and groups who demonstrate a higher value will command a higher price for their services. This will remake the FFS system into one that more closely resembles the compensation mechanisms we are familiar with in other sectors of the economy.

References

Adams, J. S. 1963. "Toward an Understanding of Inequity." *Journal of Abnormal and Social Psychology* 67 (5): 422–36.

Bartol, K.M. 1979. "Professionalism as a Predictor of Organizational Commitment, Role Stress, and Turnover: A Multidimensional Approach." *Academy of Management Journal* 22 (4): 815–21.

Berkowitz, S. M. 2002. "The Development of a Successful Physician Compensation Plan." *Journal of Ambulatory Care Management* 25 (4): 10–25.

Berwick, D. M. 1995. "Toxicity of Pay for Performance." *Quality Management in Healthcare* 4 (1): 27–33.

Bunning, R. L. 1992. "Models for Skill-Based Pay Plans." *HR Magazine* 37 (2): 62–64.

Burchell, R. C., H. L. Smith, and N. F. Piland. 2002. *Reinventing Medical Practice: Care Delivery That Satisfies Physicians, Patients and the Bottom-Line.* Denver, CO: Medical Group Management Association.

Capo, J. 2001. "Identifying the Causes of Staff Turnover." *Family Practice Management* 8 (4): 29–33.

Conrad, D. A., A. M. Sales, A. Chaudhuri, S. Liang, C. Maynard, L. Pieper, L. Weinstein, D. Gans, and N. Piland. 2002. "The Impact of Financial Incentives on Physician Productivity in Medical Groups." *Health Services Research* 37 (4): 885–906.

Croasdale, M. 2002. "Practice Must Cope as More Physicians Work Part-Time Hours." *American Medical News* 45 (39): 1–2.

Egger, E. 2000. "Nurse Shortage Worse than You Think, but Sensitivity May Help Retain Nurses." *Healthcare Strategic Management* 18 (5): 16–18.

Epstein, A. M., T. H. Lee, and M. B. Hamel. 2004. "Paying Physicians for High-Quality Care." *New England Journal of Medicine* 350 (4): 406–10.

Fishman, P. A., and E. H. Wagner. 1998. "Managed Care Data and Public Health: The Experience of Group Health Cooperative of Puget Sound." *Annual Review of Public Health* (19): 477–91.

Gaynor, M., and M. V. Pauly. 1990. "Compensation and Productive Efficiency in Partnerships: Evidence from Medical Group Practice." *Journal of Political Economy* 98 (3): 544–73.

Grib, G., and S. O'Donnell. 1995. "Pay Plans that Reward Employee Achievement—Competency-based Payment Plans." *HR Magazine* 40 (7): 49–50.

Grumbach, K., J. V. Selby, C. Damberg, A. B. Bindman, C. Quesenberry, A. Truman, and C. Uratsu. 1999. "Solving the Gatekeeper Conundrum: What Patients Value in Primary Care and Referrals to Specialists." *JAMA* 282 (3): 261–66.

Gunderman, R. B. 2004. "The Perils of Paying Academic Physicians According to the Clinical Revenue They Generate." *Medical Science Monitor* 10 (2): 15–20.

Gupta, N., and J. D. Shaw. 1998. "Let the Evidence Speak: Financial Incentives Are Effective." *Compensation and Benefits Review* 30 (2): 26, 28–32.

Herzberg, F., B. Mausner, and B. Snyderman. 1959. *The Motivation to Work.* New York: John Wiley.

Hills, F. S., T. J. Bergmann, and V. G. Scarpello. 1994. *Compensation Decision Making, 2nd Edition.* Forth Worth, TX: Dryden.

Homans, G. C. 1961. *Social Behavior: Its Elementary Forms.* New York: Harcourt, Brace and World.

Jacobs, K. 1997. "The Broad View." *The Wall Street Journal* Eastern Edition (April 10): R10.

Kaplan, R. S., and D. P. Norton. 1996. *The Balanced Scorecard.* Boston: Harvard Business School Press.

Kilborn, P. T. 1999. "Doctors' Incomes Rising Again Despite HMOs." *Cincinnati Enquirer* (April 22): A2.

Kingma, M. 2003. "Economic Incentive in Community Nursing: Attraction, Rejection or Indifference?" *Human Resources for Health* [Online publication; retrieved 5/12/05.] http://www.human-resources-health.com.

Managed Care Outlook. 1999. "Florida Blues Ditch Capitation in Favor of Fee-for-Service." *Managed Care Outlook* [Online publication; retrieved 5/21/05.] http://www.managedcaremag.com.

Mariner, W. K. 2000. "What Recourse? Liability for Managed-Care Decisions and the Employee Retirement Income Security Act." *New England Journal of Medicine* 343 (8): 592–96.

Martocchio, J. 2001. *Strategic Compensation.* Upper Saddle River, NJ: Prentice Hall.

Maslow, A. 1970. *Motivation and Personality, 2nd Edition.* New York: Harper & Row.

Mohr, V., J. Zinn, J. Angelelli, J. M. Teno, and S. C. Miller. 2004. "Driven to Tiers: Socioeconomic and Racial Disparities in the Quality of Nursing Home Care." *The Milbank Quarterly* 82 (2): 227–56.

O'Connor, J. P., D. B. Nash, M. L. Buehler, and M. Bard. 2002. "Satisfaction Higher for Physician Executives Who Treat Patients, Survey Says." *Physician Executive* 28 (3): 17–21.

Pfeffer, J. 1998. "Six Dangerous Myths About Pay." *Harvard Business Review* 76 (3): 108–19.

Rost, K. T. 2002. "What You Don't Know Can Hurt You: Why Managed Care Organizations Have a Legal Duty to Disclose the Use of Financial Incentives to Limit Medical Care." *Journal of Health Law* 35 (1): 145–69.

Simon, A. B., and A. A. Alonzo. 2004. "The Demography, Career Pattern, and Motivation of *Locum Tenens* Physicians in the United States." *Journal of Healthcare Management* 49 (6): 363–75.

Starr, P. 1982. *The Social Transformation of American Medicine*, 198–235. New York: Basic Books.

Thompson, E. 2000. "Physician Compensation Report: Docs' Income Growth Stabilizes." *Modern Healthcare* (August 7): 37–41.

Wagner, F. H., and M. B. Jones. 1994. "Broadbanding in Practice: Hard Facts and Real Data." *Journal of Compensation and Benefits* 10 (1): 27–34.

Winslow, R. 2000. "A Type of Heart Drug Wins Wide Use Owing to Small Firm's Efforts." *The Wall Street Journal* (November 17): A1.

Discussion Questions

1. In a low-budget healthcare setting (such as a local health department), what will you do to recruit new staff and to motivate current employees when competitors in the area are able to pay 30 to 40 percent more than your organization?

2. Assume that you are working as a staff nurse in a hospital and you are working under an incentive system. Do you have an obligation to disclose the nature of the compensation arrangement to patients? If so, how should this information be communicated and by whom?

3. Regardless of your personal feelings about pay for performance, what cautions will you communicate to a team that is designing an incentive system in a healthcare organization?

4. How will you design a team-based compensation system such that free riders (or "loafers") cannot take advantage of the system?

5. How can job evaluation procedures be used to determine if a healthcare organization is undercompensating its female employees?

6. What effect has managed care had on designing physician-compensation models?

7. What are the likely roles for capitation and fee-for-service reimbursement in the future?

8. For a four-person surgical group, what kind of formula may be devised to fairly and consistently measure and reward productivity? What changes may be needed if one surgeon decides to perform more office work and less surgery?

Experiential Exercises

Case   Mapleton Family Medicine is a physician group practice located in a small town (population 5,000) in the midwest about 15 miles north of a small city (population 76,000). Mapleton is an eight-physician practice, consisting of family physicians, internists, and pediatricians. The practice is owned by two of the physicians. The six other physicians are currently salaried.

The owners are concerned with productivity and quality in the practice. There is a relatively long waiting time for appointments, and a recent chart review revealed that the percentage of children who are up-to-date with immunizations has dropped. Anecdotal evidence suggests as well that at-risk persons are not routinely receiving flu and pneumonia vaccinations. Many patients have complained about having to wait up to 90 minutes in the waiting room. At this time, however, the practice is not in a position to hire another physician.

Each physician in the practice currently sees an average of 25 patients per day. The owners want this number increased to 30 patients per day without sacrificing quality of care. To reach this goal, they are thinking of moving to an incentive system, whereby physicians have a base salary equivalent to 75 percent of their current salary and have the opportunity to earn up to 125 percent of their base salary if they meet defined volume and quality goals. While the owners have not thought this system through completely, they want to set 30 patients per day as a base and, through the incentive system, encourage physicians to see up to 35 patients per day on average.

In terms of quality, the owners have considered three measures:

1. Patient satisfaction surveys
2. Child-immunization audit data
3. Patient waiting times

Quality goals will be set biannually for each physician. The expectation is that physicians who achieve these goals will earn their full salary (assuming volume is adequate), and quality measures above their goals will result in bonuses according to a pay schedule.

Case Questions

1. You have been brought in to advise the owners on their proposed compensation plan, what advice will you give them before they proceed?

2. Do you see any potential negative consequences of this plan based on the information provided? If so, how will you address these concerns?
3. How do you think the physicians in the practice will react to this plan? Should they be involved in developing the plan, and if so, how should they be involved?

Exercise   As discussed in this chapter, an organization's indirect compensation program includes a wide range of benefits and services. In this exercise, you are asked to compare two organizations' approaches to indirect compensation.

Your first task is to identify two healthcare organizations that are similar in mission or size. For example, you may select two medical group practices, two medium-size community hospitals, two nursing homes of similar size, and so forth. Your second task is to identify the senior human resources management executive, and/or the individual most closely involved in developing and implementing indirect compensation (benefits and other services) for the organization. Using the following questions as a guide, conduct an interview with this individual or individuals. Your third task is to summarize the indirect compensation offers of each organization, then report on the differences between their practices.

Questions to Guide a Compensation Comparison

1. What benefits and services are provided to all employees? What benefits and services are optional?
2. On average, what percentage of total compensation is accounted for by indirect compensation?
3. What benefits, if any, are offered only to particular groups of employees? What is the rationale for this? Does length of service affect an employee's eligibility for certain benefits?
4. How is indirect compensation administered? Which benefits are administered in-house and which are outsourced?
5. What choices are available to employees in their health insurance? If different options are available, what is the approximate number and percentage of employees electing each option?

6. Are the benefits provided by the organization perceived to be competitive with those offered by similar organizations in this market?
7. What are the most important issues, challenges, and trends facing the organization in the area of indirect compensation?
8. Organizational demographics:
   * name and purpose/mission of organization
   * number of employees
   * size (number of beds and/or other suitable measure)

CREATING AND MAINTAINING A SAFE AND HEALTHY WORKPLACE

Michael T. Ryan, Ph.D., C.H.P., and Anne Osborne Kilpatrick, D.P.A.

Learning Objectives

After completing this chapter, the reader should be able to

- identify the factors associated with safe and healthy workplaces;
- describe key steps to take in improving the safety and health of a workplace;
- understand the principles behind workplace health and safety programs;
- discuss the elements contained in a safety program; and
- define the concept of toxins, which interfere with organizational effectiveness.

Introduction

Creating and maintaining a safe and healthy workplace are concerns in all organizations, especially for healthcare institutions. To provide guidance to managers in this regard, we discuss approaches to health and safety education and suggest practical steps to follow in improving workplace safety and health. We contend that the most successful programs engage workers at all levels in the organization to anticipate and address problems in a proactive manner.

In considering the effectiveness of health and safety programs, it is useful to first consider how we think about success. Reduction in the rates of recordable injuries and illnesses is often celebrated as progress in safety excellence. While low rates of recordable injuries are often used as a measure of safety excellence or improvement, this may not be the most appropriate measure. Any goal except zero implies that some accidents are to be expected and are acceptable. The key to developing an attitude of zero injuries and accidents is for management to establish a safety-conscious work environment.

Safety in the Workplace

Maintaining a safe workplace while conforming to federal, state, and local regulations requires a comprehensive safety compliance program (ASHS 1997; AHA 1994). Such a program entails careful planning, preparation, implementation, performance tracking, and process improvement. A positive safety-conscious work environment is best established with a strong, visible commitment and active program participation from executive management down to entry-level employees. Good safety behaviors exhibited by leaders in the organization are likely to be copied; key success factors are discussed later in this chapter. Several key principles should guide the process of developing a safety program:

1. *Review carefully all rules and regulations that apply to your activities.* Pay particular attention to overlapping and seemingly conflicting requirements under different rules or regulations (Moeller 1997).

2. *Develop formal, concise, written communications that explain the organization's safety policies and that provide instructions on how to perform tasks in a safe manner.* Instructions should include specific requirements for documentation of routine activities. Methods of reporting incidents, accidents, or other unexpected circumstances should also be included in written procedures. Document all work practices and assess all tasks regarding safety and related regulatory requirements (Government Institutes 1997; Wilson 1998).

3. *Conduct formal training and retraining to routinely inform employees regarding safety issues.* Such training can include initial and refresher education on health and safety basics; special-issue seminar following an incident or accident; or new training after changes in work practices, technology, or regulatory requirements.

4. *Develop a plan to ensure buy-in throughout all levels of the organization.* Senior management must set the standard by participating in program development and being actively involved in safety training and recognition of safety performance. Throughout the organization positive safety practices must be reinforced as poor safety practices are replaced.

5. *Investigate incidents and accidents in a proactive, not punitive, fashion.* Be responsive to the facts. Incidents that do occur should be thoroughly investigated by a preestablished investigation team, including legal and technical experts. These investigations should be done for purposes of fact finding, prevention of recurrence, and satisfactory resolution of the incident at hand. Find and fix root causes, and train and retrain people accordingly.

Management's Role

Management commitment to health and safety should be visible in two ways. First, active leadership and participation are important in safety activities such as meetings, training, and celebration events. Second, leaders' involvement in setting the safety example is key to establishing a positive safety culture. Direct and indirect financial commitment to the safety program and its implementation is essential. If safety programs are to be an important part of a facility's activities, the allocation of resources is a visible way to confirm this commitment. Safety programs should be managed using the same cost, schedule, and control approaches as any other important programs within a facility. Safety should not be viewed as an add-on to someone's responsibilities or fit into the schedule of other activities. In smaller facilities it may be necessary to make safety responsibilities a part of a manager's overall duties. Care should be taken to ensure that safety receives due attention throughout the organization, no matter how large or small the entity.

A Safety Program

The first step in developing a safety program is to define, clearly and completely, all work activities that occur in all parts of the facility, as program requirements and standards will be dictated by the work activities that are formally identified and included in program considerations. Care should be taken when establishing safety standards for each work function, making sure that all identified activities are given sufficient and balanced attention. Unrealistic expectations from workers in certain areas may result in more unsafe practices or failure to obey the standards. Safety requirements that do not seem reasonable and practical are likely seen by workers as something to be followed for regulations' sake, not for the sake of ensuring worker safety. Requirements that are too rigorous may be viewed as overprotective of certain areas, leading to unnecessary work and failed implementation. Conversely, inadequate focus on some work activities may cause these areas to be underprotected.

A successful safety program embodies at least the following five characteristics:

1. *It is well written and concise.* Procedures clearly convey what work has to be done, how to perform the work safely and efficiently, and what documentation is required from the person performing the work.
2. *Its standards meet all regulatory requirements.* Regulatory agencies include but are not limited to the Occupational Safety and Health Administration (OSHA), the U.S. Environmental Protection Agency,

the Centers for Disease Control, and the U.S. Nuclear Regulatory Commission. In some cases, the responsibilities of these federal agencies are delegated to their state agency counterparts.

3. *It includes recommendations from regulatory and accrediting bodies.* Recommending bodies include but are not limited to the Joint Commission on Accreditation of Healthcare Organizations (JCAHO), the National Fire Protection Association, National Institute of Standards and Technology, the Compressed Gas Association, and various state and local agencies.

4. *It is a living program that can accommodate continual change and improvement.*

5. *It guides work activities in a positive fashion both when things are well and when incident, accident, and off-normal circumstances occur.*

Program Implementation

Safety program implementation is more likely to be supported and accepted by staff if management displays a positive attitude about the program and communicates its seriousness about following the set program requirements. Leadership not only must educate the entire workforce on the items included in the program but also must highlight the positive benefits of the program, which focuses on avoiding on-the-job injury and illness.

Four key elements must be present to ensure the successful implementation of a safety program:

1. *The chief executive officer of a healthcare institution must appoint a qualified safety director, per JCAHO's requirement.* For example, an academic medical center requires a more comprehensive program than does a small regional or rural hospital. The safety director sets program direction and goals, leads the safety committee and safety activities at the facility, and responds to success or failure in safety performance with either recognition events or process improvements.

2. *The safety committee must be an active group that continually implements program requirements, changes, and improvements.* This committee should review and attend to matters of safety in every department and every activity within the facility. It should also be involved in setting, measuring, and evaluating safety measures; reporting results; and suggesting improvements to the safety director and the organization's executive management.

3. *All work groups and departments must be involved in ensuring that safety standards are being followed in their specific areas.* Program requirements must be tailored in a way that is sensible for each area. For example, in the laundry department, the safety emphasis should

be on careful handling of material and monitoring for heat stress. These safety concerns are different in every department and area such as inpatient care. In addition, department workers can provide the safety committee and management with suggestions on how to improve the program.

4. *Work-practice modification techniques and engineering controls must be used in combination.* An example is the proper selection and use of respiratory protection, protective clothing such as gowns and gloves, and tools that help with material handling and prevent hand and foot injuries.

Program Measurement

To yield information about how the program can be improved and how it is delivering benefits and efficiencies, employee performance must be measured against the established safety requirements. Such measurements should not be punitive. If certain documentation of an incident or accident is required, those reports should be reviewed first. Evaluation may take the form of announced and unannounced inspections and topical inspections (fire, ventilation, or other systems). Inspection reports from regulatory agencies, industry-oversight organizations, and facility insurance carriers must be reviewed as well.

Measurement should not be limited to evaluation of reports and numerical data; it should include observation of work practices, practical factor demonstrations, and drills. If safety measurement becomes just a "numbers game," program effectiveness will suffer. The safety director and the safety committee must establish measures that will yield effective feedback on performance and provide improvement direction.

Continuous Safety Improvement

One way to maintain a safe workplace is to make safety a performance expectation and requirement for every employee. The perception of a punitive environment can be avoided with the establishment of a continuous quality improvement (CQI) program, an approach to improving processes and systems driven by high employee ownership and participation. Safety assessment, hazard analysis, and accident prevention are logical elements to include in a CQI program.

The Healthy Work Environment

A safe workplace is necessary, but it alone will not guarantee a healthy work environment. Classic health and safety issues do not cover the broad spectrum of the healthy workplace, which involves analytical, managerial, and leadership aspects. These two latter aspects contribute to "toxins" in the work environment that negatively affect employee health and safety and hence performance. A partial list of work environment toxins is presented in Figure 11.1.

Some organizations have focused their attention on eliminating these toxins through providing training to supervisors and linking management performance to outcomes in this area. Since 1999, the American Psychological Association has recognized organizations that have developed best practices in ensuring psychologically healthy workplaces. In Canada, a number of conferences and programs have been instituted to educate leaders on ways to implement healthy workplace practices (see, for example, Lowe 2003).

Leadership is responsible for developing and maintaining a healthy workplace free of toxins. Figure 11.2 suggests several characteristics of healthy workplaces and organizations.

FIGURE 11.1
Workplace
Toxins

- Employee fears regarding job loss
- Discrimination and harassment (e.g., racial, sexual)
- Unfair conflict (i.e., supervisor abusing his or her authority in dispute situations)
- Threats/intimidation from coworkers, supervisors, leaders
- Violence from coworkers, supervisors, leaders, patients, family
- Perception or existence of inequity (e.g., training, compensation, benefits, workload)
- Excessive stress
- Lack of privacy

- Poor or lack of communication
- Physical workplace hazards
- Poor supervisor skills
- Excessive length of work hours
- Lack of employee ownership/ accountability for their job
- Budget, service, workforce cutbacks
- Unreasonable performance goals/punishment for errors
- Employee insecurity regarding inconsistent signals about performance requirement
- Supervisor favoritism and other unequal treatment

Source: Adapted from Kilpatrick, A. O. 1995. "Organizational Ecology: Managing the Attitudes and Behaviors That Poison the Workplace Environment." Presented at the Southeastern Conference for Public Administration, July 11, Black Mountain, North Carolina.

- Efficient and effective processes and systems

- Low rates of absenteeism and turnover

- Few grievances and disciplinary actions

- High, positive, and creative energy of employees

- Existence of high worker accountability, empowerment, responsibility, and authority

- Collaboration

- Employee and team synergy

- Jobs that stretch and test worker abilities

- Conflicts are over issues, not personalities

- Participatory democracy

- Worker enthusiasm

- Presence of positive communication

- Tolerant, respectful culture

- High productivity

- Encouragement and presence of healthy competition between units and between teams

- Negotiation is practiced

- Trust is present

FIGURE 11.2

Characteristics of Healthy Workplaces

Recommendations

There are ethical and regulatory reasons to developing a safe and healthy workplace; however, having such a work environment also leads to good business (Bonnet and Yardley 2003). The Canadian Council on Integrated Healthcare (2002) conducted research on ways to reduce the $32.5 billion annual cost of workplace health and safety problems in Canada. Government, employers, and unions share in the responsibility for reducing this cost, and the research offers recommendations to this end. Such suggestions may also work for organizations in the United States:

- *Celebrate safety milestones*, such as the millionth safe work hour in which no incident or accident has occurred. Such celebrations should be part of the organization's health and safety culture. These events offer the best time to renew employees' commitment to follow the program requirements and to review the health and safety plans, procedures, and policies.

- *Create a continuous quality improvement culture*, in which employees are active participants in leading change and conceiving improvements. Such a culture ushers in adjustments to the safety program to meet changing work activities, to minimize areas of weakness, and to demonstrate and maintain regulatory compliance and organizational effectiveness. In this way, valuable human and institutional resources will be respected, conserved, and protected. This improvement culture should work in partnership with traditional elements of a safe and healthy workplace.

Summary

Maintaining a safe and healthy workplace is a major responsibility for management. Leaders have to be champions of the safety program and the workplace environment, offering support and encouragement to the safety director, the safety committee, and every employee to work together to establish, implement, and measure the program. Development of such a program must be done carefully so that the program standards in each area or department are tailored to the work activities performed within that area or department. All workers in the organization must understand the benefits of and reasons behind following safety requirements so that they do not misinterpret the program's intent as merely a regulatory tool rather than an employee-focused effort.

A workplace that is safe is not enough; it also has to be healthy to produce a productive, satisfied workforce. Again, leadership is responsible for creating and maintaining a healthy workplace and should be aware of and eliminate toxins that bring down performance, morale, and quality (for an example, see Kilpatrick 1999).

References

American Hospital Association and the National Safety Council. 1994. *Safety Guide for Health Care Institutions, 5th Edition*, edited by Linda F. Chaff. Chicago: AHA.

American Society for Healthcare Services. 1997. *Health Care Safety Management: A Regulatory Update for 1997—Professional Development Series*. Washington, DC: ASHS.

Bonnet, C., and J. Yardley. 2003. "By the Numbers." [Online publication; retrieved 2/1/03.] http://www.whru.ca/publications/papers/CHMEconomics101.pdf.

Canadian Council on Integrated Healthcare. 2002. Discussion paper on workplace health. [Online publication; retrieved 2/1/03.] http://www.ccih.ca/docs/CCIH-Discuss_Workplace.pdf.

Government Institutes, Inc. 1997. *OSHA CFRs Made Easy*. Title 29 1900–1910.END, CD-ROM version. Rockville, MD: Government Institutes, Inc.

Kilpatrick, A. O. 1995. "Organizational Ecology: Managing the Attitudes and Behaviors That Poison the Workplace Environment." Presented at the Southeastern Conference for Public Administration, July, 11, Black Mountain, North Carolina.

———. 1999. "A New Social Contract for the Next Millenium." *Journal of Public Administration and Management: An Interactive Journal* 4 (2): 165–83.

Lowe, G. 2003. "Building Healthy Organizations Requires More Than Simply Putting in a Wellness Program." *Canadian HR Reporter*. Available online at http://www.grahamlowe.ca/documents/83/.

Moeller, D. W. 1997. *Environmental Health, Revised Edition.* Cambridge, MA: Harvard University Press.

Wilson, T. H. 1998. *OSHA Guide for Health Care Facilities.* Washington, DC: Thompson Publishing Group.

Discussion Questions

1. What are the key principles to follow in developing an organizational safety program?
2. What role should management play in ensuring a safe and healthy workplace and in implementing a safety program?
3. What are workplace toxins, and what are ways to eliminate them?

Experiential Exercises

Scenario 1   An employee attends a scheduled after-hours function at which attendance is mandatory. Alcoholic beverages are served without any charge. The employee is involved in a fatal automobile accident on the drive home from the event. Is this fatality a job-related injury? What are the regulatory requirements? What management actions could have helped prevent this accident?

Scenario 2   A radiological technician, who is pregnant, does not declare her pregnancy to her employer. The supervisor wants to restrict the employee to a "low-exposure potential" assignment, which is at a lower pay level. What are the regulatory requirements? What course of action should management follow?

Scenario 3   A nurse's aid tests positive for HIV and claims it is the result of an unreported needle stick. What are the regulatory requirements? What course of action should management follow?

Scenario 4   A nurse, assigned to care for tuberculosis (TB) patients, tests positive for TB during routine, periodic testing. The nurse claims that her contraction of the disease is the result of improper ventilation maintenance in the TB care area. Combined with this assertion is a record of improper use of respiratory protection by the nurse while on duty in spite of training and retraining. What are the regulatory requirements? What course of action should management follow?

Scenario 5   Over the last several years, the rates of recordable OSHA injuries and illnesses at a large facility have stayed steady but are higher than comparable rates in similar facilities. What actions should management take to evaluate and modify these trends?

Scenario 6   One department has experienced a significant turnover among employees as well as a dramatic increase in worker's compensation claims for stress, hand and foot injuries, and back injuries. In another department, there has been a significant increase in disciplinary actions, accompanied by increased absenteeism, tardiness, and grievances. What actions should management take to evaluate and modify these trends?

12

MANAGING WITH ORGANIZED LABOR

Donna Malvey, Ph.D.

Learning Objectives

After completing this chapter, the reader should be able to

- address the relationship of organized labor and management in healthcare,
- distinguish the different phases of the labor relations process,
- describe the evolving role of unions in the healthcare workforce,
- examine legislative and judicial rulings that affect management of organized labor in healthcare settings, and
- review emerging healthcare labor trends.

Introduction

The *labor relations process* occurs when management (as the representative for the employer) and the union (as the exclusive bargaining representative for the employees) jointly determine and administer the rules of the workplace. A *union* is an organization formed by employees for the purpose of acting as a single unit when dealing with management about workplace issues, and hence the term organized labor. Unions are not present in every organization because employees must authorize a union to represent them. Unions typically are viewed as threats by management because they interfere with management's ability to make and implement decisions. Once a union is present, management may no longer unilaterally make decisions about the terms and conditions of work. Instead, management must negotiate these decisions with the union. Similarly, employees may no longer communicate directly with management about work issues but instead must go through the union. Thus, the union functions as a middleman, which is relatively expensive to maintain for both parties. Employees pay union dues, and management incurs additional costs for such things as contract negotiations and any increases in salaries and benefits negotiated by the union (Freeman and Medoff 1984). In healthcare, because labor costs generally account for 70 to 80 percent of expenditures, controlling labor costs is critically important. Thus, even if a union negotiates a minor wage or benefit increase, it will result in a significant increase in total costs. Subsequently, management has a strong incentive to keep unions out of the organization (Scott and Seers 1996). However, given the trends of unionization in healthcare, managers are increasingly forced to work with unions.

This chapter examines the phenomenon of healthcare unionization and provides direction for managing with organized labor. In addition, it discusses the possible behaviors and strategies that comprise the labor-management relationship; explains the generic labor relations process of organizing, negotiating, and administering contracts; explores developments in organizing a relatively unorganized healthcare workforce; considers the impact of labor laws, amendments, and rulings on human resources (HR) strategies and goals; and addresses the trend toward physician unions and how the changes in physician employment status will affect the growth of these unions.

Managing with organized labor involves the application and maintenance of a positive labor relations program within the organization. A productive and positive labor-management relationship can only be accomplished through integration with other HR functions. For example, employees expect management to provide environments that are clean and safe from workplace hazards and related concerns such as AIDS and hepatitis B. If management allows the environment to deteriorate, union organizers will focus on these issues (Becker and Rowe 1989; Fennell 1987). In addition, the labor relations process occurs across all levels of the organization and involves all levels of management. Upper-level management will develop objectives and strategies regarding wage rates, while mid-level managers and first-line supervisors will implement these objectives.

Developing strategies and goals to implement a positive labor relations program in healthcare requires an understanding of the generic labor relations process of organizing, negotiating, and administering contracts with a union as well as specific knowledge of emerging healthcare labor trends. A productive and positive labor-management relationship involves compromise by both parties because of the adversarial nature of the relationship. Just because a union has won the right to represent employees does not mean that management has to accept all of its terms. All parties—management, unions, and employees—have a vested interest in the success and survival of the organization; yet they also have opposing or conflicting interests. For example, unions will look toward improving the benefits package for employees, while management, faced with budget cutbacks and declining reimbursements, will have concerns about containing costs. Thus, the challenge for management is working with the union to reconcile differences in a fair and consistent manner.

As Figure 12.1 suggests, the labor-management relationship reflects a continuum of possible behaviors and strategies, ranging from the most positive or collaborative (in which management and the union share common goals oriented toward the organization's success) to the most negative or oppositional and self-serving. Even if the relationship is neutral and both parties cooperate to maintain the status quo, a variety of factors can cause the relationship to shift in either direction. For instance, restructuring, such as a merger, may create uncertainty for both the union and management and, as a result, may reposition their relationship along the continuum. However, the direction in which the relationship moves will depend largely on the knowledge and understanding of the labor relations process on both sides of the issue.

Overview of Unionization

During the 1980s and 1990s, organized labor's influence and bargaining power continued to decline and weaken as the nature of U.S. industries shifted from factories and traditional union strongholds to service and technologies (Fottler et al. 1999). This trend appears to have continued, as evidenced by the fact that organized labor has been unable to make any net gains in membership despite downward pressure on wages, increasing healthcare insurance costs, and outsourcing of service and manufacturing jobs overseas (*Christian Science Monitor* 2004).

Union membership has been declining steadily for decades. In the 1950s to 1970s, union membership represented 25 to 30 percent of the U.S. workforce. In 2000, unions represented only 16.3 million or 13.5 percent of workers in the United States. By 2003, only 15.8 million workers, representing 12.9 percent of the U.S. workforce, were union members. Unions appear to be more successful in organizing workers in the public sector than in the private sector (with the exception of state and local governments whose union membership has edged downward) and in healthcare rather than in other industries. The union rate for government or public sector workers has held steady at approximately 37.2 percent since 1983, while the rate for private-industry workers has fallen to 8.2 percent or about half over the same time period (Bureau of Labor Statistics 2000a, 2004; Scott and Lowery 1994).

The healthcare workforce of 9.8 million represents one of the largest pools of unorganized workers in the United States and a prime target for union organizers. Of the 4.3 million healthcare workers currently employed in hospitals, only 471,000 belong to a union. In addition, just 246,000 of the 5.4 million workers employed in other healthcare sectors, such as

FIGURE 12.1
Ranges of
the Labor-
Management
Relationship
in Healthcare

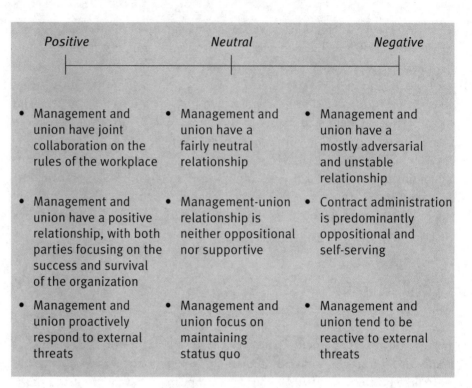

Positive	Neutral	Negative
• Management and union have joint collaboration on the rules of the workplace	• Management and union have a fairly neutral relationship	• Management and union have a mostly adversarial and unstable relationship
• Management and union have a positive relationship, with both parties focusing on the success and survival of the organization	• Management-union relationship is neither oppositional nor supportive	• Contract administration is predominantly oppositional and self-serving
• Management and union proactively respond to external threats	• Management and union focus on maintaining status quo	• Management and union tend to be reactive to external threats

nursing homes and clinics, are unionized (Bureau of Labor Statistics 2000b, 2004). Furthermore, unions in other healthcare sectors have consistently won a greater percentage of their elections than in the hospital segment or even in other industries (Scott and Seers 1996). Also, related occupations are expected to experience growth. Fifteen of the 30 fastest growing occupations are health related, and registered nurses and nursing aides, orderlies, and attendants are projected to experience greater growth during this decade than other health occupations (Hecker 2004). Even though labor surveys indicate that the demand for unions exists, healthcare unions have yet to realize significant membership increases (*Christian Science Monitor* 2004; Kearney 2003).

The Labor Relations Process

In an attempt to protect workers' rights to unionize, the U.S. Congress passed the National Labor Relations Act (NLRA) in 1935, which serves as the legal framework for the labor relations process. Although the NLRA has been amended over the years, it remains the only legislation that governs federal labor relations. The law contains significant provisions intended to protect workers' rights to form and join unions and to engage in collective bargaining. The law also defines unfair labor practices, which restrict both unions and employers from interfering with the labor relations process. The NLRA delegates to the National Labor Relations Board (NLRB) the responsibility for overseeing implementation of the NLRA and for investigating and remedying unfair labor practices. NLRB rulemaking occurs on a case-by-case basis.

Key participants in the labor relations process include (1) management officials, who serve as surrogates for the owners or employers of the organization; (2) union officials, who are usually elected by members; (3) the government, which participates through executive, legislative, and judicial branches occurring at federal, state, and local levels; and (4) third-party neutrals such as arbitrators. The process also involves three phases that are equally essential: the recognition phase, the negotiation phase, and the administration phase.

Recognition Phase

During this phase, unions attempt to organize employees and gain representation through either voluntary recognition of the union or a representation election, which certifies that the union has the authority to act on behalf of employees in negotiating a collective bargaining agreement. In rare cases, the NLRB may direct an employer to recognize and bargain with the union if evidence exists that a fair and impartial election would be impossible. During the past two decades, management strategies and tactics have become more aggressive during the recognition phase as management has endeavored to keep unions from becoming the employees' representative. For example, management may institute unfair labor practices such as filing for bankruptcy, illegally firing union supporters, and relocation. Although unions may file grievances with the NLRB over these practices and the use of any illegal or union-busting tactics, legal resolution usually occurs years after the fact and long after union elections have been held. Thus, both unions and management understand that the battle lines are drawn in the recognition phase, and both sides will be fervently engaged in shoring up support.

The desire to unionize is believed to result from three issues: wages, benefits, and employee perceptions about the workplace. Because ascertaining the desires of employees is difficult, management must rely on signals or indicators in the workplace. Table 12.1 summarizes some of the behaviors that may indicate organizing activities or the potential for organizing employees. For example, high turnover of approximately 40 percent characterizes healthcare institutions such as hospitals (Swoboda 1999). However, when employees are leaving their jobs for a local competitor, management must investigate the underlying reasons for turnover. Even simple issues, such as an increase in requests for information on policies and procedures, can indicate problems and should not be discounted.

TABLE 12.1
Warning
Indicators for
Healthcare
Organizations

Item	Increase/ Decrease	Comment
Turnover—especially to competitors	Increase	Turnover in healthcare organizations typically is much higher than in organizations in other industries because of enhanced mobility from licensing and standardization; however, if employees are moving to competing organizations in the local area, such movement may indicate dissatisfaction rather than career opportunities
Employee-generated incidents	Increase	Staff members are fighting among themselves; theft or damage to organization's property; insubordination related to routine requests by supervisors
Grievances	Increase	More grievances are being filed with the HR office compared with informal settlements of supervisors and employees
Communication	Decrease	Staff members are reluctant to provide feedback and generally become quiet when management enters the room; suggestion boxes are empty and employees are less willing to avail themselves of the "open door" system or other mechanisms to air dissatisfaction/problems
HR office informational requests	Increase	Employees are interested in policies, procedures, and other matters related to the terms and conditions of employment, and they want this information in writing; verbal responses no longer satisfy them
Off-site meetings	Increase	Employees appear to be congregating more at off-site premises
Grapevine activity	Increase	Rumors increase in number and intensity
Absenteeism and/ or tardiness	Increase	Employees are engaging in union-organizing activities prior to and during work hours

During the recognition phase, the union solicits signed authorization cards that designate the union to act as the employees' collective bargaining representative. When at least 30 percent of employees in the bargaining unit have signed their cards, the union requests the employer to voluntarily recognize the union. Voluntary recognition is rarely granted by employers, however, and occurs less than 2 percent of the time in healthcare organizations. When employers refuse voluntary recognition of the union, the union is then eligible to petition the NLRB for a representation election. In response to the petition, the NLRB verifies the authenticity of the signatures collected by the union, determines the appropriate bargaining unit, and sets a date for a secret-ballot election.

The NLRB determines which employees are eligible to be in a bargaining unit. Currently, the NLRB permits a total of eight bargaining units in healthcare settings. The implications of this number and some historical perspective are provided later in this chapter; that section summarizes legislative and judicial rulings. Although the NLRB has modified its criteria over the years, it has not changed its outlook on managerial or supervisory employees, who are ineligible for membership in a bargaining unit. Under a provision of the NLRA (29USCS 152(11), an employee is a "supervisor" if the employee has the authority, in the interest of the employer, to engage in specific activities, including responsible direction of other employees, where exercise of such authority requires the use of independent judgment. The U.S. Supreme court in the case of the *NLRB v. Kentucky River Community Care, Inc.* reached a decision about the legal question of which nurses qualify as supervisors. In its ruling on May 29, 2001, the court determined that registered nurses who use independent judgment in directing employees are supervisors and thus are exempt from being organized into collective bargaining units. This ruling is expected to have a significant impact on the ability of nurses to form unions because employers will try to claim that more registered nurses are supervisors when they direct the work of others such as practical nurses and aides.

Bargaining Units in Healthcare

Generally, the union election is scheduled to occur on workplace premises during work hours. The union is permitted to conduct a pre-election campaign in accordance with solicitation rules that are proscribed for both unions and management. For example, patient care areas such as treatment rooms, waiting areas used by patients, and elevators and stairs used in transporting patients are off limits; but kitchens, supply rooms, business areas, and employee lounges are permissible locations. During the campaign, management may not make threats or announce reprisals regarding the outcome of the election, such as telling nurses that layoffs will result if the union is elected or pay raises will be given if the union loses. Management also may not directly ask employees about their attitudes or voting intentions or those of other employees. Management is allowed, however, to conduct captive-audience speeches, which are meetings during work time to inform employees about the changes that certifying a union will mean for the organization and to persuade employees to give management another chance.

To win the election and be certified by the NLRB as representing the bargaining unit, the union must achieve a simple majority or 50 percent plus 1 of those voting. Consequently, if voter turnout is low, the decision to be unionized will be decided by less than a majority of employees eligible to vote. When the union wins the election, it assumes the duties of the exclusive bargaining agent for all employees in the unit even if those employees choose not to join the union and pay membership dues. Similarly, any negotiated agreements will cover all employees in the bargaining unit. If the union loses, however, it can continue to maintain contact with employees and provide certain representational services such as informing them of their rights. The union may lose the right to represent employees in the bargaining unit through a decertification election.

Negotiation Phase

After winning the election, the union will begin to negotiate a contract on behalf of the employees in the bargaining unit. Federal labor laws encourage collective bargaining on the theory that employees and their employers are best able to reach agreement on issues such as wages, hours, and conditions of employment through negotiating their differences. The process of negotiating this contract is referred to as *collective bargaining*. The NLRA (Section 8 [d], 1935) defines collective bargaining as follows:

> . . . the performance of the mutual obligation of the employer and the representative of the employees to meet at reasonable times and confer in good faith with respect to wages, hours and terms and conditions of employment or the negotiation of an agreement, or any question arising there under, and the execution of a written contract incorporating any agreement reached requested by either party to agree to a proposal or require the making of a concession.

The NLRA requires an employer to recognize and bargain in good faith with a certified union, but it does not force the employer to agree with the union or make any concessions. The key to satisfying the duty to bargain in good faith is approaching the bargaining table with an open mind and negotiating with the intention of reaching final agreement (NLRA, LLR 3115: 7888).

Issues for bargaining have evolved over a period of years as the result of NLRB and court decisions. Those issues are categorized as either illegal, mandatory, or voluntary (permissive). Illegal subjects, such as age-discrimination employment clauses, may not be considered for bargaining. Mandatory bargaining issues are related to wages, hours, and other conditions of employment; Figure 12.2 provides a partial list of these issues. Mandatory subjects must be bargained if they are introduced for negotiation. Voluntary, or permissive bargaining, issues carry no similar restriction. Examples of voluntary issues include strike insurance and benefits for retired employees.

Prior to bargaining, management will formulate ranges for each issue, which is similar to an opening offer, followed by a series of benchmarks that represent expected levels of settlement. Of course, management must calculate a resistance point beyond which it will cease negotiations. Fisher and Ury (1981) have developed a principled method of negotiation based on the merits or principles of the issues. The following four basic points are involved:

1. People: Separate the people from the problem
2. Interests: Focus on interests, not the positions that people hold
3. Options: Generate a variety of alternative possibilities
4. Criteria: Insist that solutions be evaluated using objective standards

According to this method, management will formulate a best alternative to a negotiated agreement for each issue. In this manner, negotiators evaluate whether the type of agreement that can be reached is better than no agreement at all. By considering mutual options for gain, the negotiator offers a more flexible approach toward bargaining and increases the likelihood of achieving creative solutions.

Collective bargaining is both a laborious and a time-consuming endeavor. Bargaining requires not only listening to others but attempting to understand the motivational force behind the dialog. Successful negotiators make every effort to understand fully what truly underlies bargaining positions and why they are so fiercely held, and they are receptive to any signals that are being communicated, including nonverbal communication such as body language (Fisher and Ury 1981).

Bargaining, as depicted in Figure 12.3, can be conceptualized as a continuum of bargaining behaviors and strategies. At one end of the continuum is concessionary bargaining, in which the employer asks the union to eliminate, limit, or reduce wages and other commitments in response to financial constraints. This type of bargaining is likely to occur when the organization is in financial jeopardy and is struggling to survive. At the

FIGURE 12.2
Mandatory
Bargaining
Issues

- Wages
- Arbitration
- Duration of agreement
- Reinstatement of economic strikers
- Work rules
- Lunch periods
- Bonus payments
- Promotions
- Transfers
- Plant reopening
- Bargaining over "bar list"
- Arrangement for negotiation
- Plant closedown and relocation
- Overtime pay
- Company houses
- Union-imposed production ceiling
- No-strike clause
- Workloads
- Cancellation of security upon relocation of plant
- Employer's insistence on clause, giving arbitrator right to enforce award
- Severance pay
- Safety
- Checkoff
- Hours
- Holidays (paid)
- Grievance procedure
- Change of payment (hourly to salary)

- Merit wage increase
- Pension plan
- Price of company meals
- Seniority
- Plant closing
- Employee physical examination
- Truck rentals
- Change in insurance carrier/benefits
- Profit-sharing plan
- Agency shop
- Subcontracting
- Most-favored-nation clause
- Piece rates
- Change of employee status to independent contractor
- Discounts on company's products
- Clause providing for supervisors' keeping seniority in unit
- Nondiscriminatory hiring hall
- Prohibition against supervisors doing unit work
- Partial plant closing
- Discharge
- Vacations (paid)
- Layoff plan
- Union security and checkoff

- Work schedule
- Retirement age
- Group insurance (health, life, and accident)
- Layoffs
- Job-posting procedures
- Union security
- Musician price list
- Change in operations resulting in reclassifying workers from incentive to straight time, cut workforce, or installation of cost-saving machine
- Motor carrier union agreement
- Sick leave
- Discriminatory racial policies
- Work assignments and transfers
- Stock-purchase plan
- Management Rights clause
- Shift differentials
- Procedures for income tax withholding
- Plant rules
- Superseniority for union stewards
- Hunting on employer forest preserve where previously granted

Note: This is a list of major items for bargaining; the list does not include subcategories

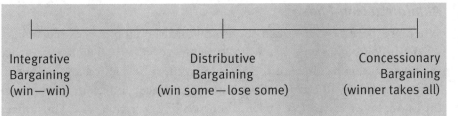

FIGURE 12.3
Collective
Bargaining
Continuum

opposite end is integrative bargaining, which seeks win-win situations and solutions that creatively respond to both parties' needs. This type of bargaining requires the trust and cooperation of both parties. In the center is distributive bargaining, which is a win-lose type in which each party gives up something to gain something else. This type of bargaining is likely when negotiations are contentious and full of conflict.

Even when both parties negotiate in good faith and fulfill the covenants of the NLRA, an agreement still may not be reached at times. When this happens, parties are said to have reached an impasse. To resolve an impasse, a variety of techniques may be implemented. These techniques involve third parties and include mediation, in which a mediator evaluates the dispute and issues nonbinding recommendations. If either party rejects the mediator's recommendations, arbitration is an alternative. Arbitrators, similar to mediators, are neutral third parties, but their decisions are legally binding. For example, arbitrators may recommend that either party's position be accepted as a final offer, or they can attempt to split the differences between the two parties' positions.

If these techniques fail to resolve the impasse, employers or the union can initiate work stoppages that may take the form of lockouts or strikes. A lockout occurs when the employer shuts down operations either during or prior to a dispute. A strike, on the other hand, is employee initiated. Lockouts or strikes can occur during negotiations and also during the life of the contract. Special provisions for these work stoppages in healthcare settings are discussed in the section below on the history of judicial and legislative rulings.

In addition, no-strike and no-lockout clauses can be negotiated in the agreement. No-strike clauses essentially prohibit strikes, either unconditionally or with conditions. An unconditional no-strike clause means that the union and its members will not engage in either a strike or work slow-down while the contract is in effect. A conditional no-strike clause bans strikes and slow-downs except in certain situations and under specific conditions, which are delineated in detail in the agreement. Comparable clauses for lockouts exist for employers.

Administration Phase

When an agreement between the union and the employer is reached, it must be recorded in writing and executed in good faith, which means that the terms and conditions of the agreement must be applied and enforced. This agreement will include disciplinary, grievance, and arbitration procedures, many of which have been discussed in other chapters. The collective bargaining agreement imposes limitations on the disciplinary actions that management may take. The right to discharge, suspend, or discipline is clearly enunciated in contractual clauses and in the adoption of rules and procedures that may or may not be incorporated in the agreement.

Management may discipline up through discharge only for sufficient and appropriate reasons and must base all procedures on due process. The union's role in the process is to defend employees and to determine the propriety of management action. The burden of proof rests with management to prove that whatever action was taken was proper and consistent with progressive discipline. If the grievance proceeds to arbitration, arbitrators will usually support management if they find evidence of progressive discipline and evidence that employees were fully aware of the standards against which their behavior was to be measured. These standards include very basic rules and regulations that outline offenses that will subject employees to disciplinary action and the extent of such action.

The heart of administering the collective bargaining agreement is the *grievance procedure*. This procedure is a useful and productive management tool that allows implementation and interpretation of the contract. A grievance must be well defined and restricted to violations of the terms and conditions of the agreement. However, other conditions may give rise to a grievance, including violations of the law or company rules, a change in working conditions or past company practices, or violations of health and safety standards.

The grievance process usually contains a series of steps. The first step always involves the presentation of the grievance by the employee (or representative) to the immediate, first-line supervisor. If the grievance is not resolved at this step, broader action is taken. Because most grievances involve an action by the immediate supervisor, the second step necessarily must occur outside the department and at a higher level; thus, the second step will involve the employee (or representative) and a department head or other administrator. Prior to this meeting the grievance will be written out, dated, and signed by the employee and the union representative. The written grievance will document the events as the employee perceived them, cite the appropriate contract provisions that allegedly had been violated, and indicate the desired resolution or settlement prospects. If the grievance is unresolved at this point, a third step becomes necessary that involves an in-house review by top management. A grievance that remains unresolved at the conclusion of the third step may go to arbitration if provided for in the contract and if the union is in agreement.

Most collective bargaining agreements restrict the arbitrator's decision to application and interpretation of the agreement and make the decision final and binding on both parties. Most agreements also specify methods for selecting arbitrators. If the union agrees to arbitration, it must notify management, and an arbitrator is jointly selected. In evaluating the grievance, arbitrators focus on a variety of criteria, including the actual nature of the offense, the past record of the grieving employee, warnings, knowledge of rules, past practices, and discriminatory treatment. Thus, a large number of factors interact, making arbitration a complex process.

An arbitration hearing permits each side an opportunity to present its case. Similar to a court hearing, witnesses, cross-examinations, transcripts, and legal counsel may be used. As with a court hearing, the nature of arbitration is adversarial. Thus, cases may be lost because of poor preparation and presentation. Generally, the courts will enforce an arbitrator's decision unless it is shown to be unreasonable, unsound, or capricious relative to the issues under consideration. Also, if an arbitrator has exceeded his or her authority or issued an order that violates existing state or federal law, the decision may be vacated. Consistent and fair adjudication of grievances is the hallmark of a sound labor-management relationship.

In healthcare settings, the strike is the most severe form of a labor-management dispute. A critical part of planning for negotiations is an honest assessment of strike potential. This involves identifying strike issues that are likely to be critical for all parties. Although estimating the impact of possible strikes, including economic pressures from lost wages and revenues, is essential, the key to a successful strike from the perspective of the union is to impose enough pressure on management to expedite movement toward a compromise. Pressure may be psychological as well as economic. In healthcare settings, the real losers in a strike are the patients and their families. During a strike, patients may be denied services or forced to postpone treatment, be relocated to another institution, or even be discharged prematurely.

Management must be aware of critical factors that affect its ability and willingness to withstand a strike. When attempting to estimate the impact of these factors, managers will evaluate several key indicators, including revenue losses, timing of the strike, and availability of replacements for striking workers. However, management must also contemplate factors that affect the union, such as the question of whether striking employees will be entitled to strike benefits, especially health benefits. If so, for how long? Both parties must also consider the impact of outside assistance to avoid or settle a strike.

A Review of Legislative and Judicial Rulings

Table 12.2 summarizes important legislative and judicial rulings and their impact on healthcare settings. As the table indicates, in recent years significant rulings have centered primarily on organizing issues, involving physicians and nurses and their eligibility for inclusion in bargaining units. In 2004, however, the onus shifted to financial issues such as new changes to the Fair Labor Standards Act, which exempted most nurses from overtime pay. Unions were also targeted with changes to the Labor-Management and Disclosure Act. Stricter reporting requirements are aimed at increased transparency and accountability for how unions spend their dues (*Harvard Law Review* 2004).

The Taft Hartley Act (Taft Hartley) amended the NLRA in 1947. The primary intent of these amendments was to strike a balance in the NLRA, because most of its protections and rights applied to workers and employers needed a means for redress. Taft Hartley also gave states federal permission to enact right-to-work laws, which essentially prohibit employees from being forced to join unions as a condition of employment. Currently, 21 states, mostly in the south and west, have enacted such laws. Unions oppose right-to-work laws in part because under the NLRA, unions are responsible for representing all employees in the bargaining unit, even those members who choose not to join the union and consequently pay no union dues. (Nonunion members of the bargaining unit are often referred to as "free riders" because they acquire all of the benefits of union membership without any cost. Meanwhile, proponents of right-to-work laws maintain that no one should be forced to join a private organization, especially if that organization is using dues money to support causes that contravene an individual's moral or religious beliefs.)

Although the NLRA, as it was initially enacted in 1935, did not exempt healthcare employees explicitly, court interpretations tended to exclude healthcare workers from its regulations, until later amendments asserted jurisdiction over a variety of healthcare institutions. Taft Hartley had a significant impact on healthcare workers because Section 2 (2) specifically excluded from the definition of "employer" those private, not-for-profit hospitals and healthcare institutions. However, the NLRB asserted jurisdiction over proprietary hospitals and nursing homes, and the 1974 Health Care Amendments, Public Law 93-360, brought the private, not-for-profit healthcare industry within the jurisdiction of federal labor law.

Approximately 2 million additional healthcare workers became eligible for representation with the 1974 Health Care Amendments (Stickler 1990). These amendments afforded stringent protections regarding work stoppages to safeguard patient care. Table 12.3 summarizes the provisions for strikes and pickets as well as impasse requirements. In drafting the 1974 amendments, the congressional committee specifically included a 10-day

Year	Legislation/Judicial Ruling	Impact on Healthcare Organizations
1947	Taft Hartley amendments to NLRA	Exempted not-for-profit hospitals from NLRA coverage, including collective bargaining
1962	Executive order #10988	Permitted federally supported hospitals to bargain collectively
1974	Healthcare amendments to NLRA	Extended NLRA coverage to private, not-for-profit hospitals and healthcare institutions; special provisions for strikes, pickets, and impasses
1976	NLRB ruling: Cedars-Sinai Medical Center, Los Angeles, CA	Ruled that medical residents, interns, and fellows (house staff) are students and excluded from collective bargaining
1989/ 1991	NLRB ruling/Supreme Court affirmation on multiple bargaining units: PL. 93-360	Expanded the number of bargaining units in acute care hospitals from three to eight
1999	NLRB Ruling: Boston Medical Center, Massachusetts	Reversed Cedars-Sinai Medical Center decision and ruled that house staff are employees, not students, and can therefore be included in collective bargaining
2001	Supreme Court decision regarding nurse supervisors: *NLRB v. Kentucky River Community Care, Inc.*	Court ruled that registered nurses who use independent judgment in directing employees are supervisors. Expected impact: limiting unions' ability to organize nurses
2003	U.S. Department of Labor adopted a rule that increases union financial reporting requirements (19 C.F.R. pts 403 and 408) to provide for transparency of union financial structures and accountability of how unions spend their dues	
2004	U.S. Department of Labor issued new rules that make most nurses ineligible for overtime pay under Part 541 of the Fair Labor Standards Act	

TABLE 12.2
Summary of Important Legislative and Judicial Rulings

TABLE 12.3

Comparison of Provisions for Strike or Picket Notification and Impasse Requirements

1974 Healthcare Amendments to the Taft Hartley Act	General NLRA Provisions
30-day "reasonable" time to picket following which a representation petition must be filed by the union with NLRB	Similar requirement
90-day notice for modifying an existing collective bargaining agreement	60-day requirement
60-day notice to FMCS* of impending expiration of existing collective bargaining agreement	30-day requirement
Following FMCS notification, contract must remain in effect for 60 days without any strikes or lockouts	30-day requirement
30-day notice of a dispute must be given to FMCS and appropriate state agency during initial negotiations	No similar requirement
The director of FMCS is authorized to appoint a board of inquiry in the event of a threatened or actual work stoppage	No similar authority
10-day written notice to employer and FMCS of strikes or pickets required of healthcare unions. (*Note:* this notice cannot occur before either (1) the end of the 90-day notice to modify the existing contract or (2) the 30-day notice in the case of an impasse during negotiations of the new contract	No similar requirement
A new Section 19 provides for an alternate, a contribution to designated 501(c)(3) charities, for the payment of union dues for persons with religious convictions against making such payments	No similar requirement

* Federal Mediation and Conciliation Service

strike and picket notice provision, a requirement that had not been applied to other industries. The committee did so to ensure that healthcare institutions would have sufficient advance notice of a strike. Furthermore, the committee report of the amendments held that a union is in violation if it struck a facility more than 72 hours after the designated notice time unless the parties agreed to a new time or the union issued a new 10-day notice. In addition, if the union does not begin the strike or other job action at the time designated in the initial 10-day notice, it must provide the healthcare facility with at least 12 hours notice before the actual beginning of the action.

Thus, the 12-hour "warning" must fall completely within the 72-hour notice period. Repeatedly serving 10-day notices on the employer also constitutes evidence of a refusal to bargain in good faith and is a violation of the NLRA.

The reprisals for violating the 10-day notice are substantial. For example, workers engaged in work stoppage in violation of the 10-day strike notice lose their status as employees and are subsequently unprotected by the NLRA provisions. Exceptions to the requirements for unions to provide notices are provided as well. If the employer has committed a flagrant or serious unfair labor practice, notices are not required. In addition, the employer may not use the 10-day notice period to essentially undermine the bargaining relationship that otherwise exists. For example, the facility can receive supplies, but it is not free to stockpile supplies for an unduly extended period. Similarly, the facility cannot bring in large numbers of personnel from other facilities for the purpose of replacing striking workers (Metzger, Ferentino, and Kruger 1984).

In 1989, an NLRB ruling established eight units for the purpose of collective bargaining in acute care hospitals: (1) physicians, (2) nurses, (3) all other professionals, (4) technical employees, (5) business office clerical employees, (6) skilled maintenance employees, (7) guards, and (8) all other nonprofessionals. Figure 12.4 provides more detail on the various occupations that fall within the eight designated categories. As with all bargaining unit determinations, supervisors are excluded from unit membership.

The American Hospital Association (1991) strongly opposed the ruling and appealed to the U.S. Supreme Court, protesting that eight units would lead to a proliferation of bargaining units in the hospital, further fragmenting healthcare collective bargaining; increasing bargaining costs; making implementation of hospitalwide policies more difficult; and ultimately inflating the cost of healthcare and rendering the bargaining process more complicated, lengthy, and subject to legal appeals and challenges. The Supreme Court disagreed, affirming the NLRB's ruling in 1991. Although little empirical evidence specifically evaluates the impact of the eight-unit ruling (Hirsch and Schumacher 1998), election activity and the union win rate increased. Table 12.4 presents election information for the period 1995 through 1999.

Developments in Organizing Physicians and Nurses

Physicians

Historically, physicians resisted union organizing for a variety of professional and philosophical reasons. In fact, much of the American Medical Association (AMA) membership views unionism in general as antithetical to profes-

FIGURE 12.4

Eight
Categories
of Workers
Specified
in NLRB
Bargaining
Rules

1. Physicians
2. Nurses:
   - registered nurses
   - graduate nurses
   - non-nursing department nurses
   - nurse anesthetists
   - nurse instructors
   - nurse practitioners
3. All professionals, except for registered nurses and physicians:
   - audiologists
   - chemists
   - counselors
   - dietitians
   - educational programmers
   - educators
   - medical artists
   - nuclear physicists
   - pharmacists
   - social workers
   - technologists
   - therapists
   - utilization review coordinators
4. Technical employees:
   - infant-care technicians
   - laboratory technicians
   - licensed practical nurses
   - operating room technicians
   - orthopedic technicians
   - physical therapy assistants
   - psychiatric technicians
   - respiratory therapy technicians
   - surgical assistants
   - x-ray technicians
5. Business office clerical employees
6. Skilled maintenance employees
7. Guards
8. All other nonprofessional employees

sionalism and unions as economic devices that extract benefits for their members at the expense of patient trust and confidence. In addition, legal challenges existed to organizing because the majority of physicians are independent contractors and technically ineligible for union membership. Only "employed" physicians, including those employed in academic settings, are authorized to bargain collectively. Physicians who practice as independent

TABLE 12.4
Summary of
Election
Activity in
Health
Services
Elections,
1995–1999

Year	Total Elections	Union Wins
1995	291	156
1996	370	205
1997	407	258
1998	486	290
1999	517	333

Source: Industrial Distribution of Representation Elections Held in Cases Closed, FY 1995–1999. Annual Reports of the NLRB.

contractors are restricted from collective bargaining by the Sherman Antitrust Act of 1980, which prohibits all business combinations that restrain free trade. Therefore, these physicians cannot legally talk with one another about price of service. Subsequently, independent contractors who engage in collective bargaining with entities such as health plans and insurers risk exposure to federal antitrust suits (Association of American Medical Colleges Executive Council 1999; Anthony and Erf 2000; Cohen 1999).

Nonetheless, the growth of "tight" managed care in the 1990s provided a powerful incentive for the rise of the physician union movement in the United States. The vast majority of physician complaints and efforts to unionize derived from corporate interference in medical decision making and coercive practices of managed care organizations (Anawis 2002; Luepke 1999). At their annual meeting in June 1999, the AMA House of Delegates approved a controversial resolution, creating a national "bargaining unit" for physicians. The bargaining unit, called Physicians for Responsible Negotiations (PRN), permitted employed physicians to bargain with health plans and insurers. The resolution was controversial because the AMA, which had traditionally opposed physician unions, reversed its position. In so doing, the AMA recognized collective bargaining as an acceptable professional mechanism for interacting with government and other third-party payers. Federal and state legislation also was proposed in support of amending antitrust laws to permit independent physicians to unionize. However, this legislation did not gain widespread support and was subsequently abandoned.

The PRN struggled for survival and recruited few members. In 2002, the AMA reduced its financial support for the PRN, only guaranteeing the union's survival through the year 2003. In March 2004, the AMA, with little press attention, severed its relationship with the PRN. It is expected that the PRN will secure affiliation with another union such as the Service Employees International Union (SEIU), which represents 1.6 million workers, including many healthcare workers (Romano 2004). Although little evidence exists to explain why the PRN was not well supported by physicians, it is possible that the loosening of managed care was a dominant factor. Increases in consumer choice and open access effectively reduced many of the physician complaints and problems that previously substantiated interest in unionizing. For example, by the late 1990s specialty physicians were regaining their status as revenue and profit generators. Still, it is also likely that physicians recognized the potential for obtaining judicial intervention. For instance, in reimbursement disputes with Aetna, physicians filed a class-action suit and won (Casalino, Pham, and Bazzoli 2004; Martinez 2003).

House Staff (Medical Residents, Interns, and Fellows) and Medical Students

In 1999, the NLRB ruled that house staff members at Boston Medical Center were employees, not students. The impact of this ruling is that house staff in private hospitals are legally entitled to bargain collectively. This determination was a reversal of a 1976 ruling for Cedars-Sinai Medical Center in Los Angeles in which house staff were classified as students (Yacht 2000). In 2001, medical residents at 525-bed Brookdale University Hospital and Medical Center in New York became the first private-sector hospital physicians in the United States to ratify a collective bargaining agreement since that right was affirmed by the NLRB (*Modern Healthcare* 2001). Opponents of house staff unionization suggest union activity will create adversarial relationships between house staff and instructors. For example, unions could negotiate resident promotions and fight against disciplinary actions and dismissal of poorly performing house staff (Levenson 1999).

Nurses

Nurses are predominantly employed in hospitals, where they represent the largest service. Nurses provide patient care 24 hours a day, 7 days a week. Consequently, they play a key role in patient care and also represent a significant labor cost. Historically, nurses have struggled with conflict among their obligation to their patients, their profession, and union representation. There are approximately 2.3 million registered nurses in the United States, and, despite uneven salary levels across the profession and widespread persistent discontent with working conditions, the majority of these nurses do not belong to a union. Approximately 18 percent are unionized (Bureau of Labor Statistics 2004; Leung 1999). In addition, because of a

2001 landmark ruling, many nurses have become ineligible for union membership because they are considered supervisors (see Table 12.2).

Unlike physicians, who appear to have had their workplace problems and needs addressed without the help of unions, nurses currently have a very different experience. As the Interview with a Nurse Activist section later in the chapter explains, nurse-management relationships are strained. National nurse shortages and pressures on hospitals to trim labor costs have led to increases in nursing workloads and hours and the potential to commit errors during longer shifts. In Massachusetts, work hours have become such a contentious issue for nurses that strikes have resulted (Kowalczyk 2004). Research affirms that for nurses to vote in favor of a union, they must believe that joining a union will help them gain greater control over patient care (Clark et al. 2000). Thus, patient care issues appear to be motivating many nurses to unionize (DeMoro 2002; Meier 2000).

Nurse activism also appears to be increasing. In 2001, United American Nurses (UAN), which has about 100,000 members and is the labor arm of the American Nurses Association (ANA), joined with the AFL-CIO, the nation's largest union. With this affiliation, the UAN looks to increase support and influence and to bring aggressiveness to organizing and other union activities. Also, some state ANA affiliates such as California and Massachusetts are opting to go it alone, charging that the UAN, with or without the AFL-CIO, is still too moderate (Bellandi 2001; Schumacher 2002). The move toward increased aggressiveness through union activism derives primarily from problems related to staffing and stress, especially managed care's pressure to reduce hospital lengths of stay. Priority issues for nurses center on patient loads, mandatory overtime, staffing cuts, "floating" to unfamiliar areas, and benefits such as wages and pensions (Meier 2000; Spetz and Given 2003).

By joining and becoming active in unions, nurses are exercising their "voice" and using other tools of unionism, ranging from election petitions and contract negotiations to work stoppages such as sick outs and strikes. Nurses are capturing the public's attention and using their influence to obtain community support (see Interview with a Nurse Activist on page 327). To date, however, aggression and activism have yielded mixed results. Efforts regarding patient safety and quality-of-care legislation have been successful at the state rather than the federal level. For example, California enacted the first law that establishes nurse-to-patient staffing ratios. This law, in effect, requires hospitals to reduce nurse workloads and improve patient safety by guaranteeing minimum nurse-to-patient ratios. This law serves as a framework for mandates in other states and at the federal level (Benko 2004). Similarly, unions have enjoyed success at the state level with mandatory overtime legislation. State laws that prohibit or limit mandatory overtime have been enacted in five states—Maine, Minnesota, New Jersey, Oregon, and Washington. However, corresponding federal legislation has not been enacted despite heavy union opposition to mandatory overtime. Unions also failed to stop revisions to the Fair Labor Standards Act, which effectively exempts most nurses from overtime pay (see Table 12.2).

Management Guidelines

This section highlights the key points to remember in labor relations.

1. *Whether a healthcare organization is union or nonunion, it should have a policy on unionism, and this policy should be communicated to current and prospective employees.* A positive labor-management relationship begins with the screening process. All prospective employees should be given information about the institution's position toward unions, including goals and strategies of fair and consistent dealings with unions. Employee handbooks and orientation represent other opportunities to communicate management's commitment to provide equitable treatment to all employees concerning their wages, benefits, hours, and conditions of employment. Furthermore, management must also communicate that each employee is important and deserving of respect and that adequate funds and management time have been designated to maintain effective employee relations (Rutkowski and Rutkowski 1984).

2. *While management must have effective policies and procedures for selection of new employees, it must also ensure proper fit of personnel with specific jobs.* Subsequently, job analyses, job descriptions, and job evaluations, as well as fair wage and salary programs, are essential for establishing a fundamental basis for fair representation. Management must not make promises that cannot be fulfilled; at the same time, it should strive to do whatever is possible to improve employee relations. Monitoring of employee attitudes through surveys is essential; otherwise, management is dependent on the union for communicating any problems or change in attitudes.

3. *Management must ensure that it is fulfilling its roles and responsibilities by providing necessary training for employees,* especially first-line supervisors who are instrumental in determining how policies are implemented and in serving as liaisons between management and employees. If these supervisors are not properly trained, grievances are less likely to be settled quickly and are more likely to escalate into substantive formal disputes. Training is especially critical in healthcare

settings because of constant and rapid changes in technology and workplace safety issues. Management's commitment to training is consistent with fair and honest treatment of employees. Similarly, if management fails to establish objective performance policies and does not ensure that they are done routinely, the labor-management relationship will be affected. Employees may perceive inequities and unfairness and experience problems of declining morale and productivity because rewards are not matched with performance.

4. *Inconsistent and unfair application of disciplinary policies and procedures can create unnecessary grievance problems.* At a minimum, the principle of just cause should guide the disciplinary process. When employees file grievances, they expect prompt attention to their requests. If management delays the process or turns a deaf ear to complaints, such actions signal to employees that management does not care about their problems and essentially cannot be trusted. Furthermore, management's credibility with employees will deteriorate, creating an imbalance in the labor-management relationship such that employees perceive the union's position as the most honest.

5. *Each phase of the labor relations process is interrelated and can affect the outcome of other phases.* For example, if the union is able to obtain representation through voluntary recognition, negotiating the collective bargaining agreement will very likely be less adversarial than if a representation election had occurred. Similarly, if the negotiations for a collective bargaining agreement are contentious, difficulties may occur in administering the contract. Thus, having a full understanding of each phase and its potential to enhance or impede the overall process of labor relations is essential.

Summary

As this chapter describes, managing with organized labor is challenging. Unionism has been declining nationally for decades, but the relatively unorganized healthcare workforce has become a target for unions. Because union membership and election activity have increased in healthcare settings, managers must devote high-level attention to the application and maintenance of a positive labor relations program that integrates HR functions. Strategies and goals to implement a positive labor relations program must be based on a solid understanding of the labor relations process and of emerging trends and legislation. The growth of nursing unions, in particular, signals major changes for HR practices and for the labor relations process.

References

American Hospital Association. 1991. "Legal Memorandum Number 16: Collective Bargaining Units in the Health Care Industry." Chicago: AHA.

Anawis, M. A. 2002. "The Ethics of Physician Unionization: What Will Happen If Your Doctor Becomes a Teamster?" *De Paul Journal of Health Care Law* 6 (1): 83–110.

Anthony, M. F., and S. Erf. 2000. "Can Physician Unionization Succeed?" *Healthcare Executive* (March/April): 50.

Association of American Medical Colleges Executive Council. 1999. "AAMC Statement on Negotiating Units for Physicians." *AAMC Reporter* 9 (2): 7.

Becker, W. L., and A. M. Rowe. 1989. "Update on Union Organization in Health Care." *Review of Federation of American Health Systems* 22 (5): 11–12, 14–16.

Bellandi, D. 2001. "Labor Flexes Muscle, United American Nurses Votes to Join AFL-CIO." *Modern Healthcare* 31 (27): 8.

Benko, L. B. 2004. "Workforce Report 2004. Ratio Fight Goes National." *Modern Healthcare* 34 (24): 23, 30.

Bureau of Labor Statistics. 2000a. "Union Membership Edges Up but Share Continues to Fall." [Online news release; retrieved 12/5/01.] http://stats.bls.gov/opub/ted.

———. 2000b. Unpublished Tabulations from Current Population Surveys, Union Membership Tables, 1999 Annual Averages. Washington, DC: U.S. Government Printing Office.

———. 2004. "Union Members in 2003." [Online news release; retrieved 7/6/04.] http://www.bls.gov/news.release/union2.nr0.htm.

Casalino, L. P., H. Pham, and G. Bazzoli. 2001. "Growth of Single-Specialty Medical Groups." *Health Affairs* 23 (2): 82–90.

Christian Science Monitor. 2004. "A Worker-Union Disconnect." *Christian Science Monitor* 96 (83).

Clark, D. A., P. F. Clark, D. Day, and D. Shea. 2000. "The Relationship Between Health Care Reform and Nurses' Interest in Union Representation: The Role of Workplace Climate." *Journal of Professional Nursing* 16 (2): 92–6.

Cohen, J. J. 1999. "Unions Are Bad Medicine for Doctors." *Academic Medicine* 74 (8): 905.

DeMoro, R. A. 2002. "What California Has Started: Staffing Ratios, Union Activism Are National Solutions to the Nurse Shortage." *Modern Healthcare* 32 (13): 26.

Fennell, K. S. 1987. "The Unionization of the Healthcare Industry: General Trends and Emerging Issues." *Journal of Health in Human Resources Administration* 10 (1): 66–81.

Fisher, R., and W. Ury. 1981. "Getting to Yes—Negotiating an Agreement Without Giving In." In *Harvard Negotiation Project*, edited by B. Patton, 21–53. Boston: Houghton Mifflin.

Fottler, M. D., R. A. Johnson, K. J. McGlown, and E. W. Ford. 1999.

"Attitudes of Organized Labor Officials Toward Health Care Issues: An Exploratory Survey of Alabama Labor Officials." *Health Care Management Review* 24 (2): 71–82.

Freeman, R. B., and J. L. Medoff. 1984. *What Do Unions Do?* New York: Basic Books.

Harvard Law Review. 2004. "Labor Law: Department of Labor Increases Union Financial Reporting Requirements." *Harvard Law Review* 117 (5): 1734–40.

Hecker, D. E. 2004. "Occupational Employment Projections to 2012." *Monthly Labor Review* 127 (2): 80–105.

Hirsch, B. T., and E. J. Schumacher. 1998. "Union Wages, Rents and Skills in Health Care Labor Markets." *Journal of Labor Research* 19 (Winter): 125–47.

Kearney, R. C. 2003. "Patterns of Union Decline and Growth: an Organizational Ecology Perspective." *Journal of Labor Research* 24 (4): 561–78.

Kowalczyk, L. 2004. "University of Pennsylvania Study Links Long Hours, Nurse Errors." *Knight Ridder Tribune Business News Washington* (July 7): 1.

Leung, S. 1999. "More Nurses Join Unions Across State." *The Wall Street Journal*, September 15.

Levenson, D. 1999. "Private Hospitals Worry NLRB Ruling Will Spark Intern, Resident Disputes." *AHA News* 35 (47): 1–2.

Luepke, E. 1999. "White Coat, Blue Collar: Physician Unionization and Managed Care." *Annals of Health Law* (8): 275–98.

Martinez, B. 2003. "Aetna to Announce Settlement with Physicians." *The Wall Street Journal Eastern Edition* 241 (100): A3.

Meier, E. 2000. "Is Unionization the Answer for Nurses and Nursing?" *Nursing Economics* 18 (1): 36–38.

Metzger, N., J. Ferentino, and K. Kruger. 1984. *When Health Care Employees Strike.* Rockville, MD: Aspen.

Modern Healthcare. 2001. "The Labor Picture." *Modern Healthcare* 31 (May).

Yacht, A. C. 2000. "Unionization of House Officers: The Experience at One Medical Center." *The New England Journal of Medicine* 342 (6): 429–31.

Petzinger, T., Jr. 1999. "A Special Report: Industry & Economics—Talking About Tomorrow—Peter Drucker: The 'Arch-Guru of Capitalism Argues That We Need a New Economic Theory and New Management Model." *The Wall Street Journal Eastern Edition* (December 31): R34.

Romano, M. 2004. "Labor Union Didn't Work." *Modern Healthcare* 34 (22): 32–34.

Rutkowski, A. D., and B. L. Rutkowski. 1984. *Labor Relations in Hospitals.* Rockville, MD: Aspen.

Schumacher, E. J. 2002. "Technology, Skills, and Health Care Labor Markets." *Journal of Labor Research* 23 (Summer): 397–412.

Scott, C., and C. M. Lowery. 1994. "Union Election Activity in the Health Care Industry." *Health Care Management Review* 19 (1): 18–27.

Scott, C., and A. Seers. 1996. "Determinants of Union Election Outcomes in the Non-Hospital Health Care Industry." *Journal of Labor Research* 17 (4): 701–15.

Spetz, J., and R. Given. 2003. "The Future of the Nurse Shortage: Will Wage Increases Close the Gap." *Health Affairs* 22 (6): 199–206.

Stickler, K. B. 1990. "Union Organizing Will Be Divisive and Costly." *Hospitals* (July 5): 68–70.

Swoboda, F. 1999. "A Healthy Sign for Organized Labor; Vote by L. A. Caregivers Called Historic." *The Washington Post*, February 27.

Discussion Questions

1. Why should management have a policy on unionism? What purpose does it serve?
2. Describe the three phases of the labor relations process. Why are all phases equally important?
3. What are some of the behaviors that may indicate to managers that organizing activities are occurring?
4. Explain why nurses have become activists in recent years. Is this trend likely to continue?

Experiential Exercises

Case   The CEO of a mid-size urban hospital was late one Friday evening, so he took a short-cut that caused him to walk by the employee lounge. He walked inside and shook his head. With all the problems of budget cuts and trying to make ends meet, he realized that there had been little money available for upkeep of non-patient areas such as the employee lounge. The carpet was dirty and worn, the coffee mugs were chipped, the wallpaper was torn, and the refrigerator groaned as it cycled on and off. The CEO decided enough was enough. The employees had worked hard and should at minimum have an employee lounge that was inviting and pleasant. He marched back to his office and called the COO to instruct her to create a weekend miracle by calling in the work crews to update and refurbish the employee lounge. He ordered new carpets, new wallpaper, and new appliances, and he wanted it all done by Monday. The CEO told the COO, "I keep telling the employees how much I appreciate their help, especially in these financially tight times, but now I am going to show them. And be sure to replace those old, chipped coffee mugs." Early on Monday morning, the CEO walked by the employee lounge. It looked terrific, and someone had already made coffee. He made a note to himself to tell the COO what a great job she had done.

When he got to his office, he found the union steward sitting on the couch. "I need to have a word with you," the union steward said. He had several words, as it turned out: He said that the CEO had violated the collective bargaining contract and that refurbishing the employee lounge should have been, at minimum, discussed with the union. The union steward spent 20 minutes complaining about violations and procedures. After he left, the CEO, called the COO and told her to put the lounge back the way it was, including the chipped coffee mugs. Then the CEO muttered to himself, "That is the last time I try to do anything nice for anyone around here. I have learned my lesson."

Case Questions

1. What is the problem in this case?
2. Would you respond in the same way? Why, or why not?
3. What, if anything, can be done at this point?

Interview with a Nurse Activist   *This interview was conducted on May 25, 2004, with the cochair of the nurses' union at a large, urban hospital in the northeast. She has more than 20 years experience as a nurse and definitely considers herself a nurse activist.*

Times have changed in nursing. The nurse activist explained that now you cannot trust management, as they will tell nurses anything just to get what they want. In her opinion, even nurses who are promoted to management cannot be trusted. "Management lies," she said. At the end of a recent negotiation, she explained, management and the union representatives did not even shake hands. There has been a loss of respect on both sides. It is ironic that at a time when management and nursing need to work together, there is a chasm of mistrust separating them. The main issues are not money, but human resources— that is, staffing, mandatory overtime, and workloads. Nurses are working harder and on longer shifts; the potential for error increases in such environments. Patient safety and quality of care are at stake. According to the nurse activist, she was 8 months pregnant and coming off of an 8-hour shift when she was ordered to work an additional 4 hours. "We are playing a game with patient safety," she said. "Management should be held accountable for what they are doing." As a result, nurses are taking to the bargaining table to hold management responsible for the staffing decisions that are threatening patient care.

Nurses are also taking their case to the public. The nurse activist routinely appears on local television and radio shows to gather support for nurses. The community is a key stakeholder. After all, she explained, patients make up the community, and they recall who actually "cared" for them during hospital visits: It was the nurse with the bedpan at 2:00AM, or it was the nurse giving comfort to the parents of a sick child. It was not management. With issues of patient safety and medication errors, nurses find it straightforward to get the community on their side in demands for staffing and work hours.

Interestingly enough, Peter Drucker, who invented the field of management study, would probably agree with this nurse activist. He cited management for not treating nurses as professionals who know their jobs. Although he acknowledged that management is under a lot of financial pressure, Drucker said that instead of telling nurses what to do, management should invite nurses to find solutions to the problems (Petzinger 1999).

Exercise 1   Think of a healthcare facility in your community, and consider its nursing situation. Then, answer the following questions:
1. Are the nurses treated as professionals? Why, or why not?
2. If given the opportunity, do you think these nurses are likely or unlikely to join a labor union in the future? Why, or why not?

Exercise 2   Refer to Table 12.1. Conduct an audit of a hospital or other healthcare organization using the indicators listed in the table. Determine if there is an increase or decrease in any of the indicators. Then, explain the possible reasons for these increases or decreases.

Exercise 3 Refer to Figure 12.1. Complete the table below by listing specific goals for the union and the organization. Once the table is completed, identify the following:

- Which goals are similar?
- Which goals have the potential for conflict?

Goal Areas	Union Goals	Organization Goals
Survival		
Growth		
Profitability		
Competitiveness		
Recruitment and retention of employees		
Motivation of employees		
Flexibility		
Decision making		
Effective use of human resources		
Communication		

NURSE WORKLOAD, STAFFING, AND MEASUREMENT

Cheryl B. Jones, Ph.D., R.N., and George H. Pink, Ph.D.

Learning Objectives

After completing this chapter, the reader should be able to

- list the factors that affect nurse workload and staffing;
- discuss the influence of nursing shortages on the deployment of nursing staff and on the ability of a healthcare organization to deliver quality patient care;
- compare and contrast the terms nurse workload and nurse staffing;
- recognize the types of licensed and unlicensed nursing personnel employed in patient care delivery, and describe how the existence of different personnel affects nurse workload and staffing decisions;
- identify three primary reasons for measuring nurse workload;
- explain how an organization's philosophy influences nurse workload and staffing decisions, and be aware of various stakeholder perspectives on staffing and workload issues;
- understand how patient classification systems are used in calculating nurse workload, and discuss the strengths and weaknesses of these systems;
- know the types of information needed to calculate nursing full-time equivalents and the process for acquiring and using this information; and
- address the impact of nurse workload and staffing on nurse stress and burnout and on the quality of patient care.

Introduction

Nurses are the "constant" in healthcare organizations—they are on the frontline and at the point of care, 24 hours a day, 7 days a week. They are the most visible faces in these highly complex organizations, where outcomes are critical and where services often are provided under difficult and unpredictable conditions. Nurses provide a critical surveillance function in healthcare organizations, particularly in hospitals, by monitoring care and safeguarding patients; thus, the availability and work of nurses affect quality of care and patient safety (Aiken et al. 2003a). Nurses are a primary determinant of patient satisfaction (Abramowitz, Cote, and Berry 1987; Greeneich 1993; Press Ganey 2003; Vahey et al. 2004), an outcome that takes high priority in a competitive healthcare environment. Clearly, having a well-trained, motivated, and appropriately deployed nursing staff complements the ability of a healthcare organization to provide effective and efficient patient care.

A critical problem for healthcare administrators is deciding how best to deploy nursing staff while considering the quality and costs of care delivered. This challenge is complicated by recurring nursing shortages and by the fierce competition for these professionals. During shortages, healthcare administrators often must take extraordinary steps (such as closing beds or hiring temporary nurses) to ensure that sufficient numbers of nurses are available to care for patients, and these steps are often taken under constrained budgets and without knowing the specific impact on patient outcomes. Managers must be aware of the implications of nurse workload and staffing decisions, particularly during times of nurse shortages, because such decisions may affect staff morale and increase turnover. A basic understanding of nurse workload and staffing issues allows managers to meet day-to-day patient care requirements as well as changing patient care demands, personnel, reimbursement, and regulations.

This chapter identifies key aspects of the nursing workload. This information aids managers in planning work, developing and implementing budgets, and staffing units or departments. The types of nursing professionals are discussed, and the terms nurse workload and nurse staffing are defined. In addition, this chapter examines the approaches used in different healthcare setting to measure nurse workload and provides the perspectives of different stakeholders on workload measurement. Nurse staffing metrics are presented, along with examples of staffing calculations.

Types of Nursing Personnel

In the United States, licensed and unlicensed nursing personnel differ in their education; knowledge, skills, and abilities; and patient care responsibilities. These differences must be taken into account when planning nurse workloads and staffing.

Licensed nursing personnel include those who work under a specific scope of practice set by state and/or national regulatory requirements (Bureau of Labor Statistics 2004). There are two types of licensed nurses: registered nurses (RNs) and licensed practical nurses (LPNs)[1]; the educational, licensure, and practice requirements for one group differ from that of the other. Healthcare organizations require proof of licensure from either type of nurses. *Unlicensed* nursing personnel provide support services to licensed nurses and other healthcare professionals. Characteristics of licensed and unlicensed nursing personnel are summarized in Table 13.1.

Healthcare organizations employ a mix of nursing personnel to meet patient care needs. The decisions about the numbers and types of nursing personnel to employ reflect an organization's philosophy about the role and importance of nursing; patient safety and satisfaction; quality of care; and the job satisfaction, perceived value, and safety of nurses and other nursing staff. In short, nurse staffing decisions represent the value that the unit, department, or organization places on the nursing practice and on patient care delivery (Van Slyck 1991). This value then is the foundation on which nurse workload decisions and nursing resources allocation are based.

Definitions and Measurement

The terms "nurse workload" and "nurse staffing" are often used interchangeably and inconsistently. For the purposes of this chapter, the following definitions will be used:

- *Nurse workload* means (1) the number of patients or patient days for which nursing care is required on a unit or within a department or organization or (2) the number of patients cared for by an individual nurse.
- *Nurse staffing* means (1) the number of nurses deployed (also called *staffing level*) or (2) the process by which the appropriate number and type of nursing personnel are deployed to satisfy nurse workload requirements.
- Nurse workload refers to a quantity of nursing services, while nurse staffing comprises the planning, budgeting, and costing aspects of providing nursing services.

A review of the literature reveals that researchers define and measure nurse staffing in different ways. These include (1) number of nursing personnel, by type of nurse; (2) type of nursing personnel hours (e.g., RN hours) as a percentage of total nursing care hours; (3) number of personnel (i.e., head count) as a percentage of total nursing staff; (4) number of FTEs (full-time equivalent) for specific nursing personnel; and (5) percent of total nursing FTEs, by type of nurse (e.g., RN FTEs) (Mark, Hughes, and Jones 2004; Seago 2001). These staffing measures focus on the staff

TABLE 13.1

Differences
Between
Licensed and
Unlicensed
Nursing Staff

	RN	LPN	Nursing Aide[a]
Educational Preparation	• 3-year diploma (hospital-based program[b]), 2-year associate degree, or 4-year baccalaureate degree	1 to 2 years of training at a technical or vocational school those certified	Varies. Some health-care organizations have mandatory training and certification require-ments; some states have a registry of
	• A few master's and doctoral programs exist for entry-level preparation		
Licensure	Issued by states; examination is required	Issued by states; examination is required	Certification by an accrediting body may or may not be required
Duties	• Provide complex nursing care to promote patient health, prevent disease, and help patients cope with illness • Observe, assess, and evaluate patient conditions • Work with patients, families, and other healthcare profes-sionals to develop and manage patient plans of care • May function independently, but often work in collaboration with physicians and other healthcare professionals		

TABLE 13.1
(continued)

	RN	LPN	Nursing Aide[a]
	• May supervise other licensed and unlicensed nursing personnel	• Provide routine nursing care	• Provide support services to licensed nurses and other healthcare professionals
Supervision Requirement	May function independently within scope of practice, or may be supervised by other RNs and, in some cases, physicians	Supervised by RN and/or physician; may also supervise other LPNs and/or unlicensed nursing personnel	Supervised by RN and/or physician; sometimes supervised by LPN

Source: Bureau of Labor Statistics, U.S. Department of Labor. 2004. Occupational Outlook Handbook, 2004–2005 Edition. [Online information; retrieved 8/29/04.] http://www.bls.gov/oco/ocos102.htm.
a. Includes nursing aides, nursing assistants, patient care assistants, and orderlies
b. The number of these programs has been in decline over the last two decades
c. Advanced practice nurses (i.e., clinical nurse specialist, nurse practitioner, nurse midwife, nurse anesthetist) require a master's or higher-level degree in nursing

levels *used* rather than the levels *needed* to provide safe care (Mark, Hughes, and Jones 2004). The relationship between nurse staffing and adverse patient events has been documented in various studies, but comparing their findings is difficult because of the inconsistencies and variation in the definition and measurement used.

There is disagreement in the nursing field as well on how to best ensure that staffing levels are adequate to meet patient care demands and keep patients safe. In 1999, California passed a nurse staffing legislation for hospitals, setting a minimum staffing requirement of 1 nurse for every 6 patients for 2004 and 1 nurse for every 5 patients beginning in 2005. These ratio requirements were established on the assumption that higher nurse staffing levels would lead to improved patient care. However, little or no evidence exists to support that the specific ratios selected are effective or that implementing these ratios yield beneficial outcomes, and whether or not nurse staffing levels should be legislated is also a topic of debate. Recognizing these arguments, California followed the 1999 staffing legislation with other bills that call for the evaluation of the previously mandated ratios and the development of staffing plans in hospitals. Other states have taken similar approaches by introducing legislation to mandate the development and implementation of specific nurse staffing plans, minimum staffing ratios, or some combination of both (American Nurses Association 2004).

In some states, nurse staffing legislation influences administrative decision making, but these laws do not cover all nursing personnel or patient care situations. In most states, nurse staffing legislation does not exist at all. As a result, administrators still struggle with several important questions:

- What numbers of nursing staff are needed to provide care for patients?
- What types of nursing staff are needed to provide care for patients?
- What mix of nursing staff is needed to provide quality care and meet patient care needs?
- What mix of nursing staff can the organization afford?
- How does the mix of nursing staff vary by patient care area?

When organizational revenues fall short of expenditure or when healthcare costs rise, labor—a large expense for healthcare organizations—often becomes a target of budget cuts. Under this scenario, nurse staffing plans that reduce the number of nurses, increase nurse workloads, or increase the number of hours worked by nurses (including overtime) may be counterproductive.

Finkler and Kovner (2002) define nurse workload as the volume of work required to deliver nursing care for a patient care unit or department.[2] Although nurse workload is often measured by unidimensional metrics such as patients or patient days, the "work" of nursing is complex, is multifaceted, and requires specialized knowledge and skills. Furthermore, nurse workload entails more than the time that staff spend with patients. The complex nature of nurses' work requires a "balance of job demands with sufficient resources (adequate staffing, time available) to plan and carry out work" (Koehoorn et al. 2002, 6).

Table 13.2 presents four scenarios to illustrate the basic components of average nurse workload. Scenario 1 shows that, given a constant nurse workload (number of patients), a decrease in nurse staffing (the number of nurses) increases the average workload (the number of patients per nurse). Scenario 2 shows that, given a constant nurse staffing, an increase in nurse workload also increases the average workload. Scenario 3 shows that average nurse workload does not change if the number of patients and the number of staff change at the same rate. Scenario 4 shows that the average nurse workload increases if the number of patients increases at a rate faster than the number of staff. These scenarios illustrate the following points: (1) an

Scenario	Nursing Workload (Number of Patients)	Nurse Staffing (Number of Nurses)	Average Nursing Workload (Number of Patients per Nurse)
1: Constant number of patients, decreasing number of nurses	25 25 25	6 5 4	4.2 5.0 6.3
2: Increasing number of patients, constant number of nurses	20 25 30	5 5 5	4.0 5.0 6.0
3: Increasing number of patients and nurses with same rate of change	20 25 30	4 5 6	5.0 5.0 5.0
4: Increasing number of patients and nurses with different rates of change	20 25 30	4 4.5 5	5.0 5.6 6.0

TABLE 13.2
Basic Components of the Average Nursing Workload

increase in the average nursing workload may be result of more patients, fewer nurses, or both and (2) the average nursing workload is not reduced by an increase in nurse staffing if the workload (number of patients) increases at a faster rate. Of course, in the real world, nursing workload is seldom constant and the work of an individual nurse usually fluctuates as patients' numbers and conditions change. Nevertheless, the average nursing workload may be considered a crude measure of the adequacy of nurse staffing.

Most healthcare organizations have formal processes related to nurse staffing that are used to reasonably, fairly, and safely address nursing workload issues. These processes include the use of committees with nursing representatives, such as quality of care and patient safety; the development and implementation of staffing policies and procedures, including standards for the number and skill mix of nursing staff; and the determination of hours-of-care requirements for different types of patients. In addition, nurse staffing issues are usually part of the collective bargaining agreement between employers and nurse unions.

Use of Measures

Nursing workload is measured for three primary reasons: (1) to inform the budgeting process; (2) to meet regulatory and accreditation standards; and (3) to inform the development, implementation, and evaluation of staffing plans. The budgeting process necessitates the calculation of nursing workload to prepare an organization's operating budget and, specifically, to determine nursing personnel requirements and costs (Finkler and Kovner 2000). The budgeting process involves decision making about the level and mix of nurse staffing, the workload that nurses will assume, and the allocation of resources.

Regulatory requirements and accreditation standards necessitate that healthcare organizations comply with regulations of the Centers for Medicare & Medicaid Services regulations and standards of the Joint Commission on Accreditation of Healthcare Organizations (JCAHO 2004). For example, in 2002, the Joint Commission instituted a staffing effectiveness requirement to which hospitals must comply for accreditation. Nursing workload systems may be used to gather staffing and outcomes data to document compliance to this requirement.

Nurse staffing plans, on the other hand, are blueprints for meeting specific patient care and regulatory requirements and for deploying nursing personnel efficiently and effectively. Staffing plans also enable managers to develop policies for reasonable work schedules, which promote a positive work environment, and for accommodating operational uncertainties and contingencies.

Nursing workload measures differ across types of healthcare settings. For example, nursing workload can be measured in terms of the number of patients or number of patient days in hospitals, in terms of the number of residents or resident days in long-term care facilities, in terms of the number of clinic visits in ambulatory clinics, in terms of the number of home visits in home health care services, in terms of the number of deliveries in maternity wards, and in terms of the number of procedures in day surgery or operating rooms (Finkler and Kovner 2000). Nursing workload measurement systems have been developed to capture nursing workload in these different settings. These systems (usually electronic) capture the variable nature of nursing care requirements across different types of patients and healthcare settings, and they are used to determine the number of nurses required to care for different types of patients (Edwardson and Giovannetti 1994). In short, information provided by these systems aids in decision making and in allocating nursing resources (O'Brien et al. 2002).

Perspectives of Stakeholders

Stakeholders view nurse workload and its measurement differently. Patients, along with their families, pay attention to these two elements because they want to receive individualized care and relevant communications about their condition and treatment (O'Brien et al. 2002). Patients' perceptions are important to healthcare organizations; however, currently no nurse workload measure or system is available that takes into account these consumers' preferences and desires.

Healthcare administrators, including patient care unit or nursing managers, are concerned about nurse workload and measurement for several reasons. First, they are responsible for allocating nursing resources—a decision that ensures patient care needs are met. For example, on a day-to-day basis, nurse managers[3] must modify staffing levels as necessary to meet nursing workload requirements. This may mean acquiring agency or per diem nursing staff to cover vacancies or to respond to unexpected (and unscheduled) variations in patient care requirements. Second, they have to balance the costs of delivering nursing care with organizational reimbursements. If the nursing staff is too large (i.e., too few patients per nurse), the costs of providing nursing services may be unnecessarily high. On the other hand, if the nursing staff is too small (i.e., too many patients per nurse), costs may be lower in the short run; however, the work under this condition may increase nursing errors, stress, burnout, dissatisfaction, absenteeism, and turnover, which likely will lead to higher costs over the long run. Thus, administrators must ensure that nursing workloads are reasonable and fair, allowing nurses to feel able to deliver the level of nursing care needed by patients.

Insurers and payers' perspective has a financial basis as well. In some cases, an increase in charges as a result of nurse workload and staffing can hike up reimbursements. An increase in overall healthcare costs because of workload and staffing also augments the costs of coverage, which are then passed along to consumers. In turn, employers and consumers need to make a decision about whether or not to retain coverage with the insurer, and if so whether to keep the same level of coverage.

Policymakers view nurse workload in terms of ensuring that nursing resources are sufficient in providing safe, effective care to communities and in meeting changing patient care demands. For example, the aging U.S. population means that more nursing resources will be needed to care for the elderly in the future, and longstanding nursing shortages in many geographic areas will increase the gap between supply and demand. Policymakers must see to it that government and industry workforce policies recognize changing demographics and support human resources adjustment, such as providing incentives to nurses and other healthcare providers to enter the geriatric care field and educating nurses and other caregivers about long-term care. In addition, policymakers must develop guidelines to ensure that nurse staffing levels are safe and do not place patients at risk of harm or injury.

Nurses view many aspects of workload and staffing in terms of how they are directly affected. These include volume of work; responsibility to their patients, themselves, and their unit; multiple, concurrent, and often competing demands on their time; their feelings of overload and inability to complete work; having to deal with the unexpected or with interruptions; their familiarity with and support of work requirements; the abilities of other caregivers with whom they are working; the degree to which the workload spills into their personal lives; the level of emotional and physical exhaustion from work; and their lack of control over workload (Gaudine 2000).

Measurement of Nurse Staffing

Nurse staffing is the numbers and types of nursing personnel employed on a patient care unit in a hospital, long-term care facility, emergency department, ambulatory clinic, or community health center. Decisions about the numbers and types of nurses employed on a patient care unit are based on (1) the patient population receiving care, (2) the education and skills possessed by nurses delivering care, and (3) an organization's philosophy about nursing and patient care delivery.

The metric for determining the numbers and types of nurses is the full time equivalent or FTE. Nursing FTE calculations are used to determine unit and departmental staffing needs and are the key input to the budgeting process. An FTE is based on the concept of one individual working full time for a year, or 40 hours a week, 2,080 hours for a 52-week period (Finkler and Kovner 2000).[4] FTE calculations include both *productive* and *nonproductive* time. Strasen (1987) defines productive time as time spent providing care and nonproductive time as time paid but not spent giving care (e.g., sick, vacation, holiday, professional development, and any other paid time off). The amount of nonproductive time is based on organizational policy and may be associated with the individual's length of service to the organization. For example, one nursing FTE's 2,080 hours of paid time may include 30 paid days off (240 hours) or nonproductive time. Thus, 2,080 hours minus 240 hours equals 1,840 hours of productive time remaining. Although the amount of benefit time may vary among organizations, only productive time is used in calculating the amount of nursing workload available to deliver care to patients. Here is another example: On a patient care unit, 1.0 FTE is equivalent to 2,080 hours paid per year. Ninety percent of the paid time is considered productive, while 10 percent is for vacation, sick time, professional development, and nonpatient care time. The calculation here is as follows: $0.90 \times 2,080$ hrs paid/FTE = 1,872 productive hours/FTE.

The prevalence of 12-hour shifts and other flexible scheduling strategies means that many nurses actually work less or greater than 40 hours per week (Strasen 1987). The number of hours worked influences the proportion of paid versus productive hours and the number of productive hours per FTE, and this must be taken into account when calculating unit FTEs (Finkler and Kovner 2000).

Nurse staffing calculations must take into account the fact that all nursing personnel do not work full time. Many nurses work part time, providing managers with some degree of flexibility in staffing a patient care unit. On any particular patient care unit, FTEs may be composed of full-time staff only, part-time staff only, or most likely a mix of full-time and part-time staff. For example, on a patient care unit where "full time" nurses work 7 days of 12-hour shifts in a 2-week pay period, the time per position exceeds 1 FTE: 12 hours/day $\times$ 7 days = 84 hours in 2 weeks / 80 hours in 2 weeks = 1.05 FTE. Alternatively, if "full time" nurses on the patient care unit work 6 days of 12-hour shifts in a 2-week pay period, the time per position is less than 1 FTE: 12 hours/day $\times$ 6 days = 72 hours in 2 weeks / 80 hours in 2 weeks = 0.90 FTE.

Various data are needed to determine nursing FTEs and staffing (Finkler and Kovner 2000):

- *Projected patient days:* A patient day is an accounting term that represents the concept of 1 patient that is cared for during a 24-hour period. An estimate of the projected number of patient days is needed to anticipate future workload needs.
- *Nursing care hours (productive plus nonproductive) per patient day:* This is time spent delivering care to patients during a 24-hour period and is generally reported as a monthly average.
- *Staffing mix:* This is the proportion of RNs, LPNs, and nursing assistants used to provide care in a 24-hour period.

An example of calculating paid nursing hours and nursing care hours per patient per day is as follows:

A patient care unit that averages 25 patients per day during a 30-day month pays for 6,000 RN hours. Of these 6,000 RN hours, 90 percent are considered productive. What are the paid nursing hours per day and per patient day? How many nursing care hours per patient day are involved?

Here are the calculations:

- 6,000 nursing hours paid per month/30 days in the month = 200 paid nursing hours per day
- 200 hours of nursing care per day / 25 patients per day = 8.0 nursing hours paid per patient per day
- 6,000 nursing hours paid per month × 90 percent productive = 5,400 nursing care hours per month
- 5,400 nursing care hours per month/30 days in the month = 180 nursing care hours per day
- 180 hours of nursing care per day / 25 patients per day = 7.2 nursing care hours per patient per day

Another important source of workload data is a patient classification or acuity system. *Patient classification systems* (either a manual, paper-and-pencil tool, or an electronic system) classify individual patient demands and nursing care requirements (Huckabay 1984) based on patient acuity or severity of illness,[5] not diagnostic category. These systems provide a standard measure of nursing care for classes of patients (generally measured in hours of nursing care required per patient day) and provide a way of matching patient needs with nursing requirements. Commercially available patient classification systems include GRASP(r), Medicus(r), and Quadramed(r), and some of these commercial products can be customized by organizations to meet their needs and integrate with other management information systems. Individual organizations also create their own patient classification systems.

The potential for patient classification systems are great because they can be used to project nurse staffing needs, develop unit budgets, establish costs for nursing services, and inform risk management and quality improvement initiatives (DeGroot 1989; Seago 2001; Van Slyck 2000). Unfortunately, patient classification systems are often not used to their potential, are generally distrusted by nurses and administrators as not reliable or valid, and, consequently, are not used for decision making. More specifically, patient classification scores are based on nurses' ratings of patients' characteristics, severity of illness, and required number and complexity of treatment interventions (Van Ruiswyk et al. 1992). Because of the way in which patient scores are obtained, some claim that nurses may actually inflate patient ratings (which is also known as acuity creep) to increase unit staffing (hence reducing nurse workload) or to prevent staff from being pulled to work on another unit that may be understaffed[6] (Malloch and Conovaloff 1999). On the other hand, some nurses believe that managers are not responsive and do not increase the number of staff when ratings suggest that more nurses are needed. Patient classification systems generally do not take into account the nurses' educational level, years of experience, or knowledge and cannot match the skills of individual nurses with the needs of individual patients. Thus, while these systems may be commonly used to estimate staffing and workload, they do not replace a manager's judgment and staff input for day-to-day or shift-to-shift staffing (Seago 2001).

Other information is needed to inform staffing assessment and measurement. Historical data help to understand variations in patient care on a unit, such as the following:

- *Average daily census* (the average number of patients cared for per day over a defined time period)—to determine a staffing standard on numbers and mix of nursing personnel by shift
- *Occupancy rate* (the number of patients divided by the number of days the unit is open)—to examine the extent to which unit capacity is reached
- *Payroll data* (including paid productive and nonproductive time)—to determine paid hours per patient day
- *Admissions, discharges, and transfers and information on short-stay patients*—to gain insight into patient turnover and work requirements
- *Temporal variations in care*—to find out factors that may affect patient admissions and requirements (for example, the flu season may increase admissions on certain units, especially on units that provide geriatric care)

Efficient nurse staffing hinges on several unit and organizational knowledge. First, knowledge of clinical policies is critical. For example, a manager who is staffing an oncology unit must be aware of the unit's clinical policy (e.g., patients on certain chemotherapeutic agents receive increased observation by registered nurses), the numbers of patients who typically receive the medication during a period of time, and the associated risks of the treatment. Second, knowledge of internal organizational changes in care delivery is needed to estimate the effect of changes in programs, procedures, or treatment protocols on staffing requirements. Third, knowledge of collective agreements is needed to ensure that staffing is in compliance with provisions agreed on in a bargaining process. Fourth, knowledge of the internal and external organizational environment, such as anticipated structural changes or policy developments, is important. Each of these pieces of information should be taken into account when calculating nurse staffing needs.

An Example of FTE and Nurse Staffing Calculations

Consider the annual nurse staffing needs for a busy, 30-bed inpatient pediatric unit at an academic health center. The nurse manager for the unit must determine the total unit workload, or nursing care hours, for the coming year using patient classification system data and patient days projected from historical data[7] (see Table 13.3). The total unit workload (W) or nursing hours can be determined based on the number of the average care hours per 24 hours (ACH) and patient days (PD) using this formula (Finkler and Kovner 2000):

$$W = \sum^{5} (PD_i \times ACH_i) = 91,300 \text{ nursing hours}$$

The number of FTEs required to staff the unit over a year is calculated and then distributed across day and night shifts. FTEs are further divided according to the types of nurses required for each shift. Here is additional information provided by a nurse manager:

- 1.0 FTE = 2,080 hours paid
- The percentage of productive nursing hours on the unit is 85 percent (an average of 1,768 productive hours /FTE)
- Nursing personnel on this unit are scheduled to work based on a staffing standard of 55 percent for the day shift and 45 percent for the night shift
- The staff mix is 75 percent RNs, 15 percent LPNs, and 10 percent nursing assistants

The overall number of FTEs required to staff this unit is determined as follows:

- 91,300 total hours of care required per year/1,768 productive hours per FTE = 51.64 FTEs for year-round nursing care coverage
- The number of nursing FTEs required to staff day and night shifts for the year is calculated as follows:
    - Days: 51.64 FTEs × 55 percent = 28.4 FTEs required to cover day shifts for the year
    - Nights: 51.64 FTEs × 45 percent = 23.2 FTEs required to cover day shifts for the year
- The type of nursing FTEs required to staff day and night shifts for the year is determined to be:
    - Days: 21.3 RN FTEs (28.4 FTEs × 75 percent), 4.26 LPN FTEs (28.4 FTEs × 15 percent), and 2.84 NA FTEs (28.4 FTEs × 10 percent)

Patient Classification Rating	Average Care Hours per 24 Hours	Projected Number of Patient Days
1	3.5	1,500
2	5.0	2,500
3	9.0	3,000
4	13.0	2,100
5	17.5	1,100

TABLE 13.3
Sample Data for a 30-bed Inpatient Pediatric Unit at an Academic Health Center

- Nights: 17.4 RN FTEs (23.2 FTEs × 75 percent), 3.48 LPN FTEs (23.2 FTEs × 15 percent), and 2.32 NA FTEs (23.2 FTEs × 10 percent)
- The 51.64 FTEs are scheduled such that nursing and shift requirements are met. Over time, if patient classification data reflect a change in nursing care requirements, the FTE and scheduling requirements may change.

The total number of FTEs needed on this unit is known, but the actual number of shifts and types of personnel needed must still be determined. Furthermore, managers must make decisions, based on the actual number of allocated FTEs, about the actual number of people to schedule for meeting ongoing requirements within their budget constraints.

In our example (see Figure 13.1, item 4), a manager may decide to staff for 9 RNs on days and 7 on nights, 2 LPNs on days and 1 on nights, and 1 nursing assistant on days and nights. Another manager may staff for 8 RNs on days and 6 on nights, 2 LPNs on days and nights, and 1 nursing assistant on days and 2 on nights. These decisions should be based on a manager's understanding of patient needs, staff availability, and organizational policy.

FTEs are likely to be filled with various combinations of full-time and part-time personnel. For example, the 21.3 RN FTEs may be made up of 22 full-time RN staff or 18 full-time RNs and 7 part-time RNs, and so forth. These decisions are necessary to determine the actual number of nursing positions that will staff the unit and, in turn, meet the unit personnel budget requirements.

FIGURE 13.1

Staffing
Calculations
for a 30-Bed
Inpatient
Pediatric Unit

Determine
1. Nursing care hours required each day
2. Number of nursing shifts per day and per week
3. Number of nursing personnel required on day and night shifts
4. Breakdown of RN/LPN/nursing assistant staffing for day and night shifts
5. Ratio of FTEs to shifts

Solution

1. An average daily nursing care requirement = 91,300 nursing care hours per year/365 days per year = 250 nursing care hours per day

2. 250 nursing care hours per day, with 12-hour shifts = 20.8 nursing shifts per 24-hour day (250 hours / 12 hours per shift)

   20.8 nursing shifts per day x 7 days per week = 145.6 nursing shifts per week

3. Using the 55 percent/45 percent standard:

   20.8 shifts × 55 percent = 11.44 nursing shifts on days

   20.8 shifts × 45 percent = 9.36 nursing shifts on nights

4. Days: 8.58 RN shifts (11.44 × 75 percent), 1.72 LPN shifts (11.44 × 15 percent), and 1.14 nursing assistant shifts (11.44 × 10 percent)

   Nights: 7.02 RN shifts (9.36 × 75 percent), 1.40 LPN shifts (9.36 × 15 percent), and 0.94 nursing assistant shifts (9.36 × 10 percent)

5. 2.48 FTEs are required to cover one shift for the entire year (e.g., 28.4 nurse FTEs are required to staff 11.44 nursing shifts during days, 23.2 nurse FTEs are required to staff 9.36 nursing shifts during nights, etc.). This means 2.48 full-time nurses must be hired to cover one 12-hour shift, 365 days of the year.

Nursing care requirements may vary by day of the week. Fewer nurses may be needed on the weekends because certain services for patient care testing and procedures are available only on weekdays. For example, the 145.6 nursing shifts per week (i.e., 20.8 nursing shifts per day × 7 days per week—see Figure 13.1, item 2) can be distributed so that there are fewer than the 20.8 nursing shifts per day on weekends and greater numbers on weekdays (Finkler and Kovner 2000), depending on unit operations.

If patient census on the unit changes over time, nursing staffing requirements may change too. In this case, it may be necessary to advocate for additional permanent or temporary nursing personnel (from unit or in-house staffing pools or outside agencies), decrease permanent FTE requirements, or ask unit staff to take vacation time and work fewer shifts. In both of these cases, the perspective and judgment of the nurse or unit manager are critical.

Returning to our example, if we divide the 51.64 FTEs required to staff the unit over a year by the 20.8 daily nursing shifts, we see that 2.48 FTEs are needed to fill each nursing shift for the year. This means that approximately 2.5 nursing staff must be hired full time (or a greater number must be hired if some work part time) to cover a 12-hour shift for 365 days (4,380 hours). The difference between hours paid to 2.48 FTEs (5,158 hours = 2.48 × 2,080 hours) and patient care hours required (4,380) takes into account the personnel needed to cover for staff days off, sick time, holidays, vacations, and so forth (Finkler and Kovner 2000).

Finally, in our example, 8.58 RN shifts (21.3 RN FTEs) are required to cover days, and 7.02 RN shifts (17.4 RN FTEs) are required to cover nights, with a patient census of 25 patients. This yields an average workload of approximately 2.9 patients per RN for the day shift and 3.6 patients per RN for the night shift.

Effects of Inadequate Workload and Staffing

Workload Stress and Burnout

Burke (2003) notes that when individuals perceive excessive workloads (that is, they feel they have too much work to complete during their work time), they become stressed and burned out, which leads to feelings of anger. Nurses in this situation are more likely to call in sick or leave the organization altogether.

Workload is one of the most significant predictors of negative health outcomes, stress, decreased job satisfaction, and burnout (Burke 2003). Burke studied the relationship between changing nurse-patient ratios and nurses' perceptions of workload, job satisfaction, psychological well-being, and effectiveness of their institutions. According to that study, nurses who are assigned high patient-nurse ratios report heavier workloads, low job satisfaction, poorer psychological health, and decreased view of hospital effectiveness. Although this study calls for further research in this area, it signifies the increased sensitivity related to the topic of nurse workload and its effect on nurse perceptions.

Healthcare administrators, especially first-line patient care unit or nurse managers, should be aware of such issues and the impact of staffing decisions on nurses' perceptions. They must be prepared to respond to nurses' concerns about workload and overload, involve nurses in establishing appropriate workloads, engage in contingency planning to deal with sudden changes in patient care needs or conditions, manage fluctuations in staffing (e.g., call outs, vacations, educational leaves), and be aware of changes in provider practices that can affect nurse workload (Prescott and Soeken 1996).

Workload data must be examined objectively and subjectively to make a case for adequate nursing resource allocation (Gaudine 2000). Providing adequate, and perhaps less costly, nursing support services can also relieve the pressure on nurses who often take on non-nursing tasks. For example, ensuring that supplies are stocked and pharmaceuticals are delivered will prevent nurses from taking time to seek out these essentials for patient care delivery. Finally, strategies should be used to give nurses as much control over their workload as is realistic to reduce their perceptions of overload (Gaudine 2000). For example, managers can ask nurses for input on the timing of patient admissions, the temporary closing of beds, and the attainment of additional nursing resources.

Poor Quality of Care

The lowest cost mix of nursing staff is not the best option if the quality of care and patient outcomes are adversely affected. Aiken and colleagues (2003b) document a relationship between nurses' educational level and patient mortality, citing that hospitals that employ higher numbers of nurses with a baccalaureate (or higher) degree have lower patient mortality rates than hospitals that employ fewer nurses with a baccalaureate (or higher) degree.

Nurse staffing has received a great deal of attention because of society's concerns about patient safety and the recent high-profile reports that cite the relationship between low nurse staffing levels and adverse patient events (Aiken et al. 2002; Kovner and Gergen 1998; Kovner et al. 2002; Needlman et al. 2002). For example, Aiken and colleagues (2003b) document that higher patient-to-nurse ratios are associated with a higher risk of mortality and failure to rescue among surgical patients. Specifically, the risk of death is 14 percent higher in hospitals where workloads or ratios are 6 or more patients per nurse and is 31 percent higher in hospitals with workloads of 8 or more patients per nurse, relative to hospitals where nurse workloads are 4 or fewer patients.

Future Directions and Challenges

Measuring nurse workload and staffing and acting on the results are issues that have occupied healthcare administrators and researchers for decades. As Edwardson and Giovannetti (1994) suggest, many thought that patient classification systems would identify the right numbers of staff to provide care for certain patients. However, these systems have proven to be problematic, especially in terms of their reliability and validity, and managers are still faced with establishing nurse workloads and calculating nurse staffing needs. Moreover, many healthcare organizations still lack the ability to free nurses from non-nursing tasks (e.g., retrieving medications from the pharmacy) that further increase the workload and do not require specific nursing knowledge to carry out (Moody 2004).

One approach for measuring nursing workload and productivity is the use of a *relative value unit* (RVU) *system* (Finkler and Kovner 2000; Graf 1992). This approach improves patient classification systems by providing a more accurate measurement of patient needs and nursing resource requirements. Patient classification systems generally rate patients on a scale—for example, from 1 to 5. However, the rating used in most patient classification systems is not to scale, such that the hours of care requirement for a patient rated 5 may not be five times greater than a patient rated 1. An RVU system assigns an acuity index value of 1 for some specific, predetermined level of patient classification. Although the choice of patient acuity level that is assigned a 1 is arbitrary, it is necessary to provide a basis for comparison. After a level is determined for a patient care unit, other patient classification levels are assigned relative values to reflect the hours of care required relative to the index. For example, if a Level 1 patient requires three hours of care per day and a Level 5 requires eight hours of care, the RVU for the Level 5 patient is 2.67 (8.0/3.0) (Finkler and Kovner 2000; Graf 1992; Moody 2004). An RVU system has advantages over patient classification systems because it takes the patient population and diagnoses into account along with the costs of providing care (Finkler and Kovner 2000; Graf 1992; Moody 2004).

Moody (2004) advocates a nursing workload approach that is grounded in human capital theory. This approach uses a nursing productivity index that takes into account nurses' knowledge, skills, and abilities (their human capital) and the patients for whom they provide care. This type of workload model is based on Peter Drucker's (1994) description of the "knowledge worker" in today's knowledge society and values nurses based on their thought processes and nursing judgments, which, although difficult to quantify, more adequately capture the complex nature of nursing work. Moody proposes that this nursing workload model capture data on patient intensity, nurse staffing, infection and error rates, organizational resources (financial and human), patient outcomes, patient ability to provide self-care, and provider outcomes. Moody also advocates for the costs of nursing turnover, which may represent 1.25 times the salary of a departing nurse (Jones 2005), to be considered in valuing nurses and their work. The details of this valuation are not provided, but the concept of valuing nursing work based on nursing knowledge, skills, and abilities is intuitively appealing.

Various nurse staffing studies have documented the important relationship between nurse staffing and patient care outcomes, yet further research is needed to explain this relationship. For example, a conceptually cogent and consistent measure of nurse staffing facilitates the comparison of findings across studies and identification of specific patient outcomes that are sensitive to changes in nurse staffing for different patient populations. Furthermore, much of the nurse staffing research is generally atheoretical. Thus, there is a dire need for theory-driven research in this area to help us understand the how and why behind the relationship between nurse staffing and patient outcomes (Mark, Hughes, and Jones 2004).

Nurse workload systems are needed that take into account short-term staffing contingencies, improve the deployment of nursing personnel, and facilitate the development of long-term staffing plans. Moreover, information systems that link nursing workloads and patient outcomes are needed to improve the quality of patient care. However, no system is likely to emerge that will replace the critical judgments of the managers who use the system and these managers' unique knowledge of nurse workload measurement, the work of nurses, clinical care processes, and the patients that nurses serve. Through such insight, healthcare administrators can proactively plan to ensure that (1) nurses are involved in decisions that affect unit operations and nurse workloads, (2) adequate nursing resources are available to provide patient care, and (3) adequate support services are in place to support nurses and relieve them of performing nonessential tasks (Burke 2003).

Summary

Nurses are key members of the healthcare team. Understanding how best to deploy nurses while balancing quality and costs is an important ongoing function for healthcare administrators that may be especially challenging during periods of nursing shortage, when adequate numbers and types of nurses are needed to ensure the delivery of safe, high-quality care to patients. This chapter provides an overview of important tools and techniques needed to calculate nursing workload and presents examples to illustrate these calculations. Utilization of these tools and techniques aids in the routine planning of patient care delivery, development of unit and organizational budgets, and the equitable distribution of nursing staff. More importantly, however, use of these practices will foster the creation of an environment that increases nurses' job satisfaction and well-being and that decreases the stress and burnout often associated with high workloads and inadequate staffing. Over the long run, sensitivity to nursing workload and staffing issues will contribute to the delivery of high-quality patient care, the formation of high-performing patient care teams, and improvements in overall organizational performance.

References

Abramowitz, S., A. A. Cote, and E. Berry. 1987. "Analyzing Patient Satisfaction: A Multianalytic Approach." *Quality Review Bulletin* 13 (4): 122–30.

Aiken, L. H., S. P. Clarke, D. M. Sloane, J. Sochalski, and J. H. Silber. 2002. "Hospital Nurse Staffing and Patient Mortality, Nurse Burnout, and Job Dissatisfaction." *JAMA* 288 (16): 1987–93.

Aiken, L. H., S. P. Clarke, J. H. Silber, and D. M. Sloane. 2003a. "Hospital Nurse Staffing, Education, and Patient Mortality." *LDI Issue Brief* 9 (2): 1–4.

Aiken, L. H., S. P. Clarke, R. B. Cheung, D. M. Sloane, and J. H. Silber. 2003b. "Educational Levels of Hospital Nurses and Surgical Patient Mortality." *JAMA* 290 (12): 1617–23.

American Nurses Association. 2004. "Background: Staffing Plans and Ratios." [Online article; retrieved 8/29/04.] http://www.nursingworld.org/GOVA/STATE/2004/staffing.pdf.

Bureau of Labor Statistics, U.S. Department of Labor. 2004. *Occupational Outlook Handbook, 2004–2005 Edition*. [Online information; retrieved 8/29/04.] http://www.bls.gov/oco/ocos102.htm.

Burke, R. J. 2003. "Hospital Restructuring, Workload, and Nursing Staff Satisfaction and Work Experiences." *The Health Care Manager* 22 (2): 99–107.

DeGroot, H. A. 1989. "Patient Classification System Evaluation: Part 2, System Selection and Implementation." *Journal of Nursing Administration* 19 (7): 24–30.

Drucker, P. F. 1994. "The Age of Social Transformation." *Atlantic Monthly* 274 (5): 53–80.

Edwardson, S. R., and P. B. Giovannetti. 1994. "Nursing Workload Measurement Systems." In *Annual Review of Nursing Research*, Volume 12, edited by J. J. Fitzpatrick and J. S. Stevenson, 95–123. New York: Springer.

Finkler, S. A., and C. T. Kovner. 2000. *Financial Management for Nurse Managers and Executives, 2nd Edition*. Philadelphia, PA: W.B. Saunders Company.

Gaudine, A. P. 2000. "What Do Nurses Mean by Workload and Work Overload?" *Canadian Journal of Nursing Leadership* 13 (2): 22–27.

Graf, C. M. 1992. "The Operating Budget." In *Budgeting Concepts for Nurse Managers, 2nd Edition*, edited by S. A. Finkler, 162–202. Philadelphia, PA: W.B. Saunders Company.

Greeneich, D. 1993. "The Link Between New and Return Business and Quality Care: Patient Satisfaction." *Advances in Nursing Science* 16 (1): 62–72.

Huckabay, L. M. 1984. *Patient Classification: A Basis for Staffing*. National League for Nursing Publications, #20. New York: NLN.

Joint Commission on Accreditation of Healthcare Organizations. 2004. "Facts About Staffing Effectiveness Standard." [Online information; retrieved 9/19/04.] http://www.jcaho.org/news+room/press+kits/facts+about+staffing+effectiveness+standards.htm.

Jones, C. B. 2005. "The Costs of Nurse Turnover, Part 2: Application of the Nursing Turnover Cost Calculation Methodology." *Journal of Nursing Administration*, in press.

Koehoorn, M., G. S. Lowe, K. V. Rondeau, G. S. Schellenberg, and T. H. Wagar. 2002. *Creating High-Quality Healthcare Workplaces.* Ottawa, Canada: Canadian Policy Research Networks and Canadian Health Services Research Foundation.

Kovner, C. T., and P. J. Gergen. 1998. "Nurse Staffing Levels and Adverse Events Following Surgery in U.S. Hospitals." *Image: Journal of Nursing Scholarship* 30 (4): 315–21.

Kovner, C. T., C. B. Jones, C. Zahn, P. Gergen, and J. Basu. 2002. "Nurse Staffing and Post Surgical Adverse Events: An Analysis of Administrative Data from a Sample of U.S. Hospitals, 1990–1996." *Health Services Research* 37 (3): 611–29.

Malloch, K., and A. Conovaloff. 1999. "Patient Classification Systems, Part 1: The Third Generation." *Journal of Nursing Administration* 29 (7/8): 49–56.

Mark, B. A., L. C. Hughes, and C. B. Jones. 2004. "The Role of Theory in Improving Patient Safety and Quality Health Care." *Nursing Outlook* 52 (1): 11–16.

Moody, R. C. 2004. "Nurse Productivity Measures for the 21st Century." *Health Care Management Review* 29 (2): 98–106.

Needlman, J., P. Buerhaus, S. Mattke, M. Stewart, and K. Zelevinsky. 2002. "Nurse-Staffing Levels and the Quality of Care in Hospitals." *New England Journal of Medicine* 346 (22): 1715–22.

O'Brien, A. J., M. Abas, J. Christensen, T. H. Nicholls, T. L. Prou, A. Hekau, and J. Vanderpyl. 2002. *Nursing Workload Measurement in Acute Mental Health Inpatient Units: A Report for the Mental Health Research and Development Strategy.* Auckland, New Zealand: Health Research Council of New Zealand.

Prescott, P. A., and K. L. Soeken. 1996. "Measuring Nursing Intensity in Ambulatory Care, Part I: Approaches to and Uses of Patient Classification Systems." *Nursing Economics* 14 (1): 14–21, 33.

Press Ganey. 2003. "Study Confirms Nursing Shortage Affects Patient Satisfaction." [Online article; retrieved 7/15/04.] http://www.press-ganey.org/scripts/news.php?news_id=57.

Seago, J. A. 2001. "Nurse Staffing, Models of Care Delivery, and Interventions." In *Making Health Care Safer: A Critical Analysis of Patient Safety Practices*, edited by K. G. Shojania, B. W. Duncan, K. M. McDonald, and R. M. Wachter. Evidence Report/Technology Assessment: Number 43. AHRQ Publication No. 01-E058. Rockville, MD: AHRQ.

Strasen, L. 1987. *Key Business Skills for Nurse Managers.* Philadelphia, PA: J.B. Lippincott Company.

Vahey, D. C., L. H. Aiken, D. M. Sloane, S. P. Clarke, and D. Vargas. 2004. "Nurse Burnout and Patient Satisfaction." *Medical Care* 42 (2, Suppl): 1157–66.

Van Ruiswyk, J., A. Hartz, C. Guse, P. Sigmann, C. Porth, and K. Buck. 1992. "Nursing Assessments: Patient Severity of Illness." *Nursing Management* 23 (9): 44–46, 48.

Van Slyck, A. 1991. "A Systems Approach to the Management of Nursing Services, Part II: Patient Classification System." *Nursing Management* 22 (4): 23–25.

———. 2000. "Patient Classification Systems: Not a Proxy for Nurse 'Busyness'." *Nursing Administration Quarterly* 24 (4): 60–65.

Notes

1. LPNs are known as licensed vocational nurses in the states of California and Texas (Bureau of Labor Statistics 2004).
2. For budgeting purposes, the patient care unit or department represents a cost center or entity for which nursing workload is determined.
3. Nurse managers are unit managers who oversee day-to-day operations of patient care units. Other healthcare administrators may serve in this capacity as well. However, because nurse managers have an understanding of clinical care processes, they commonly fill this role.
4. In a two-week pay period, 1 FTE equals 80 hours.
5. Patients, even in the same disease category or classification, and their care requirements vary.
6. Floating refers to the practice of pulling nurses from their regular unit to work on another understaffed unit.
7. Managers typically complete these calculations using spreadsheet software.

Discussion Questions

1. What are the various elements that comprise nurse workload?
2. How is nurse workload related to nurse staffing?
3. What critical data are necessary to assemble before calculating nurse staffing needs?
4. How is organizational philosophy reflected in the measurement of nurse workload?

Experiential Exercises

Exercise 1   The Michigan Nurses Association released a document entitled "The Model Case for Reducing Patient-to-Nurse Staffing Ratios in Michigan Hospitals: Two Scenarios" (to view the document, visit http://www.minurses.org/spc/index.shtml). This document presents two hypothetical cases—one of a 200-bed hospital and one of a 50-bed hospital, both of which are trying to reduce their nurse staffing ratio from 1 nurse per 5 patients to 1 nurse per 4 patients. This change in ratio is consistent with the nurse staffing ratios mandated in California. The document includes data on nurse workload, staffing, salaries, turnover, and other unit operations issues to examine the potential costs and savings associated with changing the nurse-to-patient ratio. Both cases conclude with this finding: Cost savings from a ratio change outweigh the costs of hiring more nurses. Read this document, then answer the following questions.

Exercise 1 Questions

1. If you were a manager at the 200-bed hospital, would you agree with the staffing decisions made? Justify your position.
2. Would your answer change if you were a manager at the 50-bed hospital? Justify your position.
3. In either case, what other important data sources would you examine before making a decision to decrease the nurse-patient ratio?
4. Consider that you are the chief executive officer at a hospital where it is projected that over the next two years, the nurse staffing ratio on general medical-surgical units will decrease from 1 nurse per 6 patients to 1 nurse per 4 patients. How will you estimate the costs and savings of such a change? Be sure to consider the organization's philosophy of care in your evaluation plan.

Exercise 2   The Joint Commission's staffing effectiveness standard defines staffing effectiveness as "the number, competency, and skill mix of staff in relation to the provision of needed care and treatment" (see http://www.jcaho.org/ accredited+organizations/hospitals/standards/draft+standards/staffingeffectivenessstandard0804.pdf). Most healthcare organizations must meet this requirement to receive JCAHO accreditation, and accreditation is paramount to the ability of hospitals to operate and receive reimbursement.

Exercise 2 Questions

Visit two patient care units at a local hospital, and talk to the manager in each one. Ask the following questions from each manager:

1. How has your unit implemented JCAHO's staffing effectiveness standards?
2. How have unit operations changed as a result of this implementation?
3. How has this implementation affected the quality of care delivered to patients on your unit?
4. How have the nursing staff on your unit responded to this implementation?

Following the interview, compare and contrast the two approaches followed by each manager for meeting the required staffing effectiveness standards. Is one approach better than the other? How can you use the experiences of these two unit managers to inform your own nurse workload and staffing decisions in the future?

HUMAN RESOURCES BUDGETING AND EMPLOYEE PRODUCTIVITY

Eileen F. Hamby, D.B.A., M.B.A.

Learning Objectives

After completing this chapter, the reader should be able to

- discuss the purposes and components of the labor budget,
- translate the labor budget into human resources requirements,
- determine staffing levels based on productivity standards,
- identify staffing requirements based on patient acuity levels,
- analyze employee productivity based on benchmarking,
- list the challenges in managing the labor budget,
- compare and contrast the benefits and barriers to outsourcing services, and
- explain the impact of mergers and other organizational changes on managing human resources.

Introduction

Budgeting for human resources (HR) is an important consideration when addressing the human capital needs of any organization. Because the healthcare industry is a service industry and requires people to perform the major portion of its business, the cost of the HR component usually accounts for its largest expense. Paying for appropriate manpower can be a conundrum, especially in light of the hyperturbulence in the industry and ongoing changes in reimbursement. Healthcare organizations must weigh the financial aspect of human resources carefully and ensure that they can afford the people that they hire or engage in service. HR needs differ from one organization to the next, depending on the vision, mission, goals, and objectives of the organization. The number and type of people needed in a given situation are dependent on many factors, including the skill level of the workers, the workers' familiarity with the organization, the standards the organization sets for productivity, and regulatory and accreditation requirements.

This chapter examines factors that link budgeting with human resources management (HRM) and link HRM budgeting with productivity. The components of the labor budget are enumerated, and the use of standard and nonstandard labor practices is considered from a financial standpoint.

Linking Budgeting with Human Resources Management

If an organization employs the number of staff its managers think is ideal; hires only the best candidates; and provides comprehensive benefits, high raises, and superb incentive programs, the organization will not be able to afford anything else to run its business. The total cost of human resources comprises the majority of most organizations' expenses; therefore, managers must be careful not to overspend in this area.

A budget puts the financial status of the organization into perspective, as it allows a view into projected revenues and expenses over the period of a fiscal year. This process ensures that the organization has more revenues than expenses. To plan HR activities without looking at their financial impact on the organization is negligent and is difficult to do even for the most profitable of businesses. The type and quantity of HR activities must be determined based on the fiscal priorities and allowance of the organization.

The Labor Budget

The labor budget, also known as the *salary budget*, consists of the expenses allocated for salary, wages, benefits, and other employee costs. The revenue portion of the budget is influenced by the human component. Skillful, efficient employees can usually help the facility produce more revenue. On the other hand, workers who do not perform well and who are not motivated may impede revenue growth. Using a past history of productivity and activity measures, most organizations can predict both revenue and labor costs fairly accurately. The purpose of the labor budget is to predict the following:

- Required staffing levels based on volume projections and productivity measures
- Projected expenses related to regular, overtime, and overall productive hours
- Nonproductive hour expenses related to paid time off, including vacation, sick, holiday, personal, and education and other training hours

- Expenses for benefits, including payroll taxes, insurance, and other benefits provided to employees
- Total salary, wage, and benefits costs

Healthcare organizations should develop *flexible budgets*—that is, budgets that include revenues that are dependent on volume and expenses that fluctuate with volume. Each organization needs to prepare a budget to determine its financial break-even point and the profits it needs to remain viable.

Labor Budget Terminology

A standard labor budget terminology exists, and some of these terms are defined in this section. Table 14.1 lists the most common terms used in a healthcare setting.

Salaried (exempt) employees are paid a fixed amount of income regardless of how many hours worked in a period of time. *Wage earners* (nonexempt), on the other hand, are paid per each hour worked and receive overtime pay for any hours put in over the standard 40 hours per week. Hours worked are regarded as *productive hours*, including time spent for nonbillable work (down time) such as attending meetings, making phone calls, writing correspondence and documenting patient care or incidents, and doing other nonrevenue-producing but work-related activities. *Nonproductive hours* are those that constitute time paid to the employee even when work is not produced, or in the case of nonrevenue-producing departments, these are days paid for but not worked. The paid hours of a full-time equivalent (FTE) consists of both productive and nonproductive hours. The amount of care a patient needs based on the degree or difficulty of illness—*acuity level*—must be monitored continuously to determine the required amount of FTEs.

Components of the Expense Side of the Labor Budget

The components of the expense side of the labor budget are listed below in the order in which they normally appear on a budget spreadsheet (see Figure 14.1).

- Regular hours
- Overtime hours
- Total productive hours
- Total productive FTEs
- Holiday hours
- Vacation hours
- Personal hours
- Sick time hours
- Education hours
- Total nonproductive hours
- Total nonproductive FTEs
- Total hours
- Total FTEs
- Average hourly rate
- Average overtime rate
- Total salaries and wages
- Payroll taxes, insurance, and benefits (employer share)
- Total salary, wages, and benefits

TABLE 14.1
Labor Budget
Terminology

Term	Definition
Acuity level	This is the level of caregiving difficulty that determines staffing needs (for example, because intensive care patients are sicker, higher staffing levels are needed).
Down time	These are hours spent at work that are important to the job role but do not generate revenue (for example, a respiratory therapist documenting a patient treatment is time considered "down time"; this is not billable, but it is still important for patient care).
Full-time equivalent	This is the equivalent hours of one full-time person— normally 40 hours per week. This may consist of one, two, or more employees whose working hours combined equal the hours that one full-time employee normally puts in.
Nonproductive hours	These are hours paid but not worked, including paid time off, vacation, sick, holiday, education, and personal.
Productive hours	These are hours actually worked, including down time.
Salaried employee (or exempt employee)	This is any employee who is exempt from overtime law and whose paycheck is not dependent on hours worked.
Labor (salary) budget	This includes all expenses associated with salaries, wages, and benefits.
Wage-earning employee (or nonexempt employee)	This is an employee who is not exempt from overtime law and who receives payment based on hours worked and overtime pay for time worked after 40 hours.

FIGURE 14.1
Worksheet for
Expense Side
of the Labor
Budget

Line Item	Jan	Feb	Mar	Apr	May	June	July	Aug	Sept	Oct	Nov	Dec	Total
Regular hours													
Overtime hours													
Total productive hours													
Total productive FTEs													
Holiday hours													
Vacation hours													
Personal hours													
Sick time hours													
Offsite education hours													
Total nonproductive hours													
Total nonproductive FTEs													
Total hours													
Total FTEs													
Average hourly rate													
Average overtime rate													
Total salaries and wages													
Payroll taxes, insurance, and benefits													
Total salaries, wages, and benefits													

The cost of payroll taxes includes the employer contribution to Social Security and Medicare taxes, which amount to 6.2 percent and 1.45 percent, respectively, of an employee's gross wages. Social Security has a wage cap beyond which it no longer taxes the employer or employee during the remainder of the calendar year. Unemployment compensation insurance costs 6.2 percent based on the first $7,000 of each employee's gross wages (Internal Revenue Service 2004). Workers' compensation insurance, also part of the employer's responsibility, is paid at a predetermined rate for specific employee classifications. An experience-modification rating modifies this amount by up to 50 percent less and up to 300 percent more, depending on the amount and severity of employee injuries. Employee benefits (including the employer share of Medicare and Social Security) often range between 25 percent and 35 percent of total salary.

In recent years, the cost of healthcare insurance has dramatically increased. Other benefits may include pension, child daycare, elder care, life insurance, tuition reimbursement, and travel and education. These benefits all add to the expense side of the labor budget.

Following is a step-by-step illustration of how these expense components are considered when developing a labor budget:

1. A physical therapy manager determines, through a trend analysis and new program volume projection, that next year's total volume for the department will be 100,000 procedures. In this department, all of the therapists are wage earners and are paid by the hour. No overtime is allowed. To calculate the number of hours needed to cover the projected number of procedures, knowledge of how long it takes to perform one procedure, including both productive and nonproductive hours required, is necessary. Normally, the previous year's productivity standards are used as the basis for this calculation. If the average procedure takes one-half hour, then the productivity standard is 0.50 total hours per procedure:

   100,000 procedures × 0.50 hours/procedure = 50,000 productive hours

2. The number of FTE personnel needed to perform the projected work is calculated. Based on one FTE working 40 hours per week, a year's calculation would be 2,080 hours:

   50,000 productive hours ÷ 2,080 hours/FTE = 24.04 total FTEs

3. For each FTE in the department, the following nonproductive hours will be assumed:

> Vacation—80
> Holiday—48
> Sick—80
> Personal—16
> Education—24

These nonproductive hours total 248 per FTE. Therefore,
24.04 FTEs × 248 nonproductive hours/FTE = 5962 nonproductive hours

4. Based on 2,080 hours per year, the number of nonproductive FTEs are as follows:
5962 ÷ 2080 hours/FTE = 2.87 nonproductive FTEs

5. Because the total productive hours are 50,000 and the total amount of nonproductive hours is 5,962, the total amount of productive hours is
50,000 – 5962 = 44,038 total productive hours

6. Given that there are 2,080 total hours in a year, the calculation is as follows:
44,038 total productive hours ÷ 2080 hours/year = 21.17 total productive FTEs

7. Because no overtime is permitted in the department, total productive hours equal to total regular hours

8. The average wage rate of $25.00 per hour is then multiplied by the 50,000 total hours:
$25.00 × 50,000 hours = $1,250,000 total wages

9. Given that the average payroll taxes, insurance, and benefits total 30 percent of wages, the calculation is as follows:
$1,250,000 × 30% = $375,000 payroll taxes, insurance, and benefits

10. To calculate the total salaries, wages, and benefits, add the total wages and the payroll taxes, insurance, and benefits:
$1,250,000 + $375,000 = $1,625,000 total total salaries, wages, and benefits

For 21.7 FTEs, the physical therapy department must budget $1,625,000 for salaries, wages, and benefits based on an average hourly rate of $25 per hour, and 30 percent of total salaries, wages, and benefits must be attributed to benefits.

Linking Human Resources Budgeting to Employee Productivity

HR budgeting cannot be discussed without examining worker productivity. Productivity is a critical determinant of a healthcare system's performance, and it may be defined as the physical inputs used (including labor, capital, and supplies) to achieve a given level of outcomes (Bailey et al. 1997). Productivity is the measure of how long it takes to perform a unit of service and how well it is done. The quality aspect of productivity distinguishes it from efficiency. Budgeted staffing requirements are dependent on productivity of the workers.

Managers need flexibility to make changes when warranted, but productivity standards should be set and adhered to, following the best practices in patient care and nonpatient care areas. Projecting profit is difficult without productivity standards in place.

An employee who can perform 30 procedures when the average is 15 is efficient but not productive, because the speed in which the employee is performing is likely compromising the quality of the work. However, the manager must assess whether the average of 15 is actually productive. In this assessment, managers sometimes use the average as a base and benchmark against that number. For the next budget quarter, the manager may set a goal of 16 procedures per day per employee and may then increase the number of procedures incrementally until it appears that quality may be negatively affected if any additional procedures are performed. When comparing employee productivity, the manager must compare employees who perform similar tasks or compare employees with themselves.

Inefficiencies cost the organization money. Managers can often identify inefficiencies in their areas by walking around and observing, by asking employees what is inefficient, and by evaluating budget metrics. In healthcare, the following are areas of inefficiencies that add expense to the organization:

1. *Unclear work policies and procedures.* Workplace rules are not adhered to because they are either not enforced or vague; for example, employees arrive for work on time, but leave immediately to get coffee or take an extra few minutes at break time or at lunch. Twenty minutes of waste per day × 500 employees is equivalent to over 20 FTEs worth of employees per day not working.

2. *Lack of productivity standards, or lack of monitoring of these standards.* Some organizations use hours per unit of service to set budget figures, but they do not share this information with their employees. Others do communicate the rules but fail to monitor them, so there are no repercussions for nonadherence.

3. *Inefficient use of time.* Some healthcare workers only view the service side of what they do, not the business end. They do not value time nor equate it to revenues gained or lost. For example, many clinicians write their patient notes at the end of the day, instead of at the time they are treating the patient or directly after. Some employees hold personal conversations throughout the day, instead of work.

4. *Poor work layout.* In some departments, employees have to walk down the hall for supplies, which wastes time and effort.

5. *Poor training.* Many errors are made because of poor training. Insufficient or inadequate training also causes workers to perform slower than the standard because they do not have a good grasp of what they are doing.

6. *Poor system.* Often, work processes are not evaluated to ensure that they flow in the best possible manner. This can cause employees to turn a three-step process into a five-step process.

Managing employees so that they work productively is a difficult task. Each department or functional service area should perform an audit of itself to identify where there is waste or lack of efficiency. *Multiskilling*, also known as cross-training, is a viable method of managing productivity, especially during times of seasonal fluctuations of volume (Hamby 1995). Nursing throughput, productivity, and resource utilization should all be monitored on a unit level. Although national benchmarks are helpful, variances among similar nursing units in the same facilities should identify internal best practices, and internal benchmarks should be created (Leeth 2004). Skill mix should be identified for productivity and resource utilization. Assistive personnel, also called extenders, can be used where labor shortages and cost restrictions surface (Leeth 2004). Effective in 2004, hospitals are required by the Joint Commission on Accreditation of Healthcare Organizations to establish staffing effectiveness standards and to measure their HR indicators. Long-term care and assistive living facilities are required to use these metrics starting in July 2002. Data should be collected for both direct and indirect caregivers (Mooney 2004).

Change in the productivity standard of the physical therapy department used in the earlier example can make a significant difference in the amount of total FTEs the department needs. This in turn affects the total salaries, wages, and benefits needed to be budgeted. For example, if the productivity standard is 0.4 instead of 0.5 hours per unit of service, the total hours required is 40,000 (instead of 50,000); the total FTEs is 19.23 (instead of 24.04); and the total cost of salaries, wages, and benefits is $1,300,000 (instead of $1,625,000).

This cost savings demonstrates that productivity plays a major role in the profits of the organization, a fact that makes productivity a key area to consider when budgeting. Additionally, if the reimbursement received does not cover labor and nonlabor costs, then the manager may need to reassess the services being offered.

Acuity Levels' Impact on Staffing Needs

Patient acuity is the degree of severity of illness on a given day. Traditionally, nurse staffing has been based on hours per patient day. To predict staffing levels accurately, the patient's severity variance on different hospital days must be recognized, and the staffing levels must be adjusted appropriately (Lacovara 1999). The Resource Utilization Group Classification System (RUGS) used in long-term care facilities is based on the premise that different case-mix groups of residents in nursing homes have different acuity levels, which in turn vary treatment costs. A ten-page assessment form called the Minimum Data Set is used to assess and categorize nursing home residents into 1 of 44 RUGS categories. Reimbursement is based on these RUGS categories (Adams-Wendling 2003). Kane (2004) suggests that staffing in nursing homes should be based on both the clinical and social challenges present in the job.

Providing nursing care in the intensive care unit (ICU) is quite different from providing it in a traditional medical-surgical unit. ICU patients are sicker and normally need more nursing hours per patient day of care; sicker patients in a medical-surgical unit also need an increased number of nursing hours per patient day. Each unit must be analyzed for the type and severity of patients that they treat, and nursing workloads must be adjusted according to this assessment. The same acuity assessment and staffing adjustment is needed for other healthcare professionals. The work intensity—procedures per patient day—for respiratory therapists who work in the ICU and step-down units varies from that for therapists who work on the orthopedic surgical unit. Likewise, an inpatient physical therapist (PT) who treats stroke patients needs more one-on-one time with the patient than the PT who treats orthopedic patients. Patients with comorbidities—those with multiple medical problems—also need additional treatment time, requiring additional staffing. These variations in patient care needs add expenses to the budget. Under current models of reimbursement, these additional expenses are not always recouped.

For inpatients in any setting, a daily patient classification system must be in place so that the required nursing hours can be correlated based on the intensity of care needed. Applied late in the afternoon, a patient classification system has proven to be a good predictor of need for the next day and allows nursing leaders to allocate their resources more appropriately (Flagle 2002). Information technology or a computerized system that captures census data, care hours, patient acuity, and patient activities is invaluable in formulating staffing ratios (Walsh 2003).

Carter (2004) suggests that a system that considers patient acuity, the level of staff needed to handle activities not related to volume, and patient volumes is invaluable in making staffing decisions. Physician offices have traditionally chosen units of service as a guideline for staffing. Modification of traditional levels of staffing should be adjusted to account for the requirements of new technology (Marco 2004).

Other HR Practices Related to the Labor Budget

Nonstandard Staffing

Nonstandard staffing involves the hiring of employees on a temporary or contingency basis. These employees include per diem staff, temporary agency staff, temporary pool staff, and other contingency workers. There are positives and negatives to using nonstandard employment in healthcare. On the positive side, the organization meets the current need for staffing and the patients are taken care of. In addition, the organization does not need to provide benefits to these staff. During slow times, these employees do not show up at work, preventing the organization from incurring additional labor expenses. The greatest advantage is that atypical employment allows managers to better match working time to business activity at different times of the day (Rothwell 1995).

On the negative side, however, nonstandard employees are usually very expensive. In the case of a registered nurse, the organization often pays much more than the average hourly expense of a permanent employee, especially on holidays. Quite often, nonstandard staff are less psychologically committed to the organization, which can lead to problems of motivation, communication, confidentiality, and turnover (Brewster 1995). Because of the nonpermanent nature of their jobs, these staff tend to not adhere to high-quality service standards (Brewster 1995). According to the Joint Commission (2004), nonstandard employees should attend to their work with the same detailed orientation as do permanent full-time employees. Additionally, to be in compliance with Joint Commission standards, organizations must ensure that temporary clinical staff must prove competency in the procedures they are hired to perform before they are allowed to give that service. These additional requirements drive up the staffing cost per hour. The labor cost per unit of service for both permanent and nonstandard staff for each affected functional service area must first be determined and accounted for in the budget.

Outsourcing

Outsourcing, which in healthcare has also been called contract management, is the use of services offered and performed by companies outside of the organization. The reasons for outsourcing include the following (Lanser 2003):

- Accessing expertise or capability in a given area
- Obtaining sufficient personnel in the needed area
- Accessing better technology for advanced applications
- Controlling costs
- Gaining a competitive advantage through the advantages of specialization and economies of scale

According to *Modern Healthcare*'s 25th annual outsourcing survey, in 2002, healthcare clients on a contract or outsourced basis totaled 11,000, a 9 percent increase over the previous year. In the healthcare industry, housekeeping is the most outsourced area, followed by laundry and food services. Other outsourced services include emergency department physicians and clinical and diagnostic equipment maintenance. Approximately 75 percent of hospitals outsource at least one function (Moon 2003). Some of these functions include human resources, business office administration, radiology, surgery, case management, revenue cycle management, real estate management, and information technology. Outsourcing companies are becoming more creative and offering more nontraditional contract services to better accommodate the healthcare industry's needs.

Key to the success of outsourcing is choosing a company whose organizational culture is aligned with that of the partner organization and whose outcomes focus is similar as well. The organization that will be contracting with an outsourcing company needs to set up a performance evaluation system in advance of signing the contract. The outsourcing company must be able to seamlessly integrate into the fabric of its partner organization (Lanser 2003).

Lawler, Ulrich, and Fitz-enz (2004) analyze the impact of outsourcing business processes, in particular the HR department, on the budget of both large and small organizations. The authors give examples of how major companies, such as Prudential and Bank of America, outsource the HR department, including its management function and benefits component. From a budgetary viewpoint, these companies have achieved substantial cost savings. These savings come from the fact that outsourcing firms have many customers and are able to pass on the benefits of economies of scale. For healthcare organizations and systems with many employees, business process outsourcing may be the wave of the future.

Using Labor Budget Metrics for Measurement

The success of the HR function can be measured using metrics that can be benchmarked against performance of similar organizations and against that of the organization itself. This benchmarking provides information that can help in decisions regarding whether to outsource, change certain processes within the organization, or use temporary staffing. Each healthcare facility must decide which metrics are applicable to its own needs and must gather data for the purpose of comparisons. Workload measurement and unit costing are pertinent metrics.

Lawler, Ulrich, and Fitz-Enz (2004) discuss commonly used HR and organizational metrics. The metrics for the HR department include accession rate, cost per employee hired, time to fill jobs, benefits claims response time, training hours produced, number of employees trained, HR expense per employee, and HR FTE ratio. The metrics for the organization include revenue per employee, human capital, value-added human capital, return on investment, compensation versus operating expense, healthcare costs, training cost as a percentage of payroll, voluntary separation rate, and contingent versus regular employees.

From the chief executive and chief financial officers' viewpoints of healthcare facilities, budgetary metrics are imperative so that comparisons can be made on a regular basis against other facilities within the same healthcare system, peer facilities outside the system, and within the facility. Healthcare institutions must use metrics for both the revenue and the expense sides of human resources.

The analysis of key budgetary metrics, along with reporting of the variances, is usually performed monthly in most healthcare institutions. This is done so that organizations can make necessary adjustments to be in compliance with or to adjust their budgets. Figure 14.2 presents a labor budget metrics variance worksheet with key metrics.

Actual versus budgeted amounts for the predetermined metrics are calculated and then compared. A variance of 5 percent or more in either direction requires an explanation. If the variance is positive, then the manager would like to know why so that the good result can be repeated. Alternately, if the variance is negative, then the manager would want to figure out the reason so that corrective action can be taken. Organizations that do not evaluate metrics can find themselves in a financially poor situation, which could have been foreseen. Using metrics promotes financial responsibility and accountability within the organization.

FIGURE 14.2
Worksheet
for Labor
Budget
Metrics
Variance

Month _____

Description	Budget	Actual	Percent Variance	Reason
Units of service				
Total productive hours				
Total productive FTEs				
Total nonproductive hours				
Total nonproductive FTEs				
Total hours				
Total FTEs				
Average productivity/ unit of service				
Revenue/unit of service				
Revenue per FTE				
Average hourly rate				
Average hourly rate/ unit of service				
Salaries, wages, and benefits/unit of service				
Salaries, wages, and benefits /FTE				
Total net revenues				
Total labor expenses				
Total labor expenses/ total net revenues				

Mergers, Acquisitions, and Strategic Alliances

With high performance and competitive advantage having become important factors in the success and viability of organizations, mergers, acquisitions, and strategic alliances have become increasingly attractive. Many
organizations that once were major competitors are now strategically aligned.
A merger or acquisition often results in a duplication of services, forcing
the aligned institution to make decisions on which employees to keep and

which to lay off. Although this decision is often difficult, it gives the organization an opportunity to retain only the best employees; as a result, the organization becomes stronger not only from operational and quality standpoints but also financially.

When the leadership of such a consolidation is focused on instilling a positive culture systemwide and when policies and procedures are in place that promote the well-being of all the stakeholders in that firm, the merged organization's value to its investors increases. To maximize net operating margin, a merged organization has to take advantage of its human capital, working to align its key personnel, nonstandard staff, and outsourcing partners.

Summary

This chapter extensively examines the labor budget and its components, addressing how crucial this budget is to the success and survival of an organization. Predicting future revenues and expenses is an important step in ensuring that funds will be available to pay for HR expenses. An organizational budget has a relationship with HRM, and HR budgeting has a link to employee productivity. Productivity standards have to be assessed to determine staffing requirements, and even small increases in productivity can provide substantial cost savings to an organization. Acuity levels also influence staffing needs. Nonstandard staffing and outsourcing are viable alternatives to permanent, traditional staffing. This practice offers both negative and positive outcomes. Using budget metrics is necessary to measure and compare (benchmark) an organization's performance to that of itself and of peer institutions. Such measurement is a step toward promoting best practices within the organization.

References

Adams-Wendling, L. 2003. "Clocking Care Hours with Workload Measurement Tools." *Nursing Management* 34 (8): 34.

Bailey, M. N., A. M. Garger, E. R. Bernddt, and D. M. Cutler. 1997. "Healthcare Productivity." *Brookings Papers on Economic Activity*, 143–203.

Brewster, C. 1995. "HRM: The European Dimension." *Human Resource Management: A Critical Text*, edited by J. Storey. London, England: International Thompson Publishing.

Carter, M. 2004. "The ABCs of Staffing Decisions." *Nursing Management* 35 (6): 16.

Flagle, C. 2002. "Some Origins of Operations Research in the Health Services." *Operations Research* 50 (1): 52–62.

Hamby, E. 1995. "The Use of the Multiskilled Practitioner to Manage Care." *Orthopedic Physical Therapy Clinics of North America* 4 (3): 335–50.

Internal Revenue Service. 2004. "Circular E." Washington, DC: IRS.

Joint Commission on Accreditation of Healthcare Organizations. 2004. *Comprehensive Accreditation Manual for Hospitals.* Oakbrook Terrace, IL: Joint Commission Press.

Kane, R. 2004. "Commentary: Nursing Home Staffing—More Is Necessary but Not Necessarily." *Health Services Research* 38 (2): 251.

Lacovara, J. E. 1999. "Does Your Acuity System Come Up Short?" *Nursing Management* 30 (6): 40A–43A.

Lanser, E. 2003. "Core Competencies of Successful Outsourcing." *Healthcare Executive* 18 (4): 52.

Lawler, E. E., D. Ulrich, and J. Fitz-enz. 2004. *Human Resources Business Process Outsourcing: Transforming How HR Gets Its Work Done.* San Francisco: Jossey-Bass.

Leeth, L. 2004. "Are You Fiscally Fit?" *Nursing Management* 35 (4): 42–49.

Marco, A. 2004. "The Virtual Patient Encounter—Units of Service in the Electronic Age." *Physician Executive* 30 (3): 32.

Moon, S. 2003. "Out with the Old." *Modern Healthcare* 33 (35): 28.

Mooney, M. 2004. "Stay Current with Staffing Effectiveness Standards." *Nursing Management* 35 (2): 14.

Rothwell, S. 1995. "Human Resource Planning." *Human Resource Management: A Critical Text*, edited by J. Storey. London, England: International Thompson Publishing.

Walsh, E. 2003. "Get Real With Workload Measurement." *Nursing Management* 34 (2): 38–42.

Discussion Questions

1. What is a labor budget, and why is it important in human resources management?
2. What are the benefits and drawbacks of using nonstandard employees, standard employees, and outsourced staff?
3. What are some of the reasons that certain staff members may be more productive than others?
4. Define the following terms:
   - Full-time equivalent
   - Labor budget
   - Acuity level
   - Productive hours
   - Down time
5. What is meant by the term benchmarking, and why is it important in human resources management?

6. Explain why the revenue side of the budget is just as important as the cost side when it comes to determining the quantity and quality of human resources.

Experiential Exercises

Case 1   Mr. Richards is the department manager for speech pathology services at ABC Hospital. The average productivity per visit at the department is 0.75 hours per procedure.

Case Questions

1. Based on one FTE equaling 2,080 hours and 48,000 predicted patient procedures, how many FTEs will be needed to adequately staff the department?
2. If the department productivity changes from 0.75 to 0.70 hours per procedure, what is the new number of FTEs required to staff the department?
3. What are some of the reasons that the average productivity standard in a department changes?

Case 2   XYZ Hospital is a community hospital that is not part of a larger healthcare system. This acute care hospital has 160 beds and 348 employees. Benefits given and employee pay account for 30 percent of the hospital's total salaries and wages budget. Currently, the HR function is done in house, and the chief executive officer (CEO), Ms. Jones, is evaluating whether to keep the HR function internally or outsource it.

An outsourcing company that services several large companies in the area has approached Ms. Jones, proposing that it can perform the hospital's HR function and provide benefits to each employee for a price of 28 percent of the hospital's total salary budget. As a result, employees would get better health insurance and pension benefits because of the advantages of economies of scale obtained by the business processes of the outsourcing company.

Case Question

1. What key factors should the CEO address, and what benefits should be evaluated?

CREATING CUSTOMER-FOCUSED HEALTHCARE ORGANIZATIONS

Myron D. Fottler, Ph.D., and Robert C. Ford, Ph.D.

Learning Objectives

After completing this chapter, the reader should be able to

- describe the significance of customer service in the highly competitive healthcare market,
- distinguish healthcare organizations that exhibit high levels of customer service from those that do not,
- explain the role of human resources management practices in enhancing customer service, and
- discuss six specific human resources strategies that can enhance customer service.

Introduction

The problem with human resources management (HRM) thinking is that it addresses only 50 percent of the "people equation," focusing on internal "customers" to the exclusion of external customers. The goal should be to link the external customer's requirement with the internal human capabilities, thereby optimizing the utility of both.

Consequently, the goal of the human resources (HR) function is not to make employees happy or satisfied at work; rather, its goal should be to make happy those employees who are making the external customers happy. Most healthcare organizations' mission proclaims, "People are our most important asset." Yet no one really believes such statements. What they really mean is, "People who are serving customers well are our most important asset. Others must either convert to serving customers well or leave."

Healthcare organizations have not traditionally been focused on the needs, wants, or desires of their patients/customers. As a result of their history and reimbursement sources, they have concentrated on meeting the expectations of their medical staff and third-party payers. The medical staff have historically had the power to decide where their patients would go for services, and their provider organizations have gone to great lengths to make them happy. Because third-party payers pay the bills, organizations have also spent considerable effort in satisfying them.

This limited definition of the customer has resulted in organizations focusing only on increasing market share, decreasing costs, and expanding revenues to retain the support of their third-party payers and on providing sophisticated technology and in-house amenities to satisfy their doctors. Meanwhile, the patient has been overlooked and underappreciated as the ultimate customer. Even the term "patient" implies a passive person who patiently waits for service from experts who know what that patient needs and who often provide it without consultation with or explanation to the patient.

This paradigm has led to an increasingly unhappy and vocal patient. One study commissioned by the Voluntary Hospitals of America and another survey published in *Fortune* magazine report the following consumer attitudinal trends toward healthcare organizations (*Alliance* 1998):

> Over the past five years, public trust in healthcare institutions has markedly declined, with health plans losing more ground than physicians or hospitals. The decline in trust is especially pronounced among consumers age 40 to 59; those with higher income and education levels; and those who have recently changed, added, or selected a physician or hospital. Consumers gave hospitals only a 67 percent satisfaction rating, and compared with 31 other industries, hospitals rank 27th. This placed them just above the Internal Revenue Service and 10 percentage points below the tobacco industry.

Furthermore, data from the National Coalition on Health Care (2000) indicate that 80 percent of Americans agree that hospitals have cut corners to save money, and 77 percent agree that these cuts endanger patients (Healthcare Advisory Board 1999).

None of these findings is surprising given that the services paid for by private insurers and government are not likely to reflect consumer preferences for convenience and personal control (Herzlinger 1997, 95). The increasingly involved consumer-patient and the newly evolved competitive market are forcing healthcare institutions to consider who their customers really are. They are starting to rethink the old paradigm of "take care of the doctors and third-party payers and all good things will follow" and to follow the new paradigm of "don't forget the patient as customer" (Ford and Fottler 2000). Today's medical consumers, however, have much more knowledge and access to information about the value and quality of their healthcare alternatives. They are now more savvy about what they are getting for their healthcare dollar and are increasingly involved in the decisions about how those dollars are spent. Because they have many alternative choices for their insurance coverage and healthcare providers, their voice is being heard. In addition, increasingly vocal consumer groups have changed patients' mind-set from being passive consumers into active participants in their own healthcare decisions.

Regina Herzlinger (1997, 3–4) describes this new healthcare consumer as follows:

> They want what they want, they want it fast, and they want it when they want it. Well-informed, overworked, and overburdened with child and elder-care responsibilities, they are a new breed of consumer, and their demands for convenience and control have caused many American businesses to greatly enhance their quality and control their costs . . . the consumer revolutionaries want their healthcare system to provide them with the same kinds of convenience and mastery they have found with Home Depot, *Consumer Reports*, and Nordic Track, so that their health status and costs will improve even further.

An Emerging Customer Focus

Recent Trends

No one is arguing that physicians and third-party payers are unimportant, but a lot of healthcare observers and insiders are echoing the same point: The patient is becoming increasingly critical in the success or failure of a healthcare organization. Consequently, today the patient and the patient's family are increasingly being recognized by the more successful competitors in the healthcare market as the real customers. These providers are spending increasing amounts of time and energy to convince their customers that the healthcare product they provide has both quality and value.

The results of this change in customer focus can be seen in a number of ways. First, third-party payers are more willing to pay for homeopathic treatments, acupuncture, and even chiropractic treatments, in spite of established medical practice resistance. Second, pharmaceutical companies now spend enormous sums on television and print ads to market directly to patients in hopes of influencing their use of branded drugs. This has proven to be a very effective strategy to influence doctors to prescribe certain drugs and circumvent HMO drug guidelines. Third, hospitals have begun to offer such patient amenities as chef-prepared foods, valet parking, and comprehensive single nurse care to influence the patient and family's decision to seek services from them and not from competitors.

Consumers now have access to more information through provider report cards, the Internet, and other means; however, the question remains: Why should providers be more responsive to consumers than they have been in the past? Arnold (1991) suggests that the major environmental forces leading to the increase in competition and greater provider responsiveness to consumers include excess capacity, the consumer movement, deregulation of the healthcare industry, changes to reimbursement systems, declines in occupancy rates, and corporate restructuring and diversification. Such increased competition among healthcare providers has resulted in greater interest in redesigning healthcare organizations to make them more customer focused.

An even more potent factor is the changing views of corporate America toward its role in healthcare cost management. After long relying on managed care companies as their defense against rising employee healthcare benefit costs, some U.S. employers are undergoing a fundamental change in their healthcare-cost-management strategy by turning healthcare decisions over to their employees. This idea is driven by a confluence of interacting forces, including the backlash against managed care, the popularity of 401k plans, the use of web-based information to help consumers make more informed healthcare decisions, the recent resurgence of healthcare costs (despite the efforts of managed care organizations), and a growing feeling among many that the nation's healthcare market will not work well until patients themselves hold the purse strings (Weber 1997). The new trend to let employees handle their own healthcare benefits just as they do their retirement money adds additional momentum to the growing customer involvement in healthcare decisions (Winslow and Gentry 2000). Other employers have created web sites to help employees make health benefit decisions and sign up for plans. Entrepreneurs are responding to this trend by developing web-based services that would greatly reduce the need for employers to manage this information. In addition, these entrepreneurs are more creative in providing customers with new tools to navigate the healthcare system and to take their health into their own hands (Winslow and Gentry 2000).

Corporations are also self-insuring in increasing numbers. This means that healthcare services are increasingly paid for by the corporation's own administrators, instead of the insurance companies. One of the significant advantages of self-insurance is that it allows greater flexibility in the health plans offered. When the employer manages healthcare plans, the employee has a significantly greater voice in how and what these plans provide. Employees or their union representatives need to only persuade their employer of the need to change their choices of health-care provider or health plan. Thus, the growth of self-insurance leads to patients having a louder voice in making their own healthcare decisions. This trend highlights a growing need for healthcare organizations to understand and use the successful best practices of the guest-service indus-try to gain a potential competitive advantage in this new patient-as-cus-tomer environment.

The growing trend to rank and then publicize the scores of health-care organizations is also changing the attitudes of healthcare providers about the importance of the patient as customer. Data generated by the Healthcare Advisory Board (1999) suggest that healthcare executives are beginning to respond to the patient-as-customer movement. Interviews with 321 healthcare industry executives in 1998 reveal that they agree (with a response average greater than 4.0 on a 5-point scale) with each of the following statements:

1. Consumers' new predominance in the healthcare marketplace is increasingly influencing policy, strategy, operations, and investment decisions of organizations in all segments of healthcare.
2. Healthcare organizations will provide education and readily available data to encourage and empower consumers to be direct purchasers of care.
3. Healthcare organizations will develop new products, offer more choices, and provide service enhancements to respond directly to consumer preferences.
4. Healthcare organizations will increasingly invest in feedback mecha-nisms to ensure that they are in touch with consumer needs and are meeting customer expectations.

Furthermore, national magazines such as *U.S. News and World Report* publish lists of "best hospitals," while local television and newspaper out-lets rate the best physicians in their area. Magazines in cities like Boston and Philadelphia publicize the best regional physicians and hospitals of the year (Clark 1999). The U.S. Department of Public Health rates the skilled nursing facilities in all states and posts the information on its web site; the site is updated every six months. Major clinical users track seven satisfac-tion measures, and the results are publicized in newspapers and on televi-sion (Frye 1998).

Only recently have healthcare executives begun to expand their focus to meeting the needs, wants, and desires of their patients/customers, giv-ing patients not only a positive clinical experience but also a positive health-care experience (Ford, Bach, and Fottler 1997; Fottler et al. 2000; Fottler,

Ford, and Heaton 2002; Pines and Gilmore 1998). In an environment where the patient/customer can make choices about where to seek care, it is no longer enough for a healthcare organization to just be the best medical provider at the lowest price. The organization now also needs to persuade the patient/customer that its facility is the most responsive to his or her needs and can meet his or her expectations for a total healthcare experience. The business of healthcare must transform its view of patients, from clinical material to customers with decision-making power.

Customer-Oriented Human Resources

The HR function can proactively add strategic value by enhancing the customer service capability of the organization. This capability, in turn, may enhance retention of existing customers while attracting additional customers to build market share. To enhance customer service, two preconditions must exist. First, there must be a conscious decision by key decision makers that customer service is a desirable organizational focus or agenda. Second, obstacles to customer service must be a removed; such barriers include overly bureaucratic infrastructure, too many people involved in obtaining an approval, and supervisors who are threatened by subordinate initiative. Each of these needs to be addressed if HR is to effectively enhance customer service (Ashkenas et al. 1995).

With these preconditions in place, organizations can then build an HR infrastructure that fosters and maintains customer service ethics. Key components will include the following:

- Senior leaders communicate customer service initiatives.
- Customer service role models are publicly acknowledged through multiple media.
- Evidence of customer service is explicitly applied as a criterion for hiring at all levels.
- Promotion of current staff specifically considers staff's customer service commitment and capability.
- Development of customer service skills is included in organization-wide training initiatives.
- Senior executives model customer service concepts.
- Specific organizational, departmental, and individual goals exist for customer service measures such as ensuring patient satisfaction and addressing customer complaints.
- Customer service success is measured at multiple levels using various methods and is publicized.
- Economic and noneconomic rewards for achieving customer service goals are provided and publicized.

In the following section, we examine six key HRM strategies that benchmark healthcare and customer-focused organizations have discovered as critical in meeting and exceeding their customers' expectations. Lessons learned by the hospitality industry from their guest-relations experience can be readily adopted by the healthcare industry as it moves from the old paradigm to the new paradigm. If the competitive market demands that healthcare providers treat patients as important, primary customers instead of willing bystanders to their own healthcare experience, these principles of hospitality can make the difference.

Exemplars of customer-driven organizations such as Disney, Marriott, and Southwest Airlines know that their success is based on meeting and exceeding their guests' expectations. This means that they spend considerable time and energy identifying and measuring what their guests say are the factors behind the quality and value of the service experience. The benchmark organizations manage the entire experience to the highest degree possible so that their guests' expectations are met and even exceeded. They know that the best predictor of intention to return and satisfaction with the guest-service experience can be identified and managed. They make sure that the key drivers in their guests' decision processes become the key drivers in their organizations' decision processes.

This is especially important because the service product is largely intangible. Just as benchmark hospitality organizations know that the quality and value of the service experience are in the minds of the guests, so too must healthcare organizations recognize this simple truth. Even if there is a surgical tool, an x-ray machine, or some other physical component involved in the healthcare experience, every healthcare provider knows well the significance of the intangibles. Healthcare customers expect that not only will the surgeon successfully remove the diseased organ, the surgeon will also show empathy and concern before and after the procedure. Healthcare customers also expect the operating room and the inpatient room to be sterile, the physical surroundings to be bright and tidy, the nursing staff to be responsive, and the services to be prompt.

The New Paradigm

As we have been emphasizing, a patient's determination of the quality and value of his or her total healthcare experience depends on more than the success or failure of the medical procedure or clinical service. It is derived from a holistic perception of the experience, beginning with the admission and ending with the bill payment. In a sense, this view (negative or positive) may never end, as the nature of a provider's relationship with the patient is inherently ongoing in that the customer continues to receive direct or indirect reminders (through ads and other communications) that the organization is a high-quality provider and welcomes the patient should he or she seek to return if a need arises. As it is for famous retailers (such as Nordstrom) and all hospitality businesses, the idea of repeat customers is a critical consideration for healthcare organizations as well.

Whom the organization defines as its customers determines how it makes various decisions, a consideration that drives the new paradigm. Table 15.1 summarizes the differences between the old paradigm (focus on physicians and third-party payers) and the new paradigm (focus on the patient as customer).

Customer-Focused Strategies

Following is a discussion of how the six principles of the new paradigm can be implemented in a healthcare environment. Examples from both the guest-service and healthcare industries are cited as well (Ford and Fottler 2000).

Strategy: Identify Customer Key Drivers

Principle 1: Service quality and value are always defined by the customer. Successful customer service organizations start learning about what makes their customers happy through the customers themselves. They extensively survey their customers to find out their needs, wants, expectations, and definition of a quality service experience. This knowledge then becomes the basis for organizational plans, operational strategies, and other service decisions. The key drivers should be identified by the patient/customer, not the strategic planners sitting in their isolated offices.

A firm that runs a theme park, for example, may find through its guest research that patrons like cleanliness of the park, friendliness and helpfulness of the staff, and short waits in ride and concession lines. With this knowledge, the firm can then strategically respond, putting its effort and financial resources into keeping the park clean, training employees to be pleasant and helpful, and building enough capacity to keep the waiting lines minimal. This attention to customer drivers is especially important when the customer's intention to return hinges on his or her overall satisfaction with the park.

Similarly, a healthcare organization can survey its patients. Patient key drivers may include quality of hospital food; physician's communication skills; and the staff's courtesy, warmth, and friendliness. Once these drivers are identified and their relationship to the guest's intention to return is shown, the organization can then move on to making improvements to each key driver. Such enhancements may translate into providing communication training to both physicians and staff and evaluating hospital menus.

Human Resources Strategy	Old Paradigm (Focus on Physicians and Third-Party Payers)	New Paradigm (Focus on Patients as Customers)
1. Key drivers of patient/ customer satisfaction	Clinical effectiveness and cost efficiency	Patient/customer perceptions of quality and value
2. Patient involvement in healthcare	Limited involvement	Maximum involvement
3. Organizational culture	Provider driven	Patient/customer driven
4. Staff selection and training	Focused only on clinical skills	Focused on both clinical and patient/customer service skills
5. Employee motivation	Rewards for technical proficiency	Rewards for both technical and customer service proficiency
6. Measures of effectiveness	Costs, clinical processes, and medical outcomes	Total service experience

TABLE 15.1

A Comparison Between the Old Paradigm and the New Paradigm

Joint-replacement patients at the University of Alabama at Birmingham Hospital were formerly required to arrive early in the morning for surgery and to stay long enough to receive the service and procedure they need. Now these patients are able to purchase an entire package that includes a three-night stay in redesigned rooms similar to those at high-quality hotels, preadmission one day before surgery, gourmet meals served in a communal setting with other joint-replacement patients, and specially assigned nursing staff. The hospital is so pleased with its patients' reactions to this package that it is considering providing such an amenity to patients with other diagnoses.

All of the key drivers identified by customers have implications on HRM practices such as employee selection, training, and performance appraisal. In turn, HR activities also have an effect on efforts to meet the patient/customer expectations. Because good clinical outcomes alone do not make the total healthcare experience impressive, caregivers with only technical and clinical capabilities do not make a healthcare organization competitive in a market full of consumers looking to be satisfied.

**Strategy:
Encourage
Customer
Participation**

Principle 2: Patient involvement adds value and quality to the service experience. Think of the patient as a partial employee who is responsible for coproducing the healthcare experience. Most customer service organizations know full well the value and benefits of letting their customers participate in the service experience. First, whatever customers do for themselves is one less thing that the organization has to pay someone to do for them. In other words, the patient or his or her family may be a partial substitute for employees in delivering a service.

Second, customers who coproduce the service experience are more satisfied with the outcome because they cannot criticize something that they have produced and designed to suit their own tastes and needs. For example, a person who makes his or her own salad cannot complain that the salad is not exactly what he or she wanted. Third, customers involved in a process can help supervise the actual employee. With a customer watching the moves and attitudes of the employee, the employee will tend to behave more appropriately and work more fastidiously. A loyal repeat customer can even train the employee on how to face customers or educate other customers on how to enjoy or best benefit from the service experience.

Having healthcare organizations consider the involved patient as a partial employee is a novel concept. Most physicians, employees, and organizations tend to see their patients/customers as passive and submissive objects *to whom* the experts do something, instead of *with whom*. However, the reality today is that patients want to get involved in their own care and are not shy about making demands and suggestions about how their care should be delivered. They are no longer passive or content with just waiting in bed as so-called experts circle them, making decisions about their life.

Most healthcare employees know that a patient has to be involved in his or her care at a certain point: A surgery patient has to get up and walk after the procedure, a psychiatric patient has to attend and participate in therapy, and a person with a general illness has to tell the doctor where it hurts. However, most employees are unclear on the idea of allowing patients to coproduce the healthcare experience or participate in their own wellness routine, even though enough discussion in the literature and by hospital lawyers has been done that repeatedly emphasize the value of the medical staff communicating and consulting with patients to enhance patient satisfaction. Until the patient fully comprehends and agrees to the regimen of care, the best doctors and best treatment facilities in the world will not help him or her prevent illness or get well.

Perhaps an example of how patient participation can be effective is the current practice in hospices that requires the family and loved ones to be part of making the hospice patient comfortable and content. Another example is through the use of painkiller pumps, which allows the patient to control the medication that he or she is administered. The result of this practice is often quicker healing and less discomfort for the patient and lower costs for the organization, as the patient typically uses less painkiller.

The Shouldice Hospital in Toronto, Canada, focuses on the repair of abdominal hernias (Herzlinger 1997, 159). Its operating procedures are the products of intense deliberation about patient comfort, convenience, and health status. Shouldice has an integrated operating system carefully designed so that each of its activities reinforces the others. The system purposefully places considerable demands on the patients. Meals are served only in the dining room, and the patients' rooms lack a telephone or television. Patients even prepare themselves for surgery by shaving the area to be operated on and are expected to walk from the operating room. Staff members also discourage patients from lingering in bed and demand them to engage in aerobic exercise. This system creates higher levels of patient satisfaction because patients are empowered. It also results in lower costs and higher quality than seen in general hospitals.

Principle 3: Everyone must do as, act as, and say that the customer matters. Organizational culture is generally defined as the beliefs, values, and ways of doing things that are unique to that organization and that differentiates it from others. Culture communicates to all employees what is important and what is not, what is appropriate behavior and what is not, and how people should deal with others both inside and outside the organization. In other words, culture is both "the way we do things around here" and "why we are what we are." Leaders teach and communicate the culture by what they reward, recognize, punish, and praise. They can do this not only through the formal reward and recognition systems but also through the informal stories they tell about organizational values, the heroes they create to illustrate points of importance, and the legends they perpetuate to tell what the organization stands for.

A classic illustration of this point in the guest-service industry is the legend at the Olive Garden Restaurants. When it was still trying to establish a strong customer service culture and teach it to all employees, Olive Garden encountered a portly customer named Larry. Larry wrote a letter to the president of Olive Garden to tell him of the delightful meal, the great service, and wonderful dining experience he had at one of the restaurants. Unfortunately, according to Larry, the arm chairs in the restaurant were too narrow for someone of his size, making him uncomfortable. Larry suggested that Olive Garden do something to better accommodate people like him. The president immediately responded by ordering two chairs for each restau-

Strategy: Develop a Customer-Focused Culture

rant that did not have arms (known throughout the chain as "Larry chairs") to accommodate heavier guests. This one letter and a simple suggestion gave Olive Garden not only an opportunity to better serve its customers but also an inspiring story that can be told to new employees to illustrate how dedicated the company is in providing exceptional customer service. Legends strongly communicate the cultural value of customer service.

Healthcare organizations also can use stories, legends, and heroes as an effective way of conveying the new service culture that the modern patient/customer expects. Under the old paradigm, the healthcare staff told only stories about how the hospital had responded to physicians' needs and demands or how it had sought to accommodate the expectations of an HMO. In other words, the stories, legends, and heroes were all about accommodating the needs and wants of third-party payers or physicians. The shift to following the new paradigm must be accompanied by the creation of new stories, legends, and heroes, extolling an employee who provided effective patient care or service that enhanced a patient's overall satisfaction with the healthcare experience.

For example, in one nursing home, the legend is about a nurse's aide. The aide one day discovered that an elderly resident, who had no interest in eating anything, had a passion for peanut butter milkshakes. The aide went out of her way, on her own time, to make such a concoction so that the resident would eat something. A top manager told this story in an employee gathering and recognized this person with a customer satisfaction award. This story and the subsequent satisfaction from the organization, employee, and the resident had an enormous impact on defining the culture in this nursing home: Do whatever it takes to achieve patient satisfaction.

A strong culture with the "right" values can reinforce customer service. Healthcare executives are increasingly seeking ways to identify job candidates who share their organizations' cultural values. Irvine Medical Center in California uses testing and interviews to evaluate employee hospital congruence on values such as service orientation, proactiveness, and teamwork (Eubanks 1991). The medical center has found that selecting employees who share its core values has greatly reinforced its corporate culture. These hiring practices have achieved better results than the "chit-chat" interviews and reference checks that previously were the norm. Research indicates that nurses whose values are congruent with those of their employing hospitals tend to remain in their organizations longer (Vandenberghe 1991).

Culture building should not end at the initial employee orientation; cultural values have to be reinforced. One appropriate venue for doing this is the staff retreat. One of the objectives of a retreat should be to build a customer service culture, leading employees to discuss questions such as who are our customers? what do they want? what values does the organization need to adopt to deliver what customers want? what human resources practices will nurture those values? (*Hospitals* 1991a). Neutral outside facilitators can help staff participants differentiate between their individual and institutional values and to reconcile the two when necessary.

The stronger the culture, the less necessary it is to rely on typical bureaucratic control mechanisms such as policies, procedures, and managerial directives. Because so much of the healthcare experience happens in the encounter between the patient and staff, healthcare organizations must be able to rely on staff to do the right things (i.e., exceed expectations). Culture is critically important in ensuring that these rights things happen, guiding employees even when their supervisors are not nearby. Unlike a manufacturing organization in which the production process is fairly predictable, the process of providing a healthcare experience is subject to incredible variation—that is, as many different things can happen as there are different types of people. Because defining all the possibilities is impossible, the healthcare organization must rely on its employees to understand what is expected and deliver that expectation to the customer every time. The more uncertain the task, the more employees must depend on corporate values rather than on managerial instructions, formal policies, and established procedures to guide their behavior (Davidoff and Uttal 1989).

The HR department adds considerable value to the organization when it creates a customer-focused corporate culture. This entails enhancing each employee's understanding and valuing of what patients/customers want and need (both clinically and in team service). This effort facilitates the organization's reactive responses to short-term market demands and enhances its capability to proactively track future market directions and provide appropriate services (Cespedes 1995). Initial research on the practices that have the greatest influence on creating customer-focused cultures suggests that the following HR practices play a key role (Brockbank 1999):

- Provide a free flow of information directly from external customers through the entire organization via customer focus groups, videos or DVDs, audio tapes, in-house visits, and employee involvement in market research.
- Implement comprehensive communication programs from key organizational leaders on the importance of the organization being unified on winning the hearts and minds of its external customers.
- Ensure that measurement, rewards, training, and promotions reinforce the importance of customer focus.
- Design organizational structures and physical settings that facilitate teamwork around customer requirements.

If the HR function is to be strategically proactive in healthcare organizations, HR personnel must become highly knowledgeable about external customers in terms of their needs and desires for various services. The HR competency study at the University of Michigan indicates that knowledge of competitors, customers, marketing, and sales is a critical aspect of an HR professional's knowledge base (Brockbank, Ulrich, and James 1997). Lack of integration with HR practices is a major contribution to the suboptimization of marketing activities (Ballantyne, Christopher, and Payne 1995).

The healthcare industry often does not invest in what it claims to value. Although it says that customer satisfaction and employee retention are the most important aspects of its business, the industry often fails to invest adequately in either (*Modern Healthcare* 1998). Instead, healthcare's to-do lists focus on such areas as upgrading technology, building an integrated delivery system, diversifying business lines, and reengineering business and clerical services (*AHA News* 1998). In contrast, patients care most about responsiveness, information about their case, pain management, and positive attitudes from physicians and other caregivers (Studer and Boylan 2000). As a result, top healthcare executives show that they do not give high priority to the major concerns of their customers. However, both employees and customers judge leaders not on what they say but on what they do, and what they do is focus on organizational priorities, not on customers.

Culture begins at the top; thus, a commitment to customer service should start at the executive level. The lessons of behavior taught by top managers on a continuing basis are more important than slogans and communications. The chief executive officer (CEO) and senior management must "walk the talk" of customer service if that message is to be believed throughout the organization. Reinforcement of the customer-focused culture also requires appropriate employee selection and training as discussed below.

Strategy: Select and Train Customer-Focused Employees

Principle 4: Find, hire, and train competent and caring employees.
The guest-service literature suggests that only a certain percentage of people really care about giving high-quality guest service. In his book, *Positively Outrageous Service*, Scott Gross (1991) calls employees who love to provide great service "lovers." These employees give customers a "feel good" level of service—that is, it feels good because the employee connects with the customer even for a brief period of time. Such a service encounter makes the customer feel that there is something special and memorable about the experience.

The challenge for healthcare executives is to recruit employees who can give such a service, continually train all employees in guest-service principles, and provide positive incentives to maintain and improve these principles. Gross (1991, 159) estimates that people who love to serve represent only one in ten of the available workforce. He states that these 10 percent cannot get enough of their customers; 5 percent of workers, however, want to be left alone and have a prevalent mind-set of "take 'em or leave 'em." If Gross's percentages are accurate, he raises two major challenges for healthcare executives. First, they need to develop a process that will systematically recruit and select those 10 percent who are truly committed to providing excellent service. Second, they must work even harder to teach their other employees how to provide the same quality of service that the "lovers" give naturally. In other words, the successful service organizations know how to "select the best and train the rest."

Guest-service organizations like Disney, Marriott, and Southwest Airlines know this lesson well. They spend countless dollars recruiting, selecting, and training their guest-contact employees to provide excellent customer service. They know that the impact of their service is created at the moment of truth when the customer has an encounter with the employee. Ensuring that the guest-contact person is effective in providing an excellent service experience is vital for both meeting guests' expectations and influencing their intent to return or use the service again. The important point to remember is that outstanding guest-service organizations know that the people they put in front of their guests must not only be well trained in the necessary job skills but must also have the personality, disposition, and willingness to provide a high-quality service experience.

Healthcare organizations that follow the old paradigm tend to select employees based on experience and clinical credentials only, overlooking the applicants' lack of customer service skills. Clinical skills are a definite requisite for caregivers and cannot be undermined; however, those organizations that seek to move into the new customer paradigm must also give consideration to, or develop ways to identify, potential employees who have an innate understanding of how to treat their patients as guests. Both Irvine Medical Center in California and Lutheran General Hospital in Illinois use testing and structured interviews to analyze a job applicant's fit with institutional values such as service orientation and servanthood (*Hospitals* 1991b). In addition, some hospitals and healthcare systems are now offering courses or seminars in guest relations. Such an initiative is only the beginning of the movement toward the new paradigm. The willingness of these provider organizations' management to sponsor such training is a strong statement of the value they place on this critical customer-orientation part of the healthcare employee's total responsibility.

The emergency department (ED) of INOVA Fairfax Hospital in Virginia initiated customer service training in 1994 (Mayer et al. 1998). All ED staff involved in patient contact (i.e., physicians, nurses, technicians, registration personnel, core secretaries, social workers, radiology technicians, and respiratory therapists) are required to attend an eight-hour customer service training program. The program covers basic customer service principles; teaches how to recognize patients and customers; points out service-industry benchmarking leaders; gives tips on how to recognize and manage stress, how to strengthen communication and negotiation skills, and how to be more empowered and be customer-service proactive; and discusses service transitions, service fail-safes, change management, and customer-service core competencies. Customer-service updates are offered three times a year, and attendance to these updates is mandatory. Modules on conflict resolution, advanced communication skills, and assertiveness techniques, among others, are offered in these updates.

Initial results of INOVA's efforts showed that all 14 key quality characteristics identified in the organization's customer satisfaction survey increased during the one-year study period (May 1, 1994 to April 30, 1995) (Mayer et al. 1998). The most dramatic improvements were in the likelihood of customers returning, overall customer satisfaction, and physician and nurse skills. In addition, patient complaints declined by more than 70 percent, and patient compliments increased by more than 100 percent. The clear implication of this data is that customer service training offers a competitive market advantage to healthcare institutions.

Healthcare customer service courses may explore the following issues:

- Standard operating procedures for dealing with patients/customers
- Team orientation
- Training and use of multiskilled health practitioners
- Flexibility in responding to patient/customer concerns
- Communicating with patients/customers
- Responsibility for patients/customers
- Results of focus groups with patients/customers
- Exchange of patient/customer information across organizational units
- Greeting patients/customers, and making eye contact
- Calling patients/customers by name
- Responding to patients/customers requests and concerns

An organization's reputation can aid its recruitment efforts. As authors Benjamin Schneider and David Bowen (1995, 115) note, employers who have a positive image in the community and a satisfied and motivated workforce have a deep applicant pool from which they can fish out the best. These "employers of choice" are good neighbors to the community and have established their reputation for hiring and developing people for the long term. Their mentality, according to Len Berry (1995), is to "recruit rather than save on those who leave." In other words, hold out employee selection for the better applicants and then invest in their growth and development; keep the challenged but motivated staff in their current jobs, and offer them future opportunities with the organization.

Selling a healthcare employment opportunity is like selling a healthcare experience. If the company is known for offering its people high-quality job and career opportunities, it will attract high-quality applicants and build a pool of people who prefer to work for it rather than for the competition. Quint Studer of Baptist Hospital in Florida took over a hospital with high turnover and low staff morale. Within three years, Studer's strategy of emphasizing customer service by focusing on employee selection, training, and rewards had reduced turnover by 67 percent and, according to employee satisfaction surveys, tripled the level of employee morale (Studer and Boylan 2000). Baptist Hospital became the "employee of choice" for northwest Florida.

Principle 5: Customers expect employees who are not only well trained but also have good interpersonal skills.

Strategy: Motivate Employees to Be Customer Focused

In the guest-service industry, the normal practice is to recognize and reward employees not only for their technical excellence but also for their ability to deliver guest satisfaction. In other words, a delicious, one-of-a-kind gourmet meal will not make a guest happy if it were served by someone unpleasant and insulting to the guest, or a nonturbulent, quiet plane ride will not count as an excellent trip if the flight attendant was rude to the passengers. Because the customer service aspect of the total job performance is so important, managers of guest-service organizations are evaluated on the manner with which the service was provided in addition to the quality of all the components that went into that service. These managers spend countless hours to motivate their employees to be both technically proficient and guest focused.

In the guest-service industry, there is a demonstrated statistical relationship between happy employees and happy guests (Ford and Heaton 2000). If the employees are having a fun, enjoyable experience serving the guests, they will positively influence the experience of the guests they are serving. This is a fundamental philosophy of CEO Herb Kellerman of Southwest Airlines. Managers in guest-service organizations know the importance of keeping their employees upbeat, happy, and positive so that they not only deliver the product in the way they were trained but do so in a way that promotes an exceptional service.

Traditionally, healthcare managers measured and reinforced healthcare services according to the definition of "excellent" service by other providers and accreditation agencies. Managers and their organizations were evaluated only on aggregate statistical measures or Joint Commission accreditation standards, which typically measured the organization's structure, processes, or clinical outcomes. For example, a hospital that has a below-average mortality rate, a surgeon that has a high survival rate for heart transplants, and an HMO that has a large percentage of female patients receiving mammograms were considered of higher quality than their counterparts. Thus, the reward and reinforcement mechanism were focused on these provider-dominated measures of success.

In the new paradigm, managers, staff, and organizations must be measured and rewarded on the extent to which they provide patient/customer satisfaction. Because "what gets measured gets managed," the motivation and reward systems must include measures of customer satisfaction as well as employee attitudes to ensure that the managers spend the necessary time and effort on these vital aspects of customer service.

Strategy: Measure All Aspects of the Service Experience

Principle 6: What gets measured gets managed.
Excellent service organizations, like Marriott, Disney, Nordstrom, and Southwest Airlines, send out questionnaires, interview departing guests, and pay people to sample the guest-service experience to be had in their organizations. These are highly systemic investigations that yield the necessary data for understanding and assessing the customers' perception of the quality and value of the service experience.

Asking the customer directly is especially important in healthcare for three reasons. First, the healthcare service is an intangible product that is consumed at the moment it is produced. Only the person who has undergone the experience has a complete understanding of it. Second, each patient/customer is not only different from one another, but his or her service experience also varies depending on a lot of internal and external factors. The patient/customer can deliver a personal account of any problems that arose during the service and can give a suggestion on how such problems could have been remedied and prevented in the first place. Third, managers equipped with first-hand feedback can better design measures for what is important to the patient/customer and subsequently oversee them more effectively. As a popular saying goes, what gets measured gets managed. Unfortunately, most dimensions of customer satisfaction in healthcare today are neither measured nor managed, and patients' perceptions of convenience, comfort, and service quality are ignored. The healthcare equivalent of surveys of consumer perception, like the Zagat's survey of restaurants and the J. D. Powers surveys of automobiles, have yet to appear (Herzlinger 1997, 94).

Furthermore, accreditation of hospitals and industry-developed ratings of HMOs do not appear to be highly correlated with independent surveys of user satisfaction (*Consumer Reports* 1996). Some healthcare organizations, however, are beginning to use measurement techniques to understand their patients/customers' perception of their healthcare experience. Increasingly, hospitals, healthcare centers, and even individual physician practices send out questionnaires to patients after receiving care at their facility to identify these customers' satisfaction with the service as well as the flaws in the delivery system that impede the desired level of service. More and more, the service industry is realizing the consequences of failing their customers twice (because errors in the service experience were not determined and then corrected immediately). Therefore, learning and responding to mistakes early are becoming an equally important part of pursuing the new customer-focus paradigm. Measurement tactics currently being used in healthcare include mystery shoppers, comment cards, focus groups, and other creative surveys (Ford, Bach, and Fottler 1997). The Campbell Health System in Texas reinforces its patient satisfaction data by using mystery shoppers. These shoppers report the details of their service encounters, and managers then share the feedback in a way that is meaningful and motivating for the staff (Millstead 1999).

Healthcare organizations can measure and reward superior service by establishing a base line of patient/customer satisfaction in every unit and then continually sampling patient attitudes. This approach can help to identify both problems and opportunities. Salnik Healthcare, which operates outpatient cancer centers in many states, has meticulously maintained patient records from which it has worked up detailed practice guidelines to standardize and refine the treatment of numerous types of cancer (Bianco 1998). Salnik has been able to achieve better clinical outcomes, higher levels of customer satisfaction, and lower costs of care.

The key HR task is to link customer expectations and satisfaction back to the factors that are measured in the organization's performance appraisal system. This will undoubtedly mean significant differences in the criteria for different positions. Success in meeting customer expectations should also be reinforced through economic and noneconomic rewards. An increasing number of companies (e.g., Federal Express, Best Buy, various restaurants) use internal and external "customer approved" measures as sources of employee performance appraisal information. Examples are answering a telephone within four rings or responding to an e-mail within one day. Managers establish customer service measures and goals for employees (linked to company goals). Achievement of these customer service goals is often linked to employer compensation through incentive programs. By including customer service measures in performance reviews, managers hope to produce more objective evaluations, more effective employees, more satisfied customers, and better financial performance.

Organizations also have internal customers—people who work in the facility—who can provide feedback on anyone inside the organization with whom they work and/or on whose work outputs they depend. Healthcare executives who rely on the HR department for employee selection and training services can conduct an internal customer evaluation on that department. For both administrative and developmental purposes, internal customers can provide extremely useful feedback about the value added by an employee or team of employees.

Summary

Patients today are no longer passive participants in their care; they are assertive and proactive in their search for convenient, cost-effective, high-quality, and customer focused healthcare. Furthermore, the healthcare system is now more responsive to these demands. The growth of medical savings accounts should enhance this trend (Goodman and Musgrave 1992).

Achieving competitive advantage in this hypercompetitive market requires developing organizational capabilities that are difficult for competitors to duplicate in the short run. Capabilities represent integrating and coordinating mechanisms that bring together resources and competencies that are superior to those of competitors (Henderson and Cockburn 1994). The six HR principles or strategies presented in this chapter, implemented as a total system, represent one such integrative and coordinating mechanism for achieving competitive advantage through increased customer satisfaction.

These principles are derived from the best practices of the guest-service industry and have been developed and modified over many years to be applicable to the needs of the healthcare field. Some may argue that because healthcare deals with more serious issues of life, death, and health status, their customers are not as interested in the amenities of service delivery as are customers of guest-services organizations. However, no data can support this claim, and the patients of healthcare organizations that provide both excellent clinical care and customer satisfaction will argue otherwise. These six principles are all important and indivisible, and none is more important than the others in providing superior service. The strategies must be linked together to enable the organization to achieve the level of service excellence demanded by healthcare consumers today. These principles can help the healthcare organization make the transition to the new paradigm.

Implementation of these principles, from identification of the customer's key drivers to measurement of customer-oriented employee performance, requires a champion (i.e., CEO or vice president) who will identify benchmark service organizations, cross organizational boundaries, and make total customer service the highest value in the organization. Following the principles take considerable time (several years), and success is not guaranteed. Most healthcare organizations today have made some progress toward implementing some of these principles. However, we do not know of any that have successfully implemented all strategies.

If these strategies can be successfully implemented, they would provide capabilities that can become a core competency of the organization (Prahalad and Hamel 1990). In such a case, the core competency is the collective learning about how to coordinate diverse operational skills and integrate multiple activities toward enhancing customer satisfaction. Because the process of implementing the principles requires a long-term commitment, the principles will be extremely difficult for a competitor to emulate as a short-term fix.

References

AHA News. 1998. Newsletter, May 9. Chicago: American Hospital Association.

Alliance. 1998. "Consumer Attitudes." *Alliance* (May–June): 11.

Arnold, A. 1991. "The Big Bang Theory of Competition in Healthcare." *Forum* 15 (4): 6–9.

Ashkenas, R., D. Ulrich, T. Jick, and S. Kerr. 1995. *The Boundaryless Organization: Breaking the Chains of Corporate Structures.* San Francisco: Jossey-Bass.

Ballantyne, D., M. Christopher, and A. Payne. 1995. "Improving the Quality of Service Marketing." *Journal of Marketing Management* 11 (1): 7–24.

Berry, L. L. 1995. *Oh Great Service: A Framework for Action*, 171. New York: Free Press.

Bianco, A. 1998. "Bernie Salnik's Business in Cancer." *Business Week* (June 22): 76–84.

Brockbank, W. 1999. "If HR Were Strategically Proactive: Present and Future Directions in HR's Contribution to Competitive Advantage." *Human Resource Management* 38 (4): 337–52.

Brockbank, W., D. Ulrich, and C. James. 1997. "Trends in Human Resource Competencies." Presented at the Third Conference on Human Resources Competencies, University of Michigan School of Business, Ann Arbor.

Cespedes, F. 1995. *Concurrent Marketing: Integrating Product, Sales, and Service.* Boston: Harvard Business School Press.

Clark, R. H. 1999. "Marketing Health Services." In *Healthcare Administration,* edited by L. P. Wolper, 161–82. Gaithersburg, MD: Aspen.

Consumer Reports. 1996. "How Good Is Your Health Plan?" *Consumer Reports* 61 (8): 34–35.

Davidoff, W., and B. Uttal. 1989. *Total Customer Service*, 96–97. New York: Harper.

Eubanks, P. 1991. "Hospitals Probe Applicant Values for Organizational Fit." *Hospitals* 65 (20): 36–38.

Ford, R. C., S. A. Bach, and M. D. Fottler. 1997. "Methods of Measuring Patient Satisfaction in Healthcare Organizations." *Healthcare Management Review* 22 (2): 74–89.

Ford, R. C., and M. D. Fottler. 2000. "Creating Customer-Focused Healthcare Organizations." *Healthcare Management Review* 25 (4): 18–33.

Ford, R. C., and C. P. Heaton. 2000. *Managing the Guest Experience in Hospitality*. Albany, NY: Delmar.

Fottler, M. D., R. C. Ford, V. Roberts, and E. Ford. 2000. "Creating a Healthy Environment: The Importance of the Service Setting on the New Customer Oriented Healthcare System." *Journal of Healthcare Management* 45 (2): 91–106.

Fottler, M. D., R. C. Ford, and C. P. Heaton. 2002. *Achieving Service Excellence: Strategies for Healthcare*. Chicago: Health Administration Press.

Frye, L. 1998. "Patient Services Shows How Massachusetts Hospitals Stack Up." *Boston Globe* (November 13): A1.

Goodman, J., and G. Musgrave. 1992. *Patient Power*. Washington, DC: Cato Institute.

Gross, T. S. 1991. *Positively Outrageous Service*. New York: Warner Books.

Healthcare Advisory Board. 1999. *Hardwiring for Service Excellence: Breakthrough Improvements in Patient Satisfaction*. Washington, DC: Healthcare Advisory Board.

Henderson, R., and I. Cockburn. 1994. "Measuring Competence." *Strategic Management Journal* 15 (1): 63–84.

Herzlinger, R. 1997. *Market Driven Healthcare: Who Wins in the Transformation of America's Largest Service Industry*. Reading, MA: Addison-Wesley.

Hospitals. 1991a. "Retreats Advance Corporate Culture." *Hospitals* 65 (18): 58.

———. 1991b. "Hospitals Probe Applicants' Values for Organizational Fit." *Hospitals* 65 (20): 34.

Mayer, T. J., R. J. Cates, M. J. Mastorovich, and D. L. Royalty. 1998. "Emergency Department Patient Satisfaction and Ratings of Patient and Nurse Skill." *Journal of Healthcare Management* 43 (4): 427–40.

Millstead, J. B. 1999. "Satisfying Your Customers: Mystery Shopping in Your Organization." *Healthcare Executive* 14 (3): 66–67.

Modern Healthcare. 1998. "Put up or Shut up: Study Finds Execs Not Investing in What They Claim to Value." *Modern Healthcare* 11 (28): 42.

National Coalition on Health Care. 2000. "How Americans Perceive the Healthcare System." [Online article; retrieved 6/04.] http://www. nchc.org/perceive.html.

Pines, B. J., and J. H. Gilmore. 1998. "Welcome to the Experience Economy." *Harvard Business Review* 78 (4): 97–105.

Prahalad, C. K., and G. Hamel. 1990. "The Core Competence of the Corporation." *Harvard Business Review* 68 (1): 78–90.

Schneider, B., and D. E. Bowen. 1995. *Winning the Service Game.* Boston: Harvard Business School Press.

Studer, Q., and G. Boylan. 2000. "Turning Customer Satisfaction into Bottom-Line Results." Presentation at the Baptist Healthcare Leadership Institute, July 8–9, Pensacola, Florida.

Vandenberghe, C. 1991. "Organizational Culture, Person-Culture Fit, and Turnover: A Replication in the Healthcare Industry." *Journal of Organizational Behavior* 20: 175–84.

Weber, D. 1997. "The Empowered Consumer." *Healthcare Forum Journal* (September/October): 28.

Winslow, R., and C. Gentry. 2000. "Medical Vouchers: Healthcare Trend—Give Workers Money, Let Them Buy a Plan." *Wall Street Journal* (February 8): A1, A12.

Discussion Questions

1. Why is customer service becoming more important to healthcare organizations? What are the negative implications of failing to address this issue?

2. Think about your own experience or that of a family member in receiving healthcare services. To what degree was the healthcare provider customer oriented? Why? What lessons can you derive from that experience that will help enhance your customer service in the future?

3. Describe one HR practice that can enhance customer service in healthcare. How would you go about implementing it, and what problems do you anticipate? If successfully implemented, what positive outcomes would you expect, and why?

4. If you were the CEO of a healthcare organization that is not customer oriented, how would you change the culture? What are the potential obstacles, and how would you overcome them? Provide a step-by-step plan for reforming your culture.

Experiential Exercises

Case   Robert Casey received his master's in health administration from a major healthcare management program ten years ago. Through a series of increasingly responsible positions in various healthcare organizations, he eventually was appointed as the vice president for human resources at a university medical center where he has been employed for the past six months. Soon after his appointment, the CEO stepped down and was replaced by a new CEO, who is committed to making the medical center "not only the best in clinical outcomes but also the best in customer service in the region."

Robert has been asked to prepare a plan for moving the medical center in the next three years from the 40th percentile in terms of patient satisfaction scores (as measured by the Gallup Organization) to the 90th percentile. Robert has asked your professor for advice on how human resources at the medical center can contribute to this objective. Your professor, in turn, has asked your student group to prepare recommendations. Your recommendations should include some element of cultural change in the organization, given that building a customer-oriented culture is more likely to be sustained.

Case Questions

1. What HR components will you suggest, and why?
2. How will you go about implementing changes in the components you chose? Why?
3. How will you monitor progress in achieving the new CEO's goal, and what will you be prepared to do if progress is inadequate?

Exercise   Form groups of three to five students in your class. Each student in each group should then share with his or her group one example of poor customer service. Then the group will probe that individual concerning possible sources of the poor service experience. Sources may range from lack of top management commitment to inadequate training of staff to inadequate staffing to failure to measure customer satisfaction to negative staff attitudes. The group should identify one or more managerial prescriptions for addressing each source.

All groups should report to the class (1) any commonalities they find concerning the sources of poor customer service and (2) their prescriptions for addressing these problems.

PRESENT TRENDS THAT AFFECT THE FUTURE OF HUMAN RESOURCES MANAGEMENT AND THE HEALTHCARE WORKFORCE

Bruce J. Fried, Ph.D., and Myron D. Fottler, Ph.D.

Learning Objectives

After completing this chapter, the reader should be able to

- enumerate and discuss the trends that are occurring in the healthcare marketplace, and
- list and explain the challenges in healthcare human resources management.

Introduction

Healthcare human resources management (HRM) operates within a complex external environment. When we consider the future of healthcare HRM and the healthcare workforce, therefore, we must take into consideration the trends that are specific to the healthcare industry and its workforce, the concerns that affect HRM as a whole, and the changes that will have an impact on human resources (HR) functions in the future. These three sets of issues are overlapping and interrelated.

Trends in the Healthcare Industry

Of all industries, the healthcare industry can easily be considered the most dynamic and, at least in some respects, the most unpredictable. This unpredictability is natural in that healthcare is about people and hence absorbs the changes that happen in all areas of society, including politics, the economy, immigration, and popular culture. The ten key trends that are expected to cause major changes in the healthcare industry, and consequently on its workforce, are examined below and summarized in Figure 16.1.

1.	Technological innovation
2.	Consumer mind-set of patients
3.	Focus on quality and evidence-based medicine
4.	Security and privacy
5.	New healthcare professionals
6.	Information technology and decision support systems
7.	Globalization
8.	Demographic changes (aging, diversity)
9.	Prevention and disease management
10.	Patient safety

Technological Innovation

One area that is not yet clearly understood but is geared to make an impact on healthcare is genetics. The Human Genome Project reached a turning point in April 2003 when the full human genome sequence was completed. As research continues about the hereditary and genetic factors associated with disease, more details concerning the treatment and management of disease will emerge, raising the question of what kind of education, training, and specialization do physicians and other caregivers need to respond to this new information. Genetic counseling will continue to grow as a field, but how will this profession change as a result of discovery and technological advances? What new types of personnel will be required as the field of human genetics comes out of the laboratory and into the clinical setting? It is likely that advances in genetic diagnosis and treatment will require a broad range of professionals in medical genetics, gene therapy, organ transplantation, and pharmacogenomics, among other areas. Demand for personnel in these areas will increase, and demand will continue for researchers in gene sequencing, biotechnology, functional genomics, proteomics, and microbial genetics.

The point here is that not only will personnel in genetics and research be in greater demand but also that jobs in these areas will be created. Other emerging technologies, including imaging, information technology, and telemedicine, are also poised to make an impact on the healthcare workforce, similarly generating new types of positions and specializations.

More unpredictable than the types of new jobs that may emerge as a result of technological advances is the impact of these changes on the structure and functioning of healthcare organizations. Will current organizational charts be viewed as simplistic and obsolete as new types of relationships form across organizational boundaries and new organizational forms emerge? Will current models of supervision become archaic with the advent of new information technologies and innovations?

Consumer Mind-Set of Patients

With increased availability of medical and health information on the Internet come patients and consumers who are more healthcare literate and savvy. This will lead to a healthcare environment that is driven by consumers. In the future, consumers will likely have possession of their own healthcare record and perhaps maintain their health information through a personal web site. As consumers assume an increasing share of their healthcare costs, we may begin to see customized health benefit plans designed to meet the patient's unique needs. Consequently, the healthcare workforce will need to be more attuned to consumer demands and concerns, and organizations have to improve the manner by which patients participate in their own medical decision making. See Chapter 15 for a discussion on consumer-driven healthcare.

Focus on Quality and Evidence-Based Medicine

Business pressures and the movement toward evidence-based medicine will force healthcare organizations to set quality and clinical outcomes goals, work toward achieving them, monitor them, and publicize the results. Organizations will need clinicians and teams to work together on quality improvement initiatives, and those who are trained in quality improvement methodologies will be more in demand.

Security and Privacy

Concerns over the security and privacy of medical records, heralded in large part by the Health Insurance Portability and Accountability Act of 1996, will shift focus as patient records become available or obtainable (and able to be shared) through electronic or digital means. Information technology specialists who understand the technological, legal, and ethical imperatives involved in healthcare information privacy will be sought after by every organization that embraces technology. Another issue in this area is the maintenance of personnel files. Employee files contain critical personal information, including performance appraisals, salary history, and disciplinary actions. Easy access to private information (medical or personnel records), identity theft, and other technology-driven dilemmas will plague healthcare managers and necessitate new policies and standards.

New Healthcare Professionals

The advances in technology and the changes in the way disease is treated and managed will bring about the possible reeducation and retraining of existing professionals and the birth of new healthcare professionals. New employees, as always, will need to be trained and their competencies will need to be assessed, and managers will have to determine these professionals' role and place within the organization. Existing professions will evolve in both predictable and unforeseen ways.

Information Technology and Decision Support Systems

Information technology will increasingly touch all aspects of healthcare. The era of the manual, paper medical record is ending and moving toward the age of paperless systems. Use of decision support systems will increase to help clinicians and teams to effectively use new diagnostic, surgical, clinical, and medical devices and new pharmaceuticals. Information technology literacy will be a core competency among healthcare personnel to enable them to match the technological savvy of healthcare consumers.

Globalization

The emergence of illnesses and health-related concerns over the past several decades—such as HIV/AIDS, SARS, foot-and-mouth disease, mad cow disease, and other viruses that took root in other countries—and the threat of biological and chemical terrorism in the last few years signal the effects of globalization on healthcare. This trend will lead to the disintegration of the fine line between traditional medicine and public health, requiring the healthcare workforce of all hospitals and healthcare systems to be trained in areas such as disaster management and community surveillance. Public health workers will work increasingly with physicians and other caregivers to respond to new strains of diseases and to develop new methods of treatment, and both groups will require training in and acculturation to this collaborative imperative.

Demographic Changes

The aging of the population is a clear and predictable change that will affect society overall and healthcare in particular. The demographic projections are very clear: By 2011, there will be 40 million U.S. residents in the over-65 age bracket, and by 2019 this number will grow to 50 million. The over-80 population will also see rapid growth: By 2020, the number of octogenarians will reach 7 million (U.S. Census Bureau 2004). Such rapid increases in the number of senior citizens have profound implications on the types and volume of services demanded and on the competencies required of healthcare professionals.

By 2050, the ratio of the non-white population to the white population in the United States will be 1 to 3 (see Chapter 5 for this changing racial profile). The growth in diversity of the population will demand cultural competency and sensitivity from the healthcare workforce. Healthcare organizations may meet this demand through retraining their staff on diversity issues, recruiting members of underrepresented or minority groups to join the caregiving and management team, and incorporating cultural competence education into the staff orientation and training curriculum.

Prevention and Disease Management

The aging of the population not only will mean more demand for healthcare services in general but will emphasize the geriatrics discipline and its various subfields such as chronic disease management and home health care. The concept of disease prevention, although not new, continues to regain momentum as healthcare consumers take more charge of their bodies and learn alternatives to traditional medicine. Healthcare organizations are heeding these cues, providing more preventive services and boosting their current disease management programs. New professions will likely emerge to meet this trend, and again the onus falls on healthcare organizations to provide training to current caregivers and to recruit employees that are skilled and knowledgeable in these concepts.

Patient Safety

As we learn more about medical errors and their causes, changes will likely be required in healthcare processes and information technology. Such changes affect HR practices in that staff will need to be trained in communicating outcomes (adverse or otherwise) to patients and their family, reporting incidences of errors to management, managing conflicts that arise, and other tasks within the purview of the staff's responsibilities. Training in the use and application of medical technology and in the dissemination and sharing of patient health information using electronic means is an appropriate response to this trend. Organizations also have to create a culture in which staff are not penalized for reporting errors or ostracized for committing mistakes. Such a culture encourages improvement in staff performance and morale, which then lead to fewer medical errors and higher quality. Performance evaluation criteria should include a patient safety component as well.

Developments and Practices In and Out of Healthcare

Figure 16.2 lists the current trends that healthcare executives say affect the future of human resources management. This list is derived from the responses of HR executives to a survey conducted by the Society for Human Resource Management (2004). The order in which these developments are presented below corresponds to the level of importance given to them by the survey respondents.

Rise in Healthcare Costs

The rise in healthcare costs has multiple effects not only on individual health-care organizations but also on the U.S. economy. First, it stifles economic growth—the more expensive healthcare services get, the less able people can afford them and the less willing the government and third-party payers will reimburse. Second, it results in greater tension between employers and employees, as organizations are forced to shift their healthcare costs to employees, which results in higher insurance premiums and higher copays. Third, it fuels strike actions from employees who get frustrated with the employer's attempts to cut down on organizational costs.

Focus on Domestic Safety and Security

The threat of terrorism is pushing employers to devote substantial resources to ensuring employee safety and security and to training employees on dis-aster management. Security policies are being revised and tightened, and multiple units of organizations, including HR, are involved in this process.

Use of Technology to Communicate with Employees

Developments in information and communication technology have changed the manner in which employers communicate with employees. This trend has brought out other issues such as ensuring the privacy of the information being communicated, the need for employees to learn to use the new communication methods, and the concern over security of such commu-nication tools.

Legal Compliance

Legal requirements, particularly state-level legislation, concerning employ-ment will continue to become increasingly complex and unpredictable. The globalization of the economy has resulted in the need for employers to be knowledgeable about the legal implications of recruiting and hiring employ-ees from other countries. The emergence of the European Union places particular demands on human resources, as European countries' employ-

FIGURE 16.2

Developments and Practices Inside and Outside Healthcare

1. Rise in healthcare costs

2. Focus on domestic safety and security

3. Use of technology to communicate with employees

4. Legal compliance

5. Use of technology to perform transactional HR functions

6. Global-market issues

7. Retirement and labor shortages

8. E-learning

9. Export of U.S. jobs to developing countries

10. Changing definition of family

Source: Society for Human Resource Management. 2004. *Workplace Forecast: A Strategic Outlook, 2004–2005.* Alexandria, VA: SHRM.

ment requirements in such areas as privacy, pension, and discrimination differ from those observed in the United States.

Use of Technology to Perform Transactional HR Functions

HR departments face pressures to bring value to the organization and to provide HR services in an efficient and effective manner. One approach to hitting this imperative is to use technology for a variety of functions, including training, evaluating compensation and benefits, and managing performance.

Global-Market Issues

Global insecurity and conflict are affecting all aspects of the economy, particularly businesses with an international presence. Organizations, including and especially healthcare systems, are establishing tight security measures to protect their interests, and they are coping with the economic downturn brought on by the war in Iraq and by homeland security initiatives. The oil market, which is deeply affected by the disturbance within oil-producing countries, is significantly causing fluctuations in prices as well. These global issues directly and indirectly influence the supply of healthcare workers as well.

Retirement and Labor Shortages

The aging of the population is ushering the retirement of older healthcare professionals and is consequently contributing to labor shortages. Healthcare organizations situated in locales with a high proportion of older workers may need to assess new approaches to retirement, including phased retirement.

E-learning

Training and skills development will continue to be an important part of organizations' strategies. However, training programs will increasingly be required to demonstrate their value, in terms of improving the performance of employees and showing a return on investment. Use of more efficient computer-based training modalities will continue to be popular.

Export of U.S. Jobs to Developing Countries

The debate over the appropriateness of offshoring jobs continues, especially white-collar jobs, which once seemed immune from globalization. It is unclear if exporting jobs to other countries for the purpose of cutting costs will in any way abate, although security concerns may place some limits on this practice.

Changing Definition of Family

Debates over same-sex marriage and providing benefits to domestic partners will likely continue, even as the portion of companies that offer such benefits increases. An annual survey by Business & Legal Reports states that the percentage of companies that provide domestic-partner benefits to exempt and nonexempt workers increased from 13 percent in 2003 to 19 percent in 2005 (Human Rights Campaign Foundation 2005a). Eleven percent of plant employers provided such benefits, up from 8 percent in 2003, and 7,768 companies made this benefit available in 2005 (Human Rights Campaign Foundation 2005b).

Challenges in Human Resources Management

Table 16.1 shows the generic and specific HRM challenges that face healthcare organizations today. These challenges extend beyond "people issues," requiring the development of a skilled and flexible workforce as well as a professional HR function.

Overriding the generic challenges in Table 16.1 is the need to measure the effectiveness of human resources management in achieving HR goals and objectives, emphasizing the idea that "what gets measured gets managed." Benchmarking of HR functions is crucial, requiring the determination of levels of performance on a wide range of HR areas such as employee commitment, turnover and retention, productivity, cost containment, diversity, job satisfaction, and compliance with legal regulations.

TABLE 16.1
Generic and
Specific HRM
Challenges

Specific Challenges	Generic Challenges					
Environmental	Integrating HR and Strategy	Using Technology	Enhancing Productivity	Containing Costs	Managing Diversity	Complying with Legal Standards
1. Rapid change	X	X			X	
2. The Internet revolution	X	X	X			
3. Workforce diversity	X	X	X			X
4. Evolving work and family roles	X	X	X			
5. Skill shortages	X	X	X	X		

TABLE 16.1
(continued)

Specific Challenges	Integrating HR and Strategy	Generic Challenges				
		Using Technology	Enhancing Productivity	Containing Costs	Managing Diversity	Complying with Legal Standards
Organizational						
1. Competitive position	X	X	X	X	X	
2. Organizational restructuring	X	X	X			
3. Organizational culture	X	X	X	X		
4. Outsourcing and downsizing	X	X	X			
5. Optimal recruitment and retention	X	X	X	X	X	X
6. Design of compensation systems	X	X	X			
7. Ethical behavior	X	X				X
8. Employee empowerment	X	X	X			
9. Benchmarking of the HR functions	X	X	X	X	X	X

In addition, the organization may benchmark its own outcomes against those of its competitors in areas such as cost effectiveness, market share, customer satisfaction, clinical quality, technology, profitability, and reputation in the community. Obviously, the HR function can more directly influence employee outcomes than organizational outcomes, given that the latter are affected by various external and non-HR factors. Nevertheless, determining where an organization stands on both employee and organizational outcomes relative to its competitors is a necessary prerequisite to maximizing the impact of the HR function.

Integrating Human Resources and Strategic Management

Human resources represent the single most important cost in most healthcare organizations. How effectively the organization uses and integrates its human resources with its strategy can have a dramatic effect on its ability to compete and survive in a hypercompetitive environment. The goal is to develop the organization's human resources so that its skill, knowledge, and distinctive capabilities exceed that of its competitors. Obviously, the specifics depend on the nature of the organization and its market. By assessing external factors, the organization can exploit environmental opportunities and neutralize threats.

The management of human resources should also be responsive to the market. HR functions should be focused on producing staff who are ready, willing, and able to respond to customer needs and wants in terms of quality, innovation, variety, and service excellence. As noted in Table 16.1, the above goals are not easy to achieve in light of environmental challenges such as rapid change, workforce diversity, and skill shortages. The latter, in particular, is a severe challenge because healthcare organizations do not usually educate and graduate healthcare professionals and are dependent on educational institutions to produce appropriately trained graduates. In addition, the integration of HR and strategy does not occur in a static internal environment. The organization faces continual pressure from external stakeholders to restructure, outsource, downsize, and modify its culture. While integration of HR and strategy can enhance organizational performance in the long run, there are many short-term pressures that can impede it in the real world.

Nevertheless, the benefits of such integration will include encouragement of proactive rather than reactive behavior, explicit communication of organizational goals to all stakeholders, stimulation of cultural thinking and examination of assumptions, identification of gaps between the current situation and future vision, participation of line managers, identification of HR constraints and opportunities, and creation of a common bond (Gomez-Mejia, Balkin, and Cardy 2004, 21–22).

Using Technology

Advancements in information technology have enabled healthcare organizations to take advantage of the information explosion. With computer networks, unlimited amounts of information can be stored, retrieved, and used in a variety of ways. Even in healthcare, with a long tradition of "hands-on" service, the web is transforming the way goals are accomplished. Healthcare organizations function via computer-mediated connections and are giving rise to a new generation of "virtual" workers, who work from home or wherever their work takes them. The implications for managing human resources are enormous. Information technology can be a potent weapon for lowering administrative costs, increasing productivity, speeding response times, improving decision making, and enhancing service. It is vital for coordinating activities with individuals and groups that are external to the organization. Ultimately, it supports HR efforts to link and leverage the organization's human resources to achieve competitive advantage.

This is achieved by automating routine activities, alleviating the administrative burden, reducing costs, and improving productivity. Technology may also enhance service and employee empowerment by providing line managers and employees with remote access to HR databases, supporting their HR decisions, and increasing their ability to connect with other parts of the organization. It can also expand the scope and function of the HR department, such as providing training through e-learning.

Finally, technology can assist in benchmarking the HR function against that of similar organizations. This helps to determine which areas of HR are strong or weak and what experience of others HR can learn from.

Enhancing Productivity

Obviously, the Internet can enhance employee and organizational productivity, which is defined as quantity and quality of output divided by input. Other factors also enhance productivity as noted in Table 16.1. These include flexibility in job design to accommodate different family patterns; organizational restructuring, outsourcing, and downsizing; optimal recruitment and retention policies; encouragement of a high-productivity culture; design of a compensation system to enhance motivation; employee empowerment; and benchmarking HR organizational processes and outcomes against those of other organizations.

These and other factors have been discussed throughout this book. The challenge is to find the appropriate mix of tactics that will enhance productivity without reducing organizational commitment, loyalty, and retention. Many healthcare organizations recognize that employees are more likely to choose an employer and to stay if they perceive it to offer a high quality of work life. The latter is positively related to job satisfaction, absenteeism, and turnover, which in turn are related to customer service. An exclusive focus on quantitative/accounting measures of "productivity" to the exclusion of HR considerations can reduce an organization's employee commitment, loyalty, and retention.

Containing Costs

Employees, managed care, and government insurance programs (i.e., Medicare and Medicaid) have all put pressures on healthcare organizations to lower costs and to improve efficiency. In response, organizations have tried a number of approaches, including restructuring, downsizing, outsourcing, and employee leasing. Each has had a direct impact on HR policies and practices.

There are significant potential downsides to each approach, particularly in terms of reducing employee attachment to the organization. In well-managed healthcare organizations, accounting considerations focused on short-term data should never have priority over longer-term HR considerations. Labor costs can be controlled through a compensation system that uses innovative reward structures to control labor costs and reward staff for behaviors that relate to achieving strategic goals. In addition, costs may also be contained by some combination of the following HR tactics:

- Select better candidates, which leads to the likelihood that they will stay and perform better as employees.
- Train employees to make them more efficient and productive.
- Structure work to reduce time and resources needed to deliver quality services (i.e., decentralization).
- Empower employees through reducing direct supervision and increasing span of control.
- Reinforce cultural values that emphasize service and efficiency.

Managing Diversity

A diverse workforce is becoming the norm in American businesses. Customers and employees alike have become and will continue to become more diverse. Specific diversity challenges include the following (Gomez-Mejia, Balkin, and Cardy 2004, 120–53):

- Linking affirmative action programs to employee diversity so that the two support one another.
- Identifying how each of the HR functions can contribute to the successful management of diversity.
- Reducing potential conflicts among employees that cause cultural clashes and misunderstandings.
- Developing a profile of employee groups who are less likely to be well represented in higher-level positions, and developing policies targeted to their needs.
- Implementing HR systems that assist the organization in managing diversity.

To accommodate these demographic trends, many healthcare organizations have increased their efforts to recruit and train a more diverse workforce through providing more internships to members of minority groups, flexible work-schedule options for women and older workers, phased-retirement options for older workers, diversity training programs, a culture of mutual respect, access to higher-level positions, and an environment that respects and is sensitive to different cultural beliefs.

Among the most important impediments to managing employee diversity are prejudice, resistance to change, group cohesiveness, segmented communication networks, resentment of perceived favoritism to minorities, and competition for opportunities. Managing diversity requires awareness and sensitivity to all of these factors.

Complying with Legal Standards

Much of the growth of the HR function in the past four decades is attributable to its crucial role on keeping organizations out of legal trouble. Most healthcare organizations are concerned about potential liability resulting from HR decisions that may violate laws or regulatory guidelines from the U.S. Congress, state legislators, or local governments. These laws and regulations are continually interpreted and reinterpreted in cases brought before government agencies, state courts, federal courts, and the U.S. Supreme Court.

A healthcare organization's management of its HR depends significantly on its ability to deal with government legislation and regulation. This requires keeping track of the external legal environment and developing internal systems to ensure compliance and minimize legal challenges. Establishing formal policies and internal administrative channels to address sensitive legal issues (i.e., sexual harassment) can help to reduce litigation.

Healthcare managers need to understand legal issues that affect how they manage their staff because many of their decisions are constrained to some extent by laws. They should be particularly sensitive to legal issues when making decisions about whom to hire or promote, how to compensate employees, what benefits to offer or not offer, how to accommodate employees with dependents, and how and when to terminate employees.

Legal compliance in HR practices has become increasingly more complex as a result of new employment laws, regulatory guidelines, and recent court decisions that interpret existing laws. Examples of newer employment laws are the Americans with Disabilities Act and the Family and Medical Leave Act. Court decisions relate to issues such as worker safety and sexual harassment. All of these changes have made HR decisions more difficult and risky and have increased the cost of making poor decisions.

HR managers advise and consult with departmental managers about the legal aspects of their personnel decisions. Obviously, legal compliance is not the only priority in employment decisions but should be heavily considered along with other factors such as timeliness, service quality, and productivity. Well-managed healthcare organizations go well beyond legal compliance in managing their human resources; they attempt to consistently practice the golden rule—do unto others as you would have them do unto you.

Summary

This chapter examines the present and future trends in the business and healthcare industries to determine the effects they will have on healthcare human resources management. Six generic challenges are also identified, with the overriding challenge being how best to integrate strategic management and human resources management so that the HR function becomes a full partner in the pursuit of the organization's strategic objectives.

Strategic human resources management requires that each HR function be aligned both horizontally and vertically. Horizontal alignment occurs when each HR function reinforces and supports other HR functions. For example, it would make no sense to recruit the best people and then fail to offer them opportunities for growth and advancement. Vertical alignment, on the other hand, occurs when each HR function reinforces and supports one or more strategic goals or objectives. For example, it would make no sense to have a strategic goal of providing the highest-quality service and then compensate staff below the market and/or provide little or no training. The result would be mediocre staff with high turnover as well as dissatisfied patients.

Continually monitoring and evaluating the organization's programs are critical. Such can be done using a variety of HR indicators such as absenteeism, turnover, results of attitude surveys, and customer satisfaction. Benchmarking such indicators against those of other organizations that provide similar services provides external validation concerning HR strengths and weaknesses. Such data should then be used by the organization and its staff to allow them to implement a cycle of continuous improvement.

References

Gomez-Mejia, L. R., D. B. Balkin, and R. L. Cardy. 2004. *Managing Human Resources, 4th Edition*. Upper Saddle River, NJ: Prentice-Hall.

Human Rights Campaign Foundation. 2005a. "Domestic Partner Benefits Up, Signing Bonuses Down in 2005." [Online article; retrieved 5/16/05.] http://www.hrc.org/TEmplate.cfn?Section=Home&CONTENTiD=24990&TEMPLATE=/ContentManagement/ContentDisplay.cfm.

———. 2005b. "Work Life." [Online article; retrieved 5/16/05.] http://www.hrc.org/Template.cfn?Section=Worklife.

Society for Human Resource Management. 2004. *Workplace Forecast: A Strategic Outlook, 2004–2005*. Alexandria, VA: SHRM.

U.S. Census Bureau. 2004. [Online data; retrieved 12/24/04.] http://www.census.gov/ipc/prod/97agewc.pdf.

Discussion Questions

1. Which of the specific environmental and organizational HR challenges identified in this chapter will be most important in healthcare in the next 20 years? Use your own experience in your answer.

2. Most HR executives in healthcare do not have a major responsibility for achieving top management priorities such as enhancing productivity, quality of care, cost containment, customer service, and financial performance. What do you think are some of the reasons for this gap? Outline several ways that HR departments can align themselves with their organizations' strategic goals.

3. What are the pros and cons of having a more diverse workforce? Are more diverse healthcare organizations better able to compete because of their diversity? Why?

Experiential Exercise

Case   For the past 20 years, Metropolitan Hospital celebrated the fact that 50 percent of its new hires in management positions had been women. The hospital assumed that with such a practice, women would eventually represent 50 percent of their top management executives (vice presidential level and above). But something unexpected had happened. Five years ago, the hospital became concerned that their diversity program was not producing results, because instead of seeing an increase in the number of women employed in executive positions, it was observing a decline. Talented female managers were leaving the organization, and this represented a huge drain of capable people.

To address this problem, the hospital found the Task Force on Retention and Advancement of Women in Executive Positions to pinpoint the reasons that their female executives were leaving. The task force conducted a massive information-gathering initiative, interviewing women in all levels of positions in the hospital as well as women who had left the organization. They uncovered three main areas of concern: (1) a work environment that limited opportunity for advancement, (2) exclusion from mentoring and networking, and (3) work and family issues.

In response to these findings, the hospital retooled the work environment through renewed commitment to flexible work arrangements, reduced workloads, and flextime. The hospital also developed plans for company-sponsored networking and formal career planning for women. Results of these initiatives over the past five years have shown improvements. Retention of women at all levels has risen, and turnover rates of those in management positions (just below the executive level) have been lower for women than for men. In addition, the hospital promoted the highest percentage of women as new executives (41 percent) in its history.

The hospital is now basking in its new reputation as a woman-friendly employer. This gives them external recognition in the marketplace, which helps with recruiting efforts, and enhances their reputation in the community.

Case Questions

1. How and why did the problems in Metropolitan Hospital occur in the first place?
2. How did the changes address the underlying problem?
3. What managerial actions are required to successfully implement diversity programs?

INDEX

360-degree appraisal, 230–231, 232, 236

ability and aptitude tests, 188
Accrediting Commission on Education
  for Health Services Administration, 57
ACHE (American College of Healthcare
  Executives), 116
acuity level of patients, 359, 366–367
ADA (Americans with Disabilities Act),
  73, 74, 83–85, 142–143, 413
Adair v. United States, 76
adjusted needs-based approach, 32–33
affirmative action, 113, 412
Age Discrimination in Employment Act
  (ADEA) of 1967, 73, 83, 103
agency (legal concept), 88
AHA (American Hospital Association),
  263, 317
Albemarle Paper Company v. Moody, 142
allied health professionals, 46, 53–57,
  63–64
American College of Physician
  Executives, 58
American Management Association, 95
American Medical Association, 317–319,
  319–320
American Medical Association
  Committee on Allied Health
  Education and Accreditation, 57
American Nurses Association House of
  Delegates, 93
American Psychological Association, 296
American Society of Training and
  Development (ASTD), 213
application process and forms, 176, 188
appraisals: criteria, 228–229; data gath-
  ering methods, 229, 231–237; job

analysis, role in, 139; negative views
  of, 237–239, 242; required, 225, 226;
  subordinate, 230; tips for successful,
  240–242; training in conducting,
  238–239; types, 229–231; use of, 227
aptitude tests, 188
arbitration, 104–105, 311

*Bakke v. California Board of Regents of
  the University of California,* 77–78
BARS (behavioral anchored rating scales),
  234–235
benchmarking: of HR functions, 406,
  409; of jobs, 262; of organizational
  outcomes, 409, 414; as workforce
  planning strategy, 29, 30, 32, 37
benefits, 268–269, 270–272, 359, 406
BOS (behavioral observation scales),
  235–236
broadbanding, 259–261
business strategy, 13

CAAHEP (Commission on
  Accreditation of Allied Health
  Educational Programs), 57
capitation, 273–274
Centers for Disease Control, 294
Centers for Medicare & Medicaid
  Services, 338
chronic disease management, 403
City of Chicago v. U.S., 142
Civil Rights Act of 1964, 73, 81–82, 83,
  84, 89–90, 120–121
Civil Service Reform Act, 82
clinical (organizational) outcomes, 17,
  18, 19, 401, 409, 414
clinical practice, direct, 51–52

ABOUT THE AUTHORS

Dolores Gurnick Clement, Dr.P.H., is a tenured professor in the Department of Health Administration at Virginia Commonwealth University (VCU). She holds a joint appointment in the Department of Preventive and Community Medicine in the Medical School at VCU. From 1997 through 2004, she served as associate dean of the School of Allied Health Professions. Dr. Clement earned her doctorate in health policy and administration from the University of California, Berkeley. She has investigated such areas as community health and well-being; curriculum development in allied health professions; distance learning; Medicare risk contracting with HMOs for the elderly in the areas of quality, access, and beneficiary satisfaction; patterns of diffusion; growth and survival of HMOs; and use of alternative payment strategies by various providers.

John Crisafulli, M.B.A., is a senior consultant for Ernst & Young. He has worked at various healthcare organizations, including Rex Healthcare in Raleigh, North Carolina; Children's National Medical Center in Washington, DC; and Fair Oaks Hospital in Fairfax, Virginia. He received his master's in health administration and master's in business administration from the University of North Carolina at Chapel Hill.

Rupert M. Evans Sr., FACHE, is the principal of Trepur LLC, a healthcare management and diversity consulting company. He is the immediate past president of the Institute for Diversity in Health Management, a nonprofit organization that seeks to expand opportunities for ethnic minorities in the healthcare field. Currently, he is an instructor at Rush University in Chicago and is completing a doctorate in health administration at Central Michigan University. Mr. Evans has served as president and chief executive officer of the Erie Family Health Center, and his articles have appeared in *Hospitals & Health Networks, Modern Healthcare,* and *Journal of Healthcare Management*. A well-known speaker on the subject of diversity in healthcare, Mr. Evans was named by *Modern Healthcare* as one of the top 100 "Most Powerful People in Healthcare."

Robert C. Ford, Ph.D., is a professor of management at the University of Central Florida's (UCF) College of Business Administration. At UCF, he was chair of the Department of Hospitality Management and was associate dean for Graduate and External Programs. He has authored or coauthored more than 100 articles, books, and presentations. He has published in a wide variety of academic and practitioner journals, including the *Journal of Applied Psychology, Academy of Management Journal, Organizational Dynamics, Health Care Management Review*, and *The Academy of Management Executive*. His textbooks include *Principles of Management, Organization Theory, Managing the Guest Experience in Hospitality*, and *Achieving Service Excellence*. Currently, he is dean of the Fellows of the Southern Management Association.

Myron D. Fottler, Ph.D., is professor and executive director of Health Services Administration Program at the University of Central Florida, where he teaches courses in healthcare human resources management, service management and marketing, and dissertation research. His research addresses human resources management, service management, and strategic management issues in the healthcare industry. His publications include more than 100 journal articles and 14 books. He has been active in both the Academy of Management and the Association of University Programs in Health Administration. He also serves on several editorial review boards and is a founding coeditor of *Advances in Health Care Management*, an annual research volume published by JAI/Elsevier.

Bruce J. Fried, Ph.D., is associate professor and director of the Residential Master's Degree Program in the Department of Health Policy and Administration in the School of Public Health at the University of North Carolina at Chapel Hill. He teaches in the areas of human resources management, organizational theory, and global health. He has written numerous journal articles, book chapters, commentaries, and book reviews. Dr. Fried is also coeditor of and contributor to *World Health Systems: Challenges and Perspectives*. Among his research interests are the impact of organizational factors and culture on quality in healthcare settings, healthcare workforce problems, mental health services, and global health. Dr. Fried has conducted workshops and management training courses in Eastern Europe, Asia, Latin America, and the Caribbean. He received his undergraduate degree from the State University of New York at Buffalo, his master's degree from the University of Chicago, and his doctorate from the University of North Carolina at Chapel Hill.

Eileen F. Hamby, D.B.A., M.B.A., is a tenured associate professor and regional campus coordinator for the Master of Science Program in Health Services Administration at the University of Central Florida. She received a bachelor's degree in physical therapy from Hunter College and earned a master's degree in business administration and a doctorate degree in business administration from Nova University. Dr. Hamby is a Certified Professional in Healthcare Quality (CPHQ), a Diplomate in the American Board of Quality Assurance and Utilization Review Physicians, and a licensed healthcare risk manager in the state of Florida. She has served as chief executive officer of a nursing home and a hospital. In addition, she has received the IBM Research Award from the Center for Healthcare Management for her work on patient flow management. Dr. Hamby has published many journal articles and book chapters. Her research interests include leadership, finance, human resources management, and quality management.

James A. Johnson, Ph.D., is professor at the Herbert H. and Grace A. Dow College of Health Professions at Central Michigan University and is a visiting scholar at the Medical University of South Carolina. He teaches courses in organizational behavior and development, systems thinking, and community health. Dr. Johnson's publications include 100 articles and 9 books on a wide range of healthcare issues. He is past editor of the *Journal of Healthcare Management* and was a board member of the Association of University Programs in Health Administration. Dr. Johnson currently serves on the scientific advisory board of the national Diabetes Trust Foundation and works closely with the World Health Organization. He completed his master's degree at Auburn University and his doctorate degree at Florida State University.

Cheryl B. Jones, Ph.D., R.N., is an associate professor and coordinator of the Health Care Systems's master's program in the School of Nursing at the University of North Carolina at Chapel Hill. She obtained her bachelor's degree from the University of Florida and her master's and doctorate degrees from the University of South Carolina. She has a long-standing interest in the healthcare workforce, quality of care, and the cost of care delivery. Her articles on the nursing workforce have published in numerous peer-reviewed journals, and her work on nursing turnover and the costs of nursing turnover has been cited extensively. Dr. Jones also served as senior health services researcher at the Agency for Healthcare Research and Policy. She is a member of the Southeast Regional Center for Health Workforce Studies at the Cecil G. Sheps Center for Health Services Research, where she serves as a principal investigator on two nursing workforce projects.

Bernard "Bernie" J. Kerr, Jr., Ed.D., FACHE, is an associate professor in Central Michigan University's Doctor of Health Administration (DHA) Program. Prior to this, Dr. Kerr was a Colonel in the U.S. Air Force Medical Service Corps, serving as a professional healthcare administrator for more than 20 years. He has nearly 30 years experience in the healthcare industry, including positions in public health and faculty appointments at Baylor University and East Tennessee State University. Aside from his master's degrees in public health, health administration, business administration, and information management, he holds a doctor of education degree in curriculum and instruction and the instructional process and a graduate interdisciplinary certificate in gerontology. Dr. Kerr is a Fellow in the American College of Healthcare Executives.

Anne Osborne Kilpatrick, D.P.A., is professor of health administration and policy at the Medical University of South Carolina (MUSC). She teaches health administration students at the undergraduate, master's, and doctoral levels. She served for seven years as internal consultant to MUSC's division of finance and administration to improve the culture and climate of the organization, and she helped implement a leadership institute at the Ralph H. Johnson VA Medical Center. Dr. Kilpatrick was given MUSC's Distinguished Faculty Service Award, was the first recipient of the College of Health Professions's Scholar of the Year Award, and was honored with the College's award for excellence in service. In addition, she was the recipient of MUSC's Earl B. Higgins Award for Achievements in Diversity. She has been nominated numerous times for the quality of her teaching.

Gerald R. Ledlow, Ph.D., CHE, is a corporate vice president for the Sisters of Mercy Health System's Genesis Project, which focuses on integrating and standardizing clinical, revenue, supply chain, finance, and human resource systems, applications, and functions across the 20-hospital and 81-clinic health system in 7 states. Dr. Ledlow has held numerous positions, including as founding director of the Doctor of Health Administration Program at Central Michigan University, tenured associate professor, and executive director of healthcare programs. He is an honored recipient of the National Federal Sector Managed Care Executive of the Year Award, two Regents Awards from the American College of Healthcare Executives, and the Boone Powell Award from Baylor University. Dr. Ledlow has published numerous articles and book chapters and has served as editor of four volumes of a scholarly book. He has presented at many national and regional conferences, forums, and symposia. He was a nationally registered and certified emergency medical technician. Dr. Ledlow earned a B.A. in economics from the Virginia Military Institute, an M.H.A. from Baylor

University, and a Ph.D. in organizational leadership from the University of Oklahoma.

Donna Malvey, Ph.D., is visiting assistant professor at the University of Central Florida, Cocoa Campus. She received her master's in health services administration from George Washington University, completed an administrative residency and post-graduate fellowship in hospital administration, and earned her doctorate in health services administration from the University of Alabama at Birmingham. Her area of specialization is strategic management. She was the recipient of a research award from IBM's Center for Healthcare Management for her study of flow management. Dr. Malvey is a nationally known speaker, has published extensively in the field, and is on the editorial board of the *Journal of Health Care Management Review*. She has worked in a variety of healthcare settings and has served as executive director of a national trade association that represents health professionals and as a congressional aide.

George Pink, Ph.D., is associate professor in the Department of Health Policy and Administration at the University of North Carolina at Chapel Hill (UNC), senior research fellow at the Cecil G. Sheps Center for Health Services Research at UNC; is an adjunct professor in the Department of Health Policy, Management, and Evaluation at the University of Toronto; adjunct senior scientist at the Institute for Clinical Evaluative Sciences in Toronto; and investigator in the Nursing Effectiveness Research Unit at the University of Toronto. Prior to receiving his doctoral degree in corporate finance, Dr. Pink spent ten years in health services management, planning, and consulting. He teaches courses in healthcare finance and is involved in several research projects that study hospital financial performance.

Thomas C. Ricketts, III, Ph.D., is professor of health policy and administration and director of the Health Policy Analysis Unit and the Rural Health Research Program in the Cecil G. Sheps Center for Health Services Research of the University of North Carolina at Chapel Hill. In 2003, he was named director of the Southeast Regional Center for Health Workforce Studies, one of six such centers funded by the federal government. Dr. Ricketts has been involved in the development of federal and state rules and regulations and the creation of legislation focused on the distribution of health resources and policy for rural healthcare providers. In 2004, he was appointed to a four-year term on the U.S. DHHS's National Advisory Committee on Rural Health and Human Services.

Beverly L. Rubin, J.D., serves as the senior vice president and deputy general counsel for Quintiles Transnational Corp. She has held numerous positions for Quintiles in her seven years there, including vice president of global human resources operations. Prior to that, Ms. Rubin practiced law at the firm of Moore & Van Allen, in the areas of employment, healthcare, and commercial litigation. She received her undergraduate degree from the University of Virginia and her law degree from the University of North Carolina. Ms. Rubin has published and presented extensively in the areas of human resources and healthcare litigation.

Michael T. Ryan, Ph.D., C.H.P., is an independent consultant in radiological sciences and health physics. He holds an adjunct faculty appointment at the Medical University of South Carolina, Charleston Southern University, and Texas A & M University. He earned a B.S. in radiological health physics from Lowell Technological Institute; an M.S. in radiological sciences and protection from the University of Lowell, with a scholarship from the U.S. Energy Research and Development Administration; and a Ph.D. from the Georgia Institute of Technology, where he was inducted into the Academy of Distinguished Alumni. Dr. Ryan is the editor-in-chief of *Health Physics Journal*. Appointed in 2002, Dr. Ryan currently serves as chair of the Advisory Committee on Nuclear Waste for the Nuclear Regulatory Commission.

Howard L. Smith, Ph.D., is professor at the Anderson Schools of Management at the University of New Mexico (UNM). From 1990 to 1994, Dr. Smith served as associate dean at the Anderson Schools, and from 1994 to 2004, he was dean of both the Anderson Schools and the School of Public Administration at the UNM. He has published more than 200 articles on health services, organization theory/behavior, and strategic management in journals such as the *Academy of Management Journal, Health Care Management Review, and The New England Journal of Medicine*. He has published six books on prospective payment, staff development, hospital competition, financial management, strategic nursing management, and reinventing medical practice. His most recent professional book is *Reinventing Medical Practice: Care Delivery That Satisfies Doctors, Patients and the Bottomline*. He is an active consultant both nationally and internationally.

Kristie G. Stover, M.B.A., CHE, is a research associate and adjunct instructor for the Graduate Program in Health Administration at Virginia Commonwealth University (VCU). She is also a doctoral candidate at VCU, with a concentration in health administration. Ms. Stover received her B.A. in political science from Miami University and her M.S. in healthcare management and M.B.A. from Marymount University. She is a board certified healthcare executive (diplomate) in the American College of Healthcare Executives and has experience in hospital administration particularly in research, marketing, strategic planning, and governance.

Derek van Amerongen, M.D., is vice president and chief medical officer for Humana Health Plans of Ohio in Cincinnati. Before this, he was national medical director for Anthem Blue Cross and Blue Shield. He also served as chief of obstetrics and gynecology for the Johns Hopkins Medical Services Corporation and as a faculty member for the Johns Hopkins School of Medicine. He has written and presented extensively on managed care and women's health topics. His articles and letters have appeared in such publications as *The New England Journal of Medicine, Physician Executive*, and *Health Affairs*. His book, *Networks and the Future of Medical Practice*, won the 1998 Robert A. Henry Literary Award of the American College of Physician Executives. He received his undergraduate degree from Princeton University, his M.S. in medical administration from the University of Wisconsin, and his M.D. from Rush Medical College.

Kenneth R. White, Ph.D., FACHE, is professor in and director of the Graduate Program in Health Administration at Virginia Commonwealth University (VCU). He earned his M.P.H. degree from the University of Oklahoma, his M.S. in nursing from VCU, and his Ph.D. in health services organization and research from VCU. Dr. White has extensive experience in hospital administration and consulting, particularly in the areas of leadership development, marketing, facility planning, and operations management. He is a Registered Nurse and a Fellow and Governor in the American College of Healthcare Executives. He is coauthor of *The Well-Managed Healthcare Organization, 5th Edition* and *Thinking Forward: Six Strategies for Successful Organizations*. He is a contributing author in *Advances in Health Care Organization Theory, Peri-Anesthesia Nursing: A Critical Care Approach*, and *Introduction to Health Services*.